Connectionist Approaches to Clinical Problems in Speech and Language

onnectionist Approaches to Clinical Problems in Speech and Language

Therapeutic and Scientific Applications

Edited by

Raymond G. Daniloff

School of Allied Health Professions
Louisiana State University Medical Center

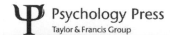
Psychology Press
Taylor & Francis Group

CEO: Lawrence Erlbaum
ice-President, Marketing: Joseph Petrowski
President, Book Production: Art Lizza
itorial: Lane Akers
es and Marketing: Robert Sidor
stomer Relations: Nancy Seitz
ulting Editor: Susan Milmoe
sistant: Stacey Mulligan
gn: Kathryn Houghtaling Lacey
oduction Manager: Paul Smolenski
 Compositor: TechBooks

as typeset in 10/12 pt. Palatino, Palatino Bold, and Palatino Italic.

d by Lawrence Erlbaum Associates, Inc., Publishers
Avenue
ew Jersey 07430

published 2012 by Psychology Press

ress   Psychology Press
ncis Group   Taylor & Francis Group
enue   27 Church Road
Y 10017   Hove, East Sussex BN3 2FA

ongress Cataloging-in-Publication Data

st approaches to clinical language problems / edited by
  Daniloff.
m.
s index.
8058-2213-5 (cloth : alk. : paper)—ISBN 0-8058-2214-3 (pbk. : alk. paper)
municative disorders.   2. Connectionism.   I. Daniloff, Raymond.

58   2001
-dc21   2001040208

Contents

Preface

Parallel and Distributed Processing (PDP), Rumelhart and McClelland (1983), was a paradigm-setting publication. It shook many professions: cognitive science, sensory psychology, linguistics, neurophysiology, computer science, engineering, education and speech pathology, and others, to their roots. It offered novel mechanisms for the explanation of brain functions. Artificial Neural Networks (ANN) inspired by PDP theory have become a preferred way to account for and test information processing of sensory data, pattern recognition, human learning, language formulation and perception, and so on.

In this volume, PDP-derived ANNs are applied to create computational linguistic characterizations of language disorders. Specifically PDP is used to explain language disorders, to plan rehabilitation strategies, and to predict the outcome of language rehabilitation.

Neuro-anatomical structures analogous to neural networks have been discovered in most sensory cortices, beginning with "barrels" of interconnected visual neurons (Hubel and Weisel, 1962), dedicated to the detection of single visual features. However, the brain is much, much larger (many orders of magnitude) than any conceivable artificial neural network. Moreover, neural networks are better designed for information processing than for central, executive decisions. Modularity theory (Fodor, 1983) maintains that "encapsulated, genetically determined and dedicated" neural networks operate swiftly and with low error to formulate streams of speech production units for speaking and streams of language units extracted from perceived speech.

Networks compute the most probable units detected and present them as their "output" to their next module in line. In fact, "computation" is a key metaphor for characterizing the formulation and perception of language, and it is ANNs that are a major factor in computing the information in verbal communication.

This assertion may be presumptuous, but it appears that ANN theory will not only dominate machine recognition of speech and language (see Trentin, et. al, Chapter 5 this volume) but will, in conjunction with other theories, explain the swiftness and accuracy of language processing during acquisition and maturation and thus form the backbone of much of language therapy in the near future.

The chapters to follow explore the implications of this assertion.

First, Norris and Hoffman present the results of a decade of their research and thinking on the clinical treatment of developmental language disorders based on a PDP-connectionist model of language learning. They compare and contrast the contributions to their model made by Piaget, Vygotsky, Bruner, Nelson, Elman, and McClelland to name but a few of the scientists who have explored the nature of developmental learning, and language in particular. They offer step-by-step explanation of their clinical intervention and the resulting changes in the child's cognitive processes during treatment. They justify their focus on the use of reading, storytelling, and dialogue as the foundation for clinical reshaping and strengthening of developmentally delayed childrens' language. Throughout, they buttress their points with references to their own extensive research and that of other authorities. Their clinical arguments are cohesive, scholarly, and cast in a readable narrative; they will answer many questions about this exciting, new therapy and provoke fresh ones.

Christman's chapter deals with some of the shortcomings of the "spreading activation," PDP modeling of phonological acquisition and phonological behaviors encountered during adult stroke and other brain trauma. In particular she points to the fact that PDP networks exemplified by ANNs have problems with achieving identification of correct language units, particularly when the network has noisy or incomplete sensory information to work on or there is too little top-down information to resolve choice of language units competing as most probable identifications. She astutely maintains that fractal (chaos) theory offers a solution to this failure in network performance. In particular, the "strange-attractor" in phase-space can be invoked as a mechanism that would nudge a network away from a nonoptimum identification toward a most appropriate solution. Her narrative is a clear, cogently argued, and exciting read for both adult and child language clinicians.

Gagnon and Martin put spreading-activation PDP networks to a clinical test by comparing results of what a computer simulation of an appropriate PDP network would predict aphasic naming disorders to be like compared with patients' actual, in-the-clinic performance. Their results closely predicted performance of human patients. The authors noted that the PDP-model therapy was effective and therefore supported spreading-activation, PDP models of disordered language processing. Also, the use of computer simulation of language processes may be a way to sharpen clinical effectiveness by pointing toward what can and cannot be expected of an aphasic client prior to treatment based on computer predictions.

Daly's chapter presents evidence of transient shifts in speech perception immediately antecedent and subsequent to epileptic seizures. These shifts can readily be explained as transient shifts in ANN thresholds, feedback, association sensitivities, and so on that resolve as the brain returns to a normal resting state following a seizure. Similarly, he discusses his data on families with inheritable, prominent, and seemingly permanent shifts in their ability to perceive and produce phonemes normally. They may well exhibit permanent physical alteration to their neural-sensory networks. Whether therapy can ameliorate such behavior is an open question.

The computer scientists in Trentin et al.'s chapter review current progress in using ANNs to perceive speech, or more specifically, to identify phonemes, words, and other immediate constituents of utterances. Factors controlling ANN performance include whether real or near real-time performance is demanded; whether speech is delivered by known or unknown speakers; whether networks are trained on a voice, by speakers of different sex, by having many or a few speakers to identify, by using none, a little, or a lot of a-priori grammatical information to inform the network, with or without efforts by speakers to talk more less clearly. They also report the successful use of differing types of networks with variable amounts of feedback, feedforward, and error-correcting paradigms. Their results demonstrate an impressive ability to analyze spoken messages in many languages. These networks currently are used in successful commercial, educational, and clinical applications, and will be refined to yield even more impressive performance in the coming decade.

Finally, Buckingham's chapter reviews the intellectual evolution of connectionism from Aristotle's analysis of the structure of cause and effect that identified such variables as contiguity, frequency of occurrence, similarity, and forces involved. This early Greek empiricism is reflected in the speculations of British empiricist thought, which gave rise to behaviorist explanations of action based on *associationist* principles. These principles were incorporated into "the artificial-intelligence" work of Weiner, McCullough, Minsky and others at MIT, and guided the construction of networks containing a few simple "perceptrons." Perceptrons mimic the function of neuron analyzer units within the ANNs; the neurons are wired into a web of multiple interconnections with neighboring perceptrons similar in fashion to axon/dendrite interconnections in real neural pathways. The author ends his chapter with a list of the theoretical shortcomings that connectionist accounts of language behavior must overcome if PDP's ANN models of language behavior are to thrive.

BIBLIOGRAPHY

1. Fodor, J. (1983) *The Modularity of Mind*. Cambridge, MA: Bradford/MIT Press.
2. Hubel, D. and Weisel, T. (1962) Receptive fields, binocular interaction and functional architecture in the cat's visual cortex. Journal of Physiology, 160, 106–154.
3. Rumelhart, D. E. and McClelland, J. L. and the PDP Research Group, eds (1986) *Parallel and Distributed Processing: Explorations in the microstructure of cognition*. Cambridge, MA: MIT Press.

Language Development and Late Talkers: A Connectionist Perspective

Janet A. Norris
Paul R. Hoffman

Tyrone plays with his toys like any other three year old. He constructs buildings and fences with his blocks, and herds his farm animals, making sure each is fed. His cars are filled with gas and repaired in his play garage. He carefully watches other children and imitates actions and events he finds interesting. He cooperates when a friend wants him to put an animal in a wagon or fill his car with gas. Tyrone appears to be a typically developing child until you notice that he is enacting these play sequences nonverbally, and in fact doesn't even vocalize. Occasionally he points, gestures, or shrugs to make his thoughts or desires known. But despite the best efforts of his parents and teachers to model language and encourage him to talk, Tyrone does not seem to grasp the concept of using language to communicate with others or to talk for his play characters.

Tyrone is described as a child with a language delay, whose development of language is not progressing typically and who lags behind developmentally in other cognitive, social, and physical dimensions. Knowing how to help Tyrone requires understanding what is needed for a child to talk to other children, adults, or even play characters. Based on this understanding, intervention can be implemented that will facilitate integration of language with cognitive and social abilities and stimulate language development and use. Connectionist models of information processing provide a useful tool for understanding how something as complex as language can develop harmoniously with cognitive, social, and physical achievements to result in normal development. They also can demonstrate how disruptions in development of this complex system result in different profiles of delay or disorder, such as the one exhibited by Tyrone.

This chapter describes how an intervention model based on principles of holistic, functional language learning can be theoretically explained using a connectionist network and principles of distributed learning. The discussion demonstrates how interrelated components of a complex network work concertedly to maximize functioning of, and refinement within and across, other components. This ongoing reconstruction of the network is used to demonstrate how changes occur within the network over time that are manifested in qualitative changes in behaviors across cognitive, social, semiotic (i.e., reference and communication), and sensory-motor domains of knowledge. These qualitative changes are described across developmental levels, beginning with those characteristic of development at birth and progressing through levels exhibited during the preschool years. Within this developmental framework, the results of disruption to synergy of the developing system will be explained, with implications for successful intervention.

DEVELOPMENT OF AN INTEGRATED NETWORK

We define a network as information processing units that exist within a system, potential interconnections between units throughout the system, and connection weights that exist between units within the system (Rumelhart & McClelland, 1986; Small, 1994). These properties of such a network allow for an infinite number of different combinations of units to be activated, inhibited, and reweighted to yield specific activation patterns within the network of units. The network is dynamic, adjusting to each new experience and each reorganization within the system. It is also constructive, building itself through its ability to change the strength of weighted connections between units, to create new links to additional units, and to selectively activate patterns, subpatterns, and associated patterns throughout the network depending on the nature of input received (Rumelhart & McClelland, 1986).

Representing Characteristics of Input

The network is designed to represent characteristics of the input it receives (Rumelhart & McClelland, 1986). This property enables a child to construct an internal representation of the physical and social world that must be achieved if environmental adaptation is to occur. Figure 1.1 is a schematic of a network, including the many aspects of an internal representation that must be constructed and integrated. The circles represent

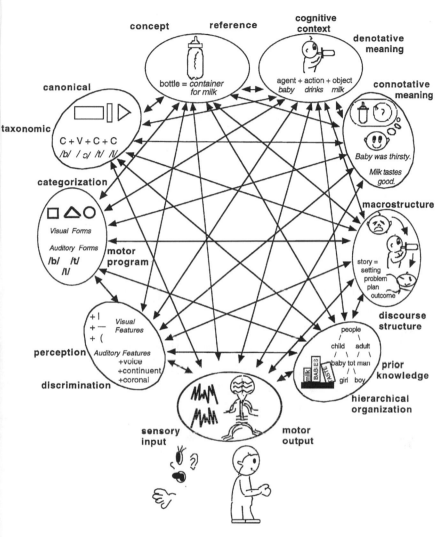

FIG. 1.1. Schematic of a network, including many aspects of an internal representation that must be constructed and integrated during development. (Reprinted with permission from Norris, JA, and Hoffman, PR (1999). The SDS developmental model of integrated functioning, Baton Rouge, LA: EleMentory.)

clusters of units that process similar information, such as sensory input or event structures. Like neurons, the units within a cluster may be wired by location within the network and/or by preset connection weights to respond to specific input, but also are modifiable to conform to the actual input received. The bottom circle of the schematic represents *sensory input* received, transmitted as patterns of wave forms of different frequencies, amplitudes, and durations. Only input for auditory and visual stimuli is profiled in this circle, but it is recognized that all sensory modalities would contribute input in similar ways. Patterns of wave forms send activation throughout the network, as shown by the double-sided arrows connecting the sensory input to each of the other locations on the network.

Some units within the network are responsive to specific wavelengths or patterns and are activated by this input, resulting in perception of a corresponding acoustic or visual feature, such as "voiced sound," or "horizontal line." Neighboring units within the cluster may be unresponsive to the input, but become activated by a different wavelength. This differential response to waveforms results in the ability of the network to discriminate between input patterns.

When the network repeatedly receives similar input, such as seeing the same objects or hearing the same words, similar perceptual patterns begin to bond, or activate together, through strong connection weights. The /b/ sound in "baby" and "bottle" are slightly different in their acoustic patterns because of the adjacent vowels and different voices speaking them on various occasions, but the similarities result in activation of many of the same units. The common units, along with those representing variations in the /b/ productions, form a *category* of perceptions that are processed as the "same." They are connected throughout the network to the same units, and activation of any variation of units within the category will result in the same response. That is, /b/ is recognized as a category of sound, and / [] / is recognized as a category of visual shape.

Because sounds and visual forms are not encountered in isolation, but rather in contexts of overlapping sounds or visual images, connections between them are also established. The network establishes patterns of connectivity corresponding to input patterns. Thus, /b/ + /a/ and /b/ + /i/ become *canonical* or "rule-like" patterns, while /b/ + /t/ do not, since this input sequence is never received by the network. Similarly, patterns of visual forms are constructed, such as /□/ + /△/, that correspond to the shapes representing the bottle.

The contexts in which sounds and visual forms are encountered are not limited to adjacent sounds and shapes. Rather, each moment of input is embedded in complex contexts of sounds and sights entering the network simultaneously and sequentially through multiple sensory modalities. An object is not seen in isolation, but rather as part of a changing complex of visual images as the object is touched, moved, or in other ways manipulated within an action-based event. Patterns of connectivity form between the images occurring simultaneously and adjacently within the event structure, as in "baby + drinks + milk." Objects and people begin to become differentiated within the event, resulting in formation of *concepts* such as "bottle." Sequences of related actions form "rule-like" patterns, or macrostructures reflecting the relationships between the action sequences within an event (i.e., baby cries, baby drinks bottle, baby goes to sleep). The many event structures experienced share components such as people, objects, and actions. These shared components form categories of knowledge that eventually become organized into hierarchies. This knowledge is then accessed by new instances of input that activate similar patterns of units.

The activation of similar patterns of units creates a cascading effect throughout the network. Any established connections between units throughout the system (i.e., sensory, perceptual, conceptual, event-structured, and so forth) are likely to reactivate each other, as indicated by the bidirectional arrows. As a result, representation of input characteristics is neither simple nor direct. Each experience is not represented exactly as it was perceived, and each experience is not represented as a discrete event. Rather, as input enters the network it is integrated with interconnections that already exist within the system. Features or characteristics of input will activate existing patterns of connectivity within the network that share those similar characteristics or features. This property enables the system to make generalizations about input it receives, allowing the child to make sense of experience (Goscheke & Koppelberg, 1991).

For example, input from a source characterized as a long, solid object with a triangular rubber tip that provides a warm, nutritious substance will activate similar clusters of units in a predictable pattern (i.e., "bottle"), so that each experience with a bottle is not an unknown and perplexing event. Despite variations in color, texture, or shape of the actual object, the representation for "bottle" will be strongly activated and the child will respond to the object in a predictable and adaptive manner. The representation is thus different from the actual object because input from the object is integrated into the existing network. This enables the specific event or experience to be interpreted according to all prior knowledge that the system has already constructed and that can be reactivated within the network (Rumelhart & McClelland, 1986). The child behaves as if he "knows something" about bottles.

The complex, simultaneous construction of the network within and across each of the components in the constellation occurs as a continuous, unending process. As a result, the child constructs representations for objects and events such as food and how it is prepared and eaten, clothing and what should be worn to conform to weather conditions, people and how they can be approached to supply needs, objects and how they can be used to accomplish goals, and an infinity of other experiences, emotions, actions, and entities that are part of human adaptation. The greater the internal representation that exists within the child's network, the more independent and self-sufficient the child becomes, therefore increasing the probability of successful adaptation. Progress toward independence is regarded as "development," and for most children it follows a predictable course (Elkind, 1974; Piaget, 1954).

Distributed Representation of Information

Representation of information does not involve assignment of a specific feature to a single corresponding unit within the network. Instead, each feature is represented by a complex activation pattern spread over many units (van Gelder, 1991). This adds flexibility to the network, enabling it to select (from possible meaningful concepts) the best fit between the input and the network representation. This distributed representation allows for different interpretations of the same input depending on the context of its occurrence and use (e.g., the rectangular object with a triangular tip is interpreted as a bottle unless the context of use is holding the nipple to pound on a drum, in which case it is reinterpreted as a drum stick). The greater the number of potential connections between units, the more flexibly and adaptively the system functions to solve problems and accomplish goals. During development, the child constructs a network of representational knowledge maximally adaptive to the social and physical environment. This is accomplished by establishing strong connection weights between units, but not rigid connections, so that flexibility of activation patterns and potential for interconnectivity between new units is assured. To demonstrate how development of such a system might occur, a merger of connectionist principles with Piagetian processes is used to talk about the emergence of such a system during early childhood.

CONNECTIONISM AND PIAGETIAN PROCESSES

Results of the development of an integrated network can be observed in changing behaviors of children, beginning in early infancy. Consider that when Tyrone was a newborn, he showed no interest in toys. Even if he would have had sufficient motor abilities to manipulate toys, he did not know what to do with them. In connectionist terms, he had no patterns of connectivity that corresponded to such play (Goscheke & Koppelberg, 1991). Seeing a toy car provided input to sensory units and activated those corresponding to colors, lines of various orientations, and motions of the object. But these visual units had no connections to other conceptual sets of units, such as those corresponding to knowledge of who drives a car or the part-to-whole relationships between car tires, car body, and the whole car. Consequently, Tyrone could only look at the car without recognition or intention. Piaget described this as a state of egocentrism, meaning the child possesses no knowledge of the world beyond immediate perceptions. Because the pattern of connectivity is based solely on sensory input, when an object, such as the car, is not directly in Tyrone's field of vision, activating the sensory units, the activation immediately ceases. Nothing within the system is in place to maintain the image, since no patterns of connectivity exist for the car as a stable concept within Tyrone's system.

But six months later, Tyrone was interested in the car. When he saw it, he responded to it as a familiar object and eagerly reached for it. When he could get it in his grasp, he knew exactly what to do with it: alternately banging it on the floor and sticking it in his mouth. When it rolled away, he reinitiated attempts to retrieve and play with it. Clearly, the network of interconnected units Tyrone had for the car had changed across time. Insights into what had changed and how this change had occurred is derived from a constructivist theory proposed by Piaget (1954), and interpreted here in terms of a connectionist model.

Assimilation and Accommodation

Piaget (1954) described learning as occurring through a process of cognitive constructivism, or building an internal system of knowledge through interactions with the environment. This construction takes place according to a process of assimilating new information into existing cognitive structures, while simultaneously making accommodations or changes in existing structures to incorporate new information or distinctions. When new information is assimilated or is successfully accommodated to existing structures, or schemas, a state of equilibrium is reached. When information cannot be integrated, a state of disequilibruim exists, resulting in cognitive dissonance.

In connectionist terms, the process of assimilation occurs when sensory input activates patterns of connectivity within already formed networks of units that match, or are a close fit for the stimuli (Goscheke & Koppelberg, 1991). That is, similar sensory input will activate the same perceptual units for color, shape, sound, or texture. Weighted connections between these units and other aspects of the network (i.e., cononical, conceptual, event-structured, and so forth) will, in turn, result in simultaneous activation of the same patterns across these internal units, thus reactivating a unified pattern or configuration of activation similar to one previously learned. The reactivation of the previously learned pattern constitutes an assimilation, or integration of new input into an already existing pattern of connectivity (McClelland & Rumelhart, 1986). Assimilation occurs for the same object or event experienced on different occasions, as when Tyrone encounters the same car each time he plays. The color, size, shape, texture, and other features associated with the car reactivate the same internal units each time it is encountered, forming a stable and reliable internal pattern of activation (i.e., a schema) for the toy.

But assimilation also occurs when objects or events that share similar perceptual features are experienced on different occasions. If a new object activates a sufficient number and strength of connections for the same units as a previously experienced object, the internal pattern corresponding to that already existing schema will be reactivated. When Tyrone is taken to a day-care center and is presented a different toy car, the experience is not new to him. Sufficient similarity in perceptual features activates many of the same units and recreates much of Tyrone's existing schema for the car. This ability to assimilate new stimuli into an existing schema enables the child to interpret new experiences as if they were familiar (Piaget, 1954). Actions associated with existing schema can be applied to the new event, and so Tyrone may bang the car and spin the wheels. Assimilation assures that what is already learned assists the child to adapt to the changing environment, so that every reaction to every object does not have to be learned as a novel event.

Every object encountered within every situation or experience is novel in many dimensions. The two cars will have perceptual differences, such as a metal finish on Tyrone's car and a plastic finish on the day-care car. Thus, only some of the units for color, size, and shape of the object will be the same, while the features that differ will activate slightly different patterns of input and connectivity (McClelland & Rumelhart, 1986). The configuration of internal activation will therefore be similar for the two cars, but not identical. To the degree that they are similar the patterns of activation will be those of the existing schema (i.e., assimilation). But the differences in color, shape, or texture will add activation from input units. These new patterns of connectivity, that did not previously exist within the system, result in a change in the internal structure of the system. The configuration maintains most of the original patterns of connectivity, but also fails to activate some subpatterns while activating new subpatterns. In Piagetian (1954) terms, an accommodation was made.

Internal structure of the schema change dynamically, allowing for the potential of different actual patterns of activation to exist as the toy car schema. As a result of this more generalized, flexible internal pattern of connectivity, the schema is "distanced" from the sensory input that created it within the system (van Gelder, 1991). The schema is not like the metal car at home, nor the plastic car at day care, nor is it like the sensory response to color, form, and motion. Rather, it is a unique internalized structure that owes its origins to all sources of input. The schema is more abstract than the real event, but represents all of the knowledge possessed by the child about the object (Piaget, 1954). The schema represents the extent to which the child "knows" the car.

When an object or other stimulus configuration is easily integrated into the child's internal system through the processes of assimilation and accommodation, then a state of equilibration is achieved (Piaget, 1954). Activation within the system settles into a stable pattern (Goschke & Koppelberg, 1991), and the child reacts as if the input is familiar or known. The child recognizes the object and knows what to do with it. However, a different state occurs when input received by the child cannot be assimilated into an existing schema, either because one doesn't exist or because the input partially fits many existing schemas, but is not a *good* fit to any. Differences may be too great or may create contradictory states within an existing schema and so the system continues in a state of changing activation or flux. In this case, a state of disequilibrium exists (Piaget, 1954), where the system is unable to settle into a solution or stable pattern (McClelland & Rumelhart, 1986). This results in a perception of stress or confusion within the system, and may be externally manifested by crying, tantrums, avoidance, or other behaviors indicative of disequilibrium. Disequilibrium is important to learning. If the system always remains in a state of equilibrium, no changes or adaptations are made, resulting in no new learning. But too much disequilibruim has an opposite, undesirable effect. If input is too novel or too advanced to process, it will be ignored and no learning will occur. Moderate levels of disequilibrium provide the stimulus for accommodations to occur and motivates change, including *expansions* and *extensions* of existing schema.

Expanding Representational Schemas

Tyrone's second encounter with the car activates, in parallel, many of the same sensory units corresponding to color, form, and motion. The connection weights previously established between these units allow for reactivation of the old pattern of connectivity (i.e., assimilation of the present experience with the car into the child's existing schema for the car). As a result of the reactivation of the old pattern, two things happen. First, reactivation of the old pattern strengthens connection weights between these units. Stronger connection weights assure that the next encounter with the object will reactivate the schema even more rapidly and reliably (McClelland & Rumelhart, 1986). Those patterns or configurations that are repeatedly and predictably activated form a schema, or a representation, of the concept of a car. The activation occurs so rapidly and automatically that the object is responded to as familiar to the child. Tyrone begins to show excitement at the sight of the car because of the state of activation it creates within his system.

Second, reactivation of the pattern of connectivity through connection weights means that response to the input need not be relearned by the system with each new encounter (van Gelder, 1991). It also means that sensory information already integrated into the pattern of connectivity requires very little attention, thus freeing the system to attend to additional bits of information or features characteristic of the car and its context of use. For example, the system can react to movement of the wheels, or color of a logo on the car, or changing orientation of lines as the car is turned. Each bit of input simultaneously activates both some of the old and many new sensory units. The overlap between activation of old units and new input allows for the existing car schema to be reconstructed, while activation of units corresponding to new colors and lines adds new units and patterns of connectivity to the car schema (Rumelhart & McClelland, 1986). The schema expands to become more complex (Muma, 1978; Norris & Damico, 1990), having stronger connection weights between more units, with a greater variety of connection weights between units. In Piagetian terms, an accommodation to the existing schema occurs, adding greater complexity and refinement to the child's knowledge of the car.

Visual input that the car provides to the system is one aspect of the network of connections that comprise the car schema. But Tyrone's experience with the car is multisensory (Lewkowicz, 1994). For example, if the car is brought to his hand, sensory input from the pressure, temperature, and spatial patterns is introduced to the system. These sensory inputs establish patterns of connectivity among units that process tactile information in the same manner as those related to visual input. At the sensory level, activated units are domain specific, so that input from the visual system activates visual units, while input from the tactile system activates tactile units. But at the level of the schema, where units and patterns of activity are distanced from the initial sensory input, connection weights are established across domains. This enables Tyrone to simultaneously "know" that the car can be seen and touched as well as mouthed, heard, and smelled. So by six months of age, the sight of the car activates motor patterns associated with touching the car, and Tyrone immediately reaches for it.

Excising Representational Schemas

Each experience with the car adds greater complexity and refinement to the patterns of connectivity for the car schema. Greater complexity is manifested as an increase in the number of units interconnected within the network. Watching, touching, manipulating, listening to, and even tasting the car adds new bits of information to the schema, so that the number of units and number of connections between them continuously increases (Adamson, 1995; van Gelder, 1991). Refinement occurs as subpatterns of connectivity within the network develop connection weights that enable a particular configuration of units to be activated independently of the whole. This results in a level of excising or separating part of the representation from the whole. For example, Tyrone might focus his attention on a wheel of the car, turning it with his finger and observing the consequences, momentarily isolating the wheel away from the car.

In connectionist terms, Tyrone's system was able to strengthen activation between units related to processing the wheel while lessening or eliminating direct activation to units related to the car body. This momentary focus on the wheel strengthens the connection weights for units specific to the wheel, and these strengthened weights enable that aspect of the car to exist within the schema as a separate subschema (McClelland & Rumelhart, 1986). At the same time, connections between units for the wheel and units for the body remain interconnected, readily reactivated by a shift in the input patterns (e.g., a shift in attention). In this manner, the part and the whole simultaneously exist, and either can be focused on (i.e., activated) independently without actually disengaging from the other.

Extending Representational Schemas

Patterns of connectivity for single objects develop as they are in focus or being manipulated. But in actuality, no object is ever experienced in isolation. Rather, objects are always part of a larger event in which the object, the person(s) handling it, and other objects are simultaneously part of the scene (Nelson, 1996). Furthermore, a scene is never experienced as a static event, but rather dynamically as actions and changing states move the event forward. The actual minimum level of input to the child's system is an event, comprised of a series of at least two actions with a beginning and an end point.

The event representation is much like the object schema. All input from objects and people present in the scene simultaneously activate units as a whole (Adamson, 1995; Seidenberg & McClelland, 1989). The system does not yet have differential patterns of internal connectivity for the car versus the hand holding it. The undifferentiated scene enters the system and establishes patterns of activation for the whole. The car and the hand are invariant in this activation pattern, perceived as one object. But as the event progresses, perception changes. The child drops the car, setting up a perceptual contrast between the hand and the car. At this moment they clearly are perceived as two separate objects. Activations within the network correspondingly begin to divide, with strong subpatterns of connectivity for the hand and for the car. Similar subpatterns for all other entities within the scenes of the event are also forming based on what appears to be an invariant whole and what entities are in contrast (Gibson, 1969). Subpatterns comprise the schemas.

Simultaneity of input within the event also causes merging subpatterns of connectivity to form strong connection weights with each of the other subpatterns within the event (McClelland & Rumelhart, 1986). For example, as Tyrone manipulates the car, he might begin to bang it on a table. The table and car appear to be an invariant whole as the car touches the table, but in the next scene objects appear in contrast to each other as they move apart (Gibson, 1969). The contrast sets up subschematic patterns of connectivity for respective objects within the whole pattern of activation. But Tyrone's banging of the car on the table also generated input that would introduce activation to both the car and table schemas in parallel. Further parallel input was generated from actions Tyrone executed (i.e., grasping, thrusting, pulling) to produce the banging, and from sounds, feels, and sights that occurred as a consequence of the banging.

Input from these multiple sources enters the system simultaneously and shares many overlapping units (Adamson, 1995; Lewkowicz, 1994). Tyrone touches the car as he grasps it, so that the schema for grasping and the schema for car share overlapping units. The car and table make contact that is observed by Tyrone, so that schema for those objects share overlapping units. Tyrone's motions and the corresponding presence and absence of banging sounds also share overlapping units with the car and table. Thus, within the system, simultaneous subpatterns of strong activation for the car, table, action, and sound are interconnected through patterns of connectivity within overlapping units. Together they exist as a large configuration of activation within the system. As a resut, the whole is not merely the sum of the parts, but rather an entire configuration of connected, overlapping, and differentially weighted units (Rumelhart & McClelland, 1986). This configuration is different from its component parts, enabling Tyrone to know it as a unified event and not a collection of discrete concepts. Thus, representational schemas for each component of experience are extended to include potential interconnections to all of the others (Muma, 1978; Norris & Damico, 1990). The extended event representation maintains the potential to reactivate the interconnected pattern. The next time Tyrone has the car, he will be more likely to seek the table and reinitiate the banging sequence. Extended representations, or event representations, provide us with knowledge of how objects are used in relationship to each other within meaningful events, and provide the means to carry out sequences of actions or behaviors needed to participate in events such as eating, dressing, or playing (Nelson, 1985, 1996).

CONSTRUCTING COGNITIVE, SOCIAL, AND SEMIOTIC KNOWLEDGE

Component parts of any event can be viewed as emerging from four domains of knowledge that the system must construct (see Fig. 1.2). Knowledge of objects and their characteristics is most closely associated with

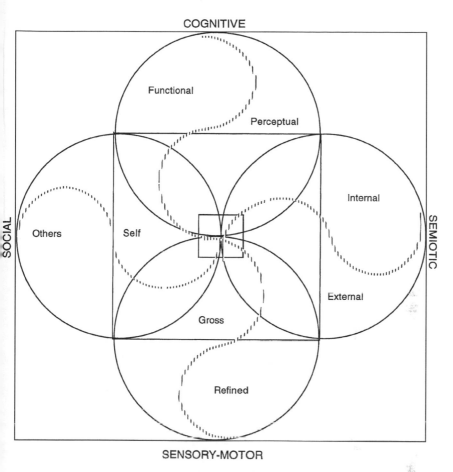

FIG. 1.2. Schematic of the relationship among the four domains of knowledge (i.e., cognitive, social, semiotic, and sensory-motor) and their subsystems that must be constructed within each event representation. (Reprinted with permission from Norris, JA, and Hoffman, PR (1999). The SDS developmental model of integrated functioning, Baton Rouge, LA: EleMentory.)

cognitive development, or the ability to form schemas and construct internal representations of the external world (Piaget, 1954). Knowledge of sensory information (e.g., input to the system) and gross and fine motor response (e.g., output from the system) are related to the ability to form schemas and construct internal representations of categorical perceptions and planned motor movements that allow for volitional control of sensory and motor processes (Massaro, 1987). Knowledge of self and the relationship to others is most closely associated with social development, or the ability to form schemas and construct internal representations for people and their thoughts, motives, beliefs, and behaviors (Mahler, Pine, & Bergman, 1975). Knowledge of associations between representations and signs, including sounds, gestures, indications, pictures, and words, is most closely associated with semiotics, or the ability to use signs to refer to information constructed by the system (Charon, 1992).

In every experience, cognitive, sensory-motor, social, and semiotic domains are inherent components and interact to result in normal development and functioning. Within the network of representations, information from these domains must be integrated and function synergistically, as one coherent and coordinated system. We can theoretically describe, and clinically assess, each domain separately, as in viewing knowledge about objects as cognitive, and knowledge regarding how to maintain a conversation as social. But we learn about objects and their functions by watching others use them, and listening to their suggestions as we try to use the objects. The more we can use language (semiotic domain) to maintain interaction (social domain), the more we learn about objects (cognitive domain). Thus, domains are not separate, but rather integrated and reciprocal in their influences on each of the others (Nelson, 1996; Norris, 1992).

Knowledge in each domain is constructed by the system, forming schemas for an infinite array of information that must be represented. The process of forming schemas is the same for all types of information. Each domain initiates this construction process from input received through the sensory system. Each domain constructs schemas for concepts or abilities within that domain. Each domain forms patterns of interconnection across schemas that form events. And, each domain forms patterns of interconnections across domains that integrate cognitive, sensory-motor, social, and semiotic knowledge and functioning within the system. Inadequate development within any of these aspects of development, or poor interconnections across domains, results in development that is different from a typical learning system, such as that observed in Tyrone.

SITUATIONAL-DISCOURSE-SEMANTIC: DEVELOPMENT MODEL

Obviously, a system that must develop, integrate, and coordinate so many aspects of functioning is extraordinarily complex. To be usable as a model of development, assessment, and intervention, a few principles and properties can be delineated to guide observations and decision making. One model that can be used for this purpose is the Situational-Discourse-Semantic (SDS) model (see Table 1.1) proposed by Norris and Hoffman (1993), adapted to account for early acquisitions and functioning, and therefore called the Situational-Discourse-Semantic: Development (SDS:D)

TABLE 1.1
Developmental and Descriptive Continuum of Language Levels
Distributed Across the Situational, Discourse, and Semantic Contexts of
the SDS Model. *Source:* Adapted with Permission from J. A. Norris and
P. R. Hoffman, Whole Language Intervention for School-Age Children,
p. 32, 1993, Singular Publishing Group

	Situational *Representing*	*Discourse* *Organizing*	*Semantic* *Processing*
	Decontextualized [Words and Ideas, No Visual Support]		
X	Logical Hypothetical Knowledge	Interactive *(multiple topics interwoven)*	Meta-Knowledge *(conscious knowledge)*
IX	Symbolic Imagined Experience	Complex *(parallel perspectives)*	Analogy *(associate old to new)*
VIII	Relational Rules and Directions	Compound *(two or more episodes or topics)*	Evaluation *(opinion, judgment)*
VII	Decentered Observed Experience	Complete *(compare/contrast/appraise)*	Inference *(prior knowledge)*
VI	Egocentered Own Past Experience	Plan or Purpose *(problem/solution)*	Interpretation *(deduce from cues)*
	Contextualized [Visual or Multisensory Support]		
V	Logical Low Support Sensory Cues	Reactive Sequence *(cause/effect)*	Attribution *(characteristics, emotions)*
IV	Symbolic Replicas, Pictures	Ordered Sequence *(time/procedures)*	Description *(action relationships)*
III	Relational Event-Related Action Real Objects	Listing *(topic maintained)*	Labeling *(naming, imitation)*
II	Decentered Attention or Action: Objects or People	Collection *(associated topics or actions)*	Indication *(points, gestures, sounds)*
I	Egocentered Own Body: Direct Sensory Input	Discrete *(isolated actions or facts)*	Reaction *(reflexive response)*

Reprinted with permission from Norris, JA, and Hoffman, PR (1999). The SDS developmental model of integrated functioning, Baton Rouge, LA: EleMentory.

model (Norris & Hoffman, 1997). This model describes integration of cognitive, social, and semiotic domains, accounting for changing characteristics across time and across activities.

Situational Context

In a connectionist network, organizing properties will cause changes to occur across three dimensions, designated as situational, discourse, and semantic contexts in the SDS:D model (Norris & Hoffman, 1993). The situational context describes what the system is capable of representing. This could be real objects, pictures or other symbolic representations of objects, or knowledge expressed in words. Developmentally, as the system constructs internal representations for the physical and social environment, representations progressively separate from the original input. The situations that the child can represent and adapt to are increasingly more displaced. In Piagetian terms, egocentrism is reduced (Piaget, 1954).

Recall that in early infancy, activation of units is primarily generated from direct sensory input, with no internal structures available to assimilate or accommodate information. When sensory input is removed, processing of information ceases. But as schemas, event representations, concepts, and linguistic representations develop, processing becomes less dependent on sensory input (Clark, 1993). Instead, the system increasingly receives as much or more activation from internal representations as it does from sensory stimulation. Thus, situations in which learning and functioning occur are increasingly displaced from direct sensory experience and from a personal or egocentered perspective. The situational context increasingly comprises representations existing within the system rather than sensory-motor input received from the external physical surroundings (McClelland & Rumelhart, 1986).

Figure 1.3 profiles the continuum of change within the situational context that emerges developmentally. At the most egocentered level, the child is aware of the physical and social world only when people or objects directly impact the child's sensory system (Piaget, 1952, 1954). The child is unaware of the separation of self from objects or others (Mahler, Pine, & Bergman, 1975). But with greater internalization of representations, the child's thought becomes increasingly decentered. Objects and people are recognized as meaningful apart from the child. Gradually, the child responds to external representations of reality, such as pictures or toys. Even greater development yields a state where internal representations create reality, so that words generate the situational context and actual physical surroundings must be largely ignored, as when listening to a story. Goldilocks and her three bears are not present in the physical context, but only in a mental context created from words.

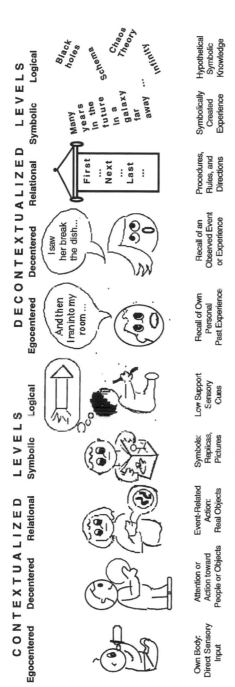

FIG. 1.3. Profile of the continuum of change within the situational context that emerges developmentally, from the most contextualized and egocentered to the most decontextualized and displaced or logical. (Reprinted with permission from Norris, JA, and Hoffman, PR (1999). The SDS developmental model of integrated functioning, Baton Rouge, LA: EleMentory.)

17

Results of changes in organization are apparent in developments within cognitive, social, semiotic, and sensory-motor domains (see Table 1.2). Thus, in the cognitive domain displacement progresses from knowledge of physical objects to representational objects. Likewise, in the social domain displacement progresses from failure to separate self from others to creating representations of the world from the perspective of other people and cultures. In the semiotic domain, displacement progresses from reacting only to immediately present stimuli, through talking about things present in the physical environment, and finally to highly decontextualized talk that itself creates the cognitive and social environment (Vygotsky, 1962; Westby, 1985). In the sensory-motor domain, displacement progresses from a level of responses consisting of repetition of reflexive movements, to imitation of other's actions and roles (Holdgrafer & Dunst, 1986; Piaget, 1954).

Clearly, changes in development result in the creation of very different realities for children with increasing age and experience. The situational context describes the nature of the environment that the child is able to represent and function within. But creation of a representational situational context is not the only outcome of the organizing principles of a connectionist network. Not only does knowledge become more displaced from an egocentered status, it also becomes more elaborate and complex in its organization. In the SDS:D model, this type of organization is referred to as discourse context.

Discourse Context

In a connectionist model, input to the network is organized according to existing schemas and their interconnections. Recall that a newborn only attends to stimuli as long as it directly activates sensory units. While learning begins intra-utero (Vihman, 1999), schemas at this stage are unelaborated, comprised of relatively disconnected units unstructured by expansions, excisions, or extensions. With increasing development, schemas become interconnected through experience into event representations (Nelson, 1996). Different objects that serve common roles within the event begin to group together and share patterns of connectivity to each other and to other parts of the event (Nelson, 1985, 1996). For example, cereal is eaten, but so are fruit, vegetables, and meats. These all become interconnected because of their overlapping relationships to hunger, the highchair, spoons, bowls, and bibs. As a consequence, an organization governed by topic begins to be imposed on edible objects, and the child performs similar event-related actions with each of these objects. Similarly, perceptually dissimilar objects such as the spoon and the cereal become linked to each other through extensions to form an event representation.

TABLE 1.2
Profile of Development Observed within the Situational, Discourse,
and Semantic Contexts that Occur in Cognitive, Social, Semantic,
and Sensory-Motor Domains

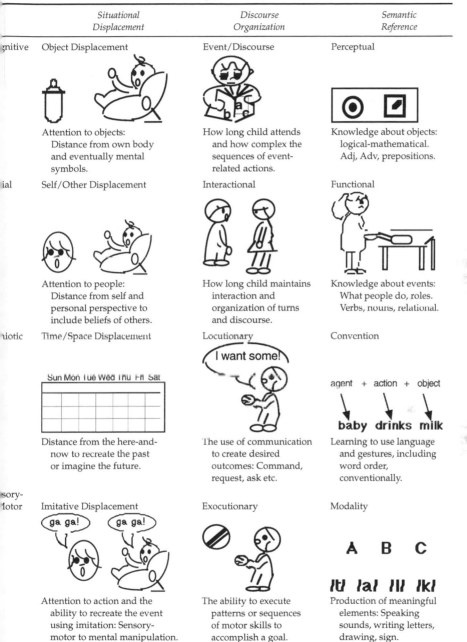

	Situational Displacement	*Discourse Organization*	*Semantic Reference*
gnitive	Object Displacement	Event/Discourse	Perceptual
	Attention to objects: Distance from own body and eventually mental symbols.	How long child attends and how complex the sequences of event-related actions.	Knowledge about objects: logical-mathematical. Adj, Adv, prepositions.
ial	Self/Other Displacement	Interactional	Functional
	Attention to people: Distance from self and personal perspective to include beliefs of others.	How long child maintains interaction and organization of turns and discourse.	Knowledge about events: What people do, roles. Verbs, nouns, relational.
iotic	Time/Space Displacement	Locutionary	Convention
		I want some!	agent + action + object
			baby drinks milk
	Distance from the here-and-now to recreate the past or imagine the future.	The use of communication to create desired outcomes: Command, request, ask etc.	Learning to use language and gestures, including word order, conventionally.
sory-lotor	Imitative Displacement	Exocutionary	Modality
	ga ga! ga ga!		A B C
			/t/ /a/ /l/ /k/
	Attention to action and the ability to recreate the event using imitation: Sensory-motor to mental manipulation.	The ability to execute patterns or sequences of motor skills to accomplish a goal.	Production of meaningful elements: Speaking sounds, writing letters, drawing, sign.

As a result, a temporal sequence of actions begins to form, such as grasping the spoon, scooping cereal from the bowl, eating the cereal, and banging the spoon on the highchair tray. Additional development yields organization by factors including causality, problem-solution, and moral, as profiled along the continuum of the discourse context presented in Table 1.1.

These patterns of organization are manifested across domains as seen in Table 1.2. Cognitively, events are engaged in with greater elaboration and organization. Daily routines are performed in a sequenced, goal-directed manner, play is structured into organized events, and stories begin to exhibit narrative structure. Socially, patterns of interaction initially are noninclusive of others, and only gradually become inclusive, initiated and structured by the child to conform to needs and expectations implied by social context. In the semiotic domain, organization progresses from production of unintentional, reflexively occurring behaviors to those purposefully generated to achieve goals and finally intentionally designed to achieve specific differentiated outcomes, or locutionary acts, such as informing, requesting, protesting, entertaining, or commanding (Norris, 1992, 1995). Within the sensory-motor domain, organization progresses from short bursts of unpatterned sound or movement to bilateral coordination of movements to accomplish complex oral-motor and fine/gross motor movements (Elkind, 1974; Stark, 1979).

Changes in patterns of connectivity within a connectionist network result in creation of increasingly more extended and organized internal representations (Clark, 1993). This organization is manifested across domains and throughout the continuum of situational contexts represented within the network. That is, an event such as playing with toys (e.g., a contextualized/symbolic level of the situational context) can be organized as simply as a single discrete action, or with the complexity of an extended interactive event. The relationship between situational and discourse contexts is dynamic and interactive (Norris & Hoffman, 1993). This same principle is also true of the semantic context of the SDS:D model.

Semantic Context

In connectionist models, internal representations are originally formed through establishment of weighted connections between units receiving input from the sensory-motor system. Hence, the initial representation for an object or action within the network is minimally distanced from sensory input. The representation is iconic, comprised of patterns of sensory input such as frequency, duration, or amplitude of a visual or auditory image along with innate perceptual units activated by these signals (Charon,

1992; Lewkowicz, 1994). At this level, no meaning is assigned. However, processes of assimilation and accommodation soon create more complex representations increasingly distanced from the perception. Generalized concepts are formed based on perception of the object and its role within an event. These concepts refine as new input is assimilated on a "best fit" basis (Rosch, 1978). Even greater perceptual distance is realized through expansion, excision, and extension. Representations are continuously recombined in new ways to accommodate new contexts of use (remember the knife used to pry open the paint can). Prior knowledge becomes increasingly important to making interpretations regarding the meaning and function of objects, actions, and words or other semiotic reference to specific representations.

Table 1.1 profiles the continuum of change within the Semantic Context that occurs when representations are refined and recombined. Figure 1.4 demonstrates the relationship of these increasingly more complex levels of processing to the structure of the network. Beginning with undifferentiated reactions to stimuli, internal representations develop that allow the child to indicate what is noticed, label objects based on perceptions, describe relationships between objects and people, and gradually form interpretations, inferences, and evaluations by combining and recombining representations within the network (Blank, Rose, & Berlin, 1978; Norris & Hoffman, 1993).

Table 1.2 designates how this refinement is manifested across domains. Within the cognitive domain, knowledge gained through explorations of objects progresses from response to perceptual input, to abstract knowledge of perceptual features such as color, number, size, or dimension, through abstract analysis of thought (Piaget, 1954; Van Kleeck, 1994). Within the social domain, knowledge about the function of objects as they are used by people to attain goals is refined, progressing from undifferentiated action schemes, toward concepts and language that refer to knowledge of how people use, know, feel, judge, and interpret their world (Moore & Dunham, 1995). Within the semiotic domain, the conventions of communication become increasingly refined, including use of words, word order, gestures, intonation, and other essential elements to refer to and share meaning (Vygotsky, 1962). In the sensory-motor domain nonreferential movements of the vocal mechanism become modified and integrated with meaning to develop a phonological system that governs production of speech (Stark, 1979).

This understanding of the changes that occur within situational, discourse, and semantic contexts across cognitive, social, semantic, and sensory-motor domains can be used to examine development. To accomplish this, we will follow the development of Tyrone from early infancy.

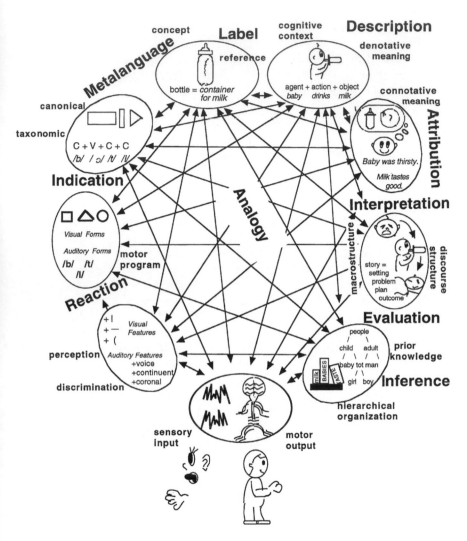

FIG. 1.4. Schematic of the network with the ten levels of the semantic context imposed. The situational context is determined by the input presented to the child (i.e., real objects, pictures, decontextualized words), as well as the ability of the child to process the input (i.e., the degree to which the network has formed). The discourse context is organized at the level of the macrostructure of this figure. (Reprinted with permission from Norris, JA, and Hoffman, PR (1999). The SDS developmental model of integrated functioning, Baton Rouge, LA: EleMentory.)

EGOCENTERED, DISCRETE, AND REACTIVE: DEVELOPMENT FROM 0 TO 1 MONTH

The world experienced by the newborn is very different from one experienced by the older child or adult. Absence of a network of integrated knowledge about the physical and social world limits how an infant can respond and what is interpreted from experience. With minimal internal representations for objects, people, actions, or emotions, experience is limited to sensory-motor perceptions, intra-utero learning, and schema genetically formulated (Uzgiris, 1983; Uzgiris & Hunt, 1975; Vihman, 1999). The task of the newborn is to begin to construct an interconnected network of information by establishing weighted connections between units and processing input from individual sensory systems (e.g., visual, auditory, olfactory, tactile-proprioceptive, or gustatory), while simultaneously integrating input from units across these modalities to form coherent representations of the experience. Evidence indicates, though not without controversy, that the newborn's perceptual experience is one of perceptual unity (Meltzoff & Kuhl, 1989; Stern, 1985), with primarily amodal qualities such as duration, beat, rhythm, intensity, and shape that can be specified by every sense (Adamson, 1995). From holistic perception, the infant must abstract component parts while unifying the whole with increasing complexity. The abilities demonstrated by the newborn across domains (i.e., cognitive, social, semiotic, and sensory-motor) within the Situational, Discourse, and Semantic Contexts is profiled in Table 1.3.

Situational Context

Newborns are very active learners, as their systems respond to multisensory input and begin the process of establishing and weighting connections between units throughout the system to represent the input. However, lack of an internal representation for the external source of input causes infants to appear to be passive learners. For example, Tyrone's lack of internalized schemas for objects, sounds, or people encountered in the environment results in an inability to attend or respond to the stimulus unless it is presented in his immediate sensory field (Uzgiris, 1983). Thus, the immediate sensory field defines the situational context from Tyrone's perspective. Situational characteristics at this level reflect a lack of displacement (i.e., an egocentered state) (Piaget, 1952, 1954), manifested as no attention to objects unless they are touching or very near; no understanding of self as separate from other people (Mahler, Pine, & Bergman, 1975); no displacement of stimuli in time and space from the moment of its occurrence; and no ability to repeat sensory-motor behaviors, except those occurring reflexively (Piaget, 1954). Infants at this stage

TABLE 1.3
Abilities Demonstrated by the Newborn (0 to 1 Month of Age) Across the
Cognitive, Social, Semiotic, and Sensory-Motor Domains Profiled within
the Situational-Discourse-Semantic Contexts of the
SDS: Development Model

	0–1 Month Level Ia		
	Situational Egocentered Displacement	Discourse Discrete Event Organization	Semantic Reaction Reference
Cognitive	Object Displacement Objects noticed only when touching or very near the child; not viewed as separate from the child.	Event/Discourse No organization imposed so each moment of stimulation is a discrete event.	Perceptual Reflexive response to stimuli; no recognition or meaning attached.
Social	Self/Other Displacement People responded to only when touching or very near child; no separation of self from others.	Interactional Adults initiate and respond to engage child in turn-taking.	Functional Undifferentiated action; include motion associated with source of stimuli.
Semiotic	Time/Space Displacement Reactive to immediately present sensory and proprioceptive stimuli; no attempt to reestablish or maintain.	Locutionary Adult imputes meaning to unintentional reflexive behaviors.	Convention Undifferentiated, vegetative, reflexive, and inconsistent.
Sensory-Motor	Imitative Displacement Child repeats own reflexive schemes.	Exocutionary Short, rapid bursts of sound or movement unpatterned sequence.	Modality Gross and simple. Vocal=open vocal tract; Little oral closure, lingual, or mandible movement.

Reprinted with permission from Norris, JA, and Hoffman, PR (1999). The SDS developmental model of integrated functioning, Baton Rouge, LA: EleMentory.

(as well as some older children with severe processing problems) seem oblivious to nearly all sights and noises in their environment unless those entities directly physically impact the child. When interactions do occur, they activate sensory units but no internal representations, and so Tyrone does not perceive these objects or people to be separate from himself. They are merely part of the immediate sensory experience. The situational context of his learning is restricted to his own sensory-motor perceptions.

Discourse Context

Similarly, lack of an event representation makes it impossible for Tyrone to maintain activation after the input is discontinued, a state necessary to result in organization within the discourse context. Once a schema is formed and begins to acquire overlapping relationships of units with other schema linked by action or association within an event representation, attention to the source of the input can be maintained and even controlled (Tronick, 1982). Tyrone could reach for the object, and once touched could grasp it, once grasped could bang it, and so forth. But without interconnection of units, the newborn would not be able to impose organization on the experience, rendering it a discrete event. Once input ceases, activation abruptly ends (Uzgiris, 1983). Similarly, although Tyrone's mother might engage him in turn-taking with the object, alternately presenting it and waiting for him to react, Tyrone would have no ability to structure these turns or reinitiate interactions once his mother discontinued the play (Adamson, 1995; Brazelton & Tronick, 1980). Without an event representation, Tyrone could only react to the presence of input unintentionally, responding reflexively to each occurrence with no recognition or discrimination (see Fig. 1.5). Infants at this stage, and older children with difficulty activating interconnections between related objects and actions, respond to stimulil with only momentary attention and are distracted by any sounds or sights that randomly occur within the environment. Without internal activation of a sequence of actions, each instance of attention to an object is isolated (Holdgrafer & Dunst, 1986). The most salient sensory input is attended to, rather than topically related information.

Semantic Context

Semantically, lack of schemas (i.e., limited or no connection of units at the levels of concept, event structure, macrostructure, prior knowledge) provide no means by which the child can refer to an internal representation of the input. Tyrone does not have words to say "That's bright!" nor does he have an internal representation for brightness. Response is therefore limited to those innate connections that result in reflexive reactions, such as a startle response to bright or unexpected objects (Brazelton & Tronick, 1980; Holdgrafer & Dunst, 1986; Scoville, 1984). Input activates those units that maintain an innate connection within the system, both for perceptual and functional features of stimuli. Perceptually, sensory features such as color, form, and motion are activated, and Tyrone would react with a

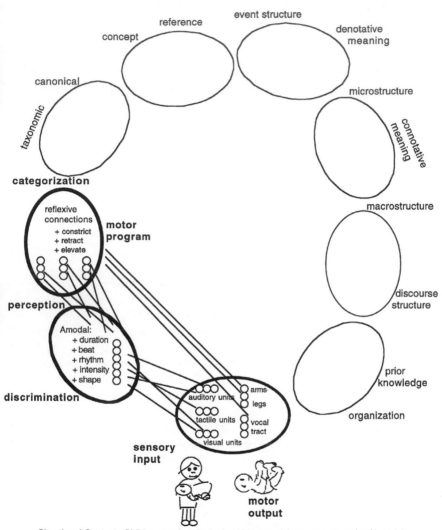

Situational Context: Child responds reflexively within caregiving events organized by adult.
(Contextualized-Egocentered)

FIG. 1.5.   Sensory input from ongoing stimuli activates innately connected perceptual units from 0 to 1 month of age. These basic units are primarily amodal and can be specified by every sense. With few internal connections between units at higher levels, the activation cannot be maintained or repeated by the child once external stimulation ceases. Response is limited to innate connections that result in reflexive reactions, with no recognition or meaning attached. (Reprinted with permission from Norris, JA, and Hoffman, PR (1999). The SDS developmental model of integrated functioning, Baton Rouge, LA: EleMentory.)

reflexive response with no recognition or meaning attached to stimuli. If Tyrone was in physical contact with the bright object, his actions would be undifferentiated with no functional knowledge of use of the object as an adult would perceive it. All modes of response would consist of reflexive actions, such as visual-motor arm, body, or head movements, and auditory-vocal unpatterned sounds and undifferentiated cries (Holdgrafer & Dunst, 1986; Sander, 1977; Scoville, 1984).

Vocalizations are not semantic at this stage of development (Stark, 1979). Connections between units within the network are present at birth and reflexive. Input entering the network, whether input is auditory, visual, or tactile, activates perceptual units for frequency, amplitude, or duration of input (Stern, 1985). Input also activates functional units for motions or actions associated with the input, including vocal movements used to produce auditory input (Field, Woodson, Greenberg, & Cohen, 1982; Meltzoff & Moore, 1983). All of these units are simultaneously activated, establishing patterns of connectivity within and across modes of information (Adamson, 1995). These activated units in turn send excitation to interconnected units, especially those controlling the motor movements recognized as reflexes. Thus, the pattern of connectivity is relatively primitive at this stage of development, with simultaneously occurring input units adding, strengthening, and modifying connection weights for corresponding perceptual and functional feature units. These in turn spread activation to units controllling undifferentiated reflexive motor responses.

Disruptions to Synergistic Development

In normal development, there is relative synergy across contexts and domains, with developments in one domain (i.e., social or motor development) having a reciprocal positive effect on another (i.e., cognitive or communicative development). This indicates that the child is constructing internal representations for many aspects of knowledge that must be integrated for the system to develop normally. But when there is disruption within one component of the system, the entire system is affected. Recall that domains are not separate and independent in the representations for objects and events that they construct. Rather, through expansion, excision, and extension, direct and indirect connections form beween all domains in an interactive and reciprocal relationship. Assume that for Tyrone, connections within the cognitve domain developed typically. He produced momentary (discourse) reflexive startles, eyeblinks, and movements (semantic) in response to sounds, objects, and other stimuli occurring within several inches of his own body (situational). Similar typical development also was noted in social development, as Tyrone engaged in undifferentiated action (semantic) when his parents initiated interaction (discourse) by talking to and touching him in play and caregiving (situational). He was physically capable of producing and hearing his own vocalizations and unpatterned bursts of sound, repeating these reflexive schemes (sensory-motor). But differences from typical development occurred within the semiotic domain, specific to vocalizations.

Complex interconnections required to attach vocalizations to social and cognitive events depend on integrity of the child's system and its ability to establish patterns of connectivity between units across sensory modes, existing representations, and cognitive-social-semiotic domains. For example, reflexive vocalization should form interconnections between motor movements used to produce verbal symbols in later development. These interconnections should link auditory features corresponding to sounds, and visual and tactile stimuli present when sounds are produced (Field, Woodson, Greenberg, & Cohen, 1982; Meltzoff & Moore, 1983). But if the child's system fails to send sufficient excitatory activation on to other units because of structural or physiological differences or timing delays within units, then connections cannot be formed (Tallal et al., 1996). As a consequence, connection weights for motor movements are not strengthened, expanded, and refined. They are not activated by sight of a stimulus, such as Tyrone's car, nor the sound of the speech of others, such as imitation of his mother's vocalizations. The normal process that establishes speech as an intergral part of interacting with others about objects is disrupted, and so production of vocalizations decreases. As a consequence, with increasing age, Tyrone may fail to develop conventions of language, with his vocalizations remaining unpatterned, undifferentiated, or absent despite appropriate development in other areas.

Forming the complex interconnections between units also depends on the social and physical environment to provide input to activate patterns of units. Problems may occur if Tyrone is provided limited opportunities to form patterns of connectivity. Parents interacting with newborns are typically highly responsive, imputing meaning and communicative purpose to the most unintentional behaviors such as burps or startle responses (Lewis, 1987; Sander, 1969). Parents treat these behaviors as if they were turns within conversations and respond by looking, touching, and talking to infants. These reactions provide opportunities for multiple sources of sensory input to interconnect within the child's system. As the child begins to produce vocalizations purposefully, parents support primitive attempts at communication by quieting while the child vocalizes and talking as the child quiets, imitating the sounds made by the child, interpreting the child's meaning and providing food, comfort, or stimulation to correspond to assumed needs, and responding in consistent ways to recognizable patterns (Bates, Camaioni, & Volterra, 1975; Murray & Trevarthen, 1986).

Failure of Tyrone's system to appropriately send or time activation for sounds to other units results in development of a differently functioning system (Tallal et al., 1996). While Tyrone produces cries and other sounds (sensory-motor), these vocalizations do not reliably connect to social and cognitive input simultaneously received by the system (situational). In contrast, responses of other reflexes, such as hand movements, startles, and eyeblinks do send activation to units throughout the system. As a consequence, Tyrone's parents begin responding to his movements, startles, and eyeblinks (discourse) before vocalizations even occur. As these nonverbal cues are more frequently reacted to than to his speech sound productions, a negative cycle of sound production is initiated (Lojkasek, Goldberg, Marcovitch, & MacGregor, 1990; Mahoney & Powell, 1988).

At initial stages of development, vocalizations would continue to be produced. Global responses such as cries and fussing would be enhanced because they tend to be long in duration and events precipitating them (i.e., wet diapers, hunger) also are extended. These long durations would provide time and a continuous flow of input, enabling the system to establish connection weights between units representing features of crying integrated with units representing the state of hunger or wetness. Similarly, other co-occurring stimuli, such as parents responding to cries, would add further complexity to the developing network of interconnected units attached to the crying reflex. Thus, the crying response to environmental stimulation would be expected to continue to occur with frequency, and to expand in pattern of production and contexts of occurrence as the network expands.

But more subtle vocalizations, such as production of unpatterned sounds that are short in duration and associated with more momentary events (i.e., a tickle, mother's voice) would suffer from any delays or deficits in activation related to their production or perception. For example, if Tyrone's mother gently tickled his tummy to elicit a response, and Tyrone reacted immediately with a reflexive contraction of the trunk, movement of arms and legs, and opening of his eyes, followed by a delayed vocalization, then connections that formed between units in the network would adhere to a similar pattern. Connection weights for a delayed vocal response would be further strengthened, while those for nonverbal response occurring simultaneously with the stimulation would be strengthened. Tyrone's mother, anticipating a response to her tickle, would begin to react at the first sign of Tyrone's reaction, which in this case would be motor movement. Consequently, the connection weights between Tyrone's behavior and further input from the social environment would be strongest for his motor reactions, and somewhat weaker for vocalizations that occurred milliseconds later. The difference would be very slight at first, but if this pattern was repeated many times across days, weeks, and months, effects on patterns of connectivity within the network and relative weights between units for movement compared to units for vocalization would begin to gain significance. Furthermore, without noticing it, Tyrone's parents are being trained by his system to respond to his movements more immediately than his sounds, and they begin to subconsciously attend more to motor responses. By the end of the first month of life, Tyrone's developmental course is progressing differently.

EMERGING SCHEMATA: DEVELOPMENT
FROM 1 TO 4 MONTHS

Each of the situational, discourse, and semantic properties profiled within the SDS:D continua change with development across cognitive, social, semiotic, and sensory-motor domains (see Table 1.4). If the system is functioning synergistically, so that the network integrates information across modalities, subschema form to establish part-to-whole relationships, and schemata are linked by time, space, or action to form coherent event representations, then typical development will be noted and the child will demonstrate behaviors consistent with developmental expectations in all areas (Nelson, 1985, 1986; Rumelhart, 1980). Each developmental advance results from changes that occur as new patterns of connectivity between units form. These changes result in qualitative changes throughout the system. In Piagetian terms, a new equilibration operates as the system constructs new means for representing and adapting to the environment (Piaget, 1954).

Situational Context

Life for the newborn is fairly predictable, with the same events recurring repeatedly within and across days of early life. The first occurrence, or episode, sets up a schema, or pattern of connectivity between all of the sources of input received (Nelson, 1996). As the same objects, actions, participants, and consequences are present during frequently occurring events such as nursing, diapering, bathing, and sleeping, the episodes combine. Frequent multisensory input is received from these predictable objects and actions that begin to form integrated event representations (Adamson, 1995). That is, appearance of the diaper becomes integrated with the feel of the material on the skin and contrasting feelings of wet or dry. Once these event representations are formed, input entering the system activates these existing patterns of connectivity and corresponding motor patterns are networked within the event representation. The child will respond to new input according to patterns of behaviors established

TABLE 1.4
Abilities Demonstrated between 1 and 4 Months of Age Across
the Cognitive, Social, Semiotic, and Sensory-Motor Domains Profiled
within the Situational-Discourse-Semantic Contexts of the
SDS:Development Model

	1–4 Months Level Ib		
	Situational Egocentered Displacement	Discourse Discrete Event Organization	Semantic Reaction Reference
Cognitive	Object Displacement Objects noticed and reacted to with attention, excitement, or distress when within immediate environment.	Event/Discourse Coordination of schemes: look & reach, hear & look, touch & grasp, grasp & bang.	Perceptual Anticipatory reaction to stimuli: react before sound or motion occurs.
Social	Self/Other Displacement People watched and reacted to within immediate vicinity; child is responsive to others.	Interactional Controlled reaction sustained briefly; watches and responds within turn-taking interactions.	Functional Predictable action to familiar event.
Semiotic	Time/Space Displacement Reactive to immediately present sensory and proprioceptive stimuli; no attempt to reestablish or maintain an activity or event.	Locutionary No intentionality but adult interprets changes in response as meaningful.	Convention Differentiated action and cries; response to stimuli consistent although idiosyncratic.
Sensory-Motor	Imitative Displacement Repeats own behavior that has been imitated by someone else.	Executionary Patterned sounds produced repetitively, irregularly distributed.	Modality Crude and simple. Vocal=crude syllables initiated by closure, velar stop /g/.

Reprinted with permission from Norris, JA, and Hoffman, PR (1999). The SDS developmental model of integrated functioning, Baton Rouge, LA: EleMentory.

from previous experiences. Input is no longer considered as novel or unknown, but rather as familiar and functional (see Fig. 1.6) (Lamb, 1981; Mahler, Pine, & Bergman, 1975). Activation of input units spreads across the event representation and activates the next action in the event sequence, causing it to occur. This activation is observed in behaviors of the child toward an object present in the immediate environment. The behaviors

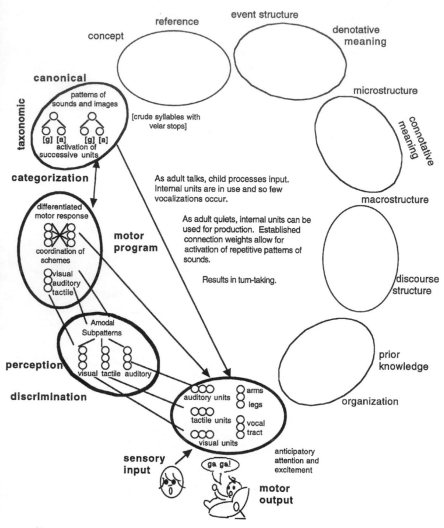

FIG. 1.6. Emergent event representation forming between 1 and 4 months. Perceptually unified, amodal structure now becoming differentiated as sensory-motor experience creates patterns of connectivity within sensory modalities and between units across modalities. Consistent patterns of co-occurring input from multiple sources integrate to form differentiated schema, resulting in primitive, preconceptual meaning. (Reprinted with permission from Norris, JA, and Hoffman, PR (1999). The SDS developmental model of integrated functioning, Baton Rouge, LA: EleMentory.)

become anticipatory, with objects reacted to with attention, excitement, or distress depending on past learning (cognitive) (Holdgrafer & Dunst, 1986; Lewis, 1987; Scoville, 1984). The sight of the diaper may elicit attention or leg kicking. Similarly, the child becomes responsive to people when they approach, and not merely reactive to adult initiations (social) (Lewis, 1987; Scoville, 1984). People are watched as they near the child, and changes in behavior such as body and limb movements or vocalizatons occur in the presence of a familiar person (semiotic) (Fogel, Diamond, Langhorst, & Demos, 1982; Wolff, 1969; Holdgrafer & Dunst, 1986).

Discourse Context

Multisensory integration of input within episodes and events also results in changes in organization of experiences (Nelson, 1986). One manifestation of this is a coordination of behaviors that at birth occurred independently. Piaget (1952) referred to this as the coordination of schemes, so that seeing an object elicits an attempt to touch it, and hearing an object elicits a directional turn toward the source of the sound (Lockman, 1986; Morehead & Morehead, 1974). Coordination occurs as the amodal undifferentiated internal structure develops specific subpatterns of connectivity for different sources of sensory input (auditory versus visual or tactile) and simultaneously strengthens connection weights for those that co-occur. Social interactions reveal similar changes in organization, including controlled reactions that are briefly sustained as adults talk to the infant, and participation in turn-taking interactions (Adamson, 1995). That is, the child responds by quieting as the adult talks, and then by moving and vocalizing as the adult quiets (Lewis, 1987; Scoville, 1984). This pattern occurs as the adult's interactions provide input to the child that activates the emerging event representation, and activation stimulates motor responses from the child through connections between auditory and motor schemata within the child's event representation. When input is not dominating the processing within the network (i.e., when the adult quits talking), units are available to activate internal schemata, and so the child takes a turn. The parent cooperates in this learning, interpreting any behavior produced by the child as meaningful and relevant (Schaffer, 1977).

Semantic Context

Modification of reflexive behaviors through addition and reweighting of connections generated through experiences results in a change in the behaviors. Experiences for which representations develop are no longer responded to reflexively because patterns of connectivity are changed. The result is the emergence of behaviors that are differentiated, so that the sight of the parent elicits a different response than the sight of a rattle. A mother's voice that at birth may have elicited a startle now elicits a smile (Wolff, 1987). The modified representations also result in responses that are more controlled and patterned because of increasing weights established between units within event representations. Responses are consistent, but idiosyncratic to the child (Fogel, Diamond, Langhorst, & Demos, 1982) because the child's reflexive responses are those which are modified, and these have not yet been reorganized and refined to resemble the conventions of others.

Vocalizations at this stage are produced in accord with representations for vocalizations that have begun to form internally. Therefore, the input-output cycle no longer represents a simple chain of connections between input and reflexive output. Rather, activated perceptual and functional features differentially spread activation to internal representations that best fit those patterns of activation. Representations may include activation of units that are not actually present in the sensory input but have been present in earlier experiences with similar stimuli (Rumelhart & McClelland, 1986). Thus, the representation is slightly different from the actual input. Similarly, vocalizations produced in response to input are no longer reflexive, but rather are different for varying sources of input. Differentiated representations for stimuli activate differentiated patterns of vocalization, so that parents begin to identify different types of cries and vocalizations (hunger versus demands or discomfort; pleasure versus drowsy) (Ramey, Beckman-Bell, & Gowen, 1980; Snow, 1984). Semantically, a primitive and presymbolic system of referring to meaning is beginning to form.

Tyrone's Atypically Developing System

Between one and four months of age, Tyrone continued to develop typically in the cognitive domain. When his bottle, favorite toy, or other familiar object was present in the immediate environment (situational), he reacted to it with attention or excitement before it neared (semantic) and showed coordination of his sensory-motor schemes by looking and reaching at the sight of the object, or by hearing and looking for the source of the sound (discourse). Socially, he also progressed as expected, watching and attending to his mother during caregiving and social play (situational), taking his turns with body movements, smiles, and some sounds when mother paused (discourse). Semiotically, nonverbal responses were more frequent, consistent, and patterned than vocalizations. Cumulative effects of his less immediate perception of and response to sound throughout the first month resulted in fewer connections and weaker connection weights to auditory information within Tyrone's network than what would be expected in normal development. Consequently, gestures and other nonverbals are more consistently interpreted as meaningful communications during caregiving and play and attended to more frequently by parents. Connections between these responses continue to strengthen and expand through direct and indirect connections to units throughout the network.

In contrast, connections for vocalizations continue to be established with a delay in timing between occurrence of an event and the vocal reaction. Delayed responding was strengthened throughout the first month of development, increasing the probability that the delay would continue or increase with further learning. Additionally, connections to situational, discourse, and semantic elements of the developing system are different in their pattern of activation than would be expected in normal learning. In typical learning, when vocalization occurs without a delay, a touch or other input from the caregiver develops simultaneous connections with the vocalization. Vocalization by one month of age becomes an immediately occurring response to presence of the mother (Mahler, Pine, & Bergman, 1975; Wolff, 1987). Presymbolic meaning (i.e., connectivity associated with the mother) and presymbolic vocal reference (i.e., connectivity associated with sound patterns) would be developing as an integrated representation. But the weak or delayed connections in Tyrone's system result in touch or sight of the mother eliciting vocalization less reliably. Thus, vocalization occurs less frequently and contingently during turn-taking interactions. Failure to vocalize means parents have fewer opportunities to interpret these productions as meaningful, and so patterns of vocalization will fail to develop differentially in response to different stimuli. These differences in Tyrone's system will result in further disruptions to development during the next substage of infancy.

EMERGENCE OF REPRESENTATIONAL MEANING: DEVELOPMENT FROM 3 TO 8 MONTHS

In infancy, a few weeks of development result in remarkable changes in abilities of the child. Between 3 and 8 months of age, event representations and schemas that represent objects, people, actions, and other features of the environment increase in number, complexity, and interconnectivity. The system is no longer limited to sensory-motor perceptions. Rather, the input activates connections to internal representations and consequently begins the process of distancing thought and response from the immediate perception (see Table 1.5).

TABLE 1.5
Abilities Demonstrated between 3 and 8 Months of Age Across
the Cognitive, Social, Semiotic, and Sensory-Motor Domains Profiled
within the Situational-Discourse-Semantic Contexts of the
SDS: Development Model

	3–8 Months Level IIa		
	Situational Decentered Displacement	Discourse Collection Organization	Semantic Indication Reference
Cognitive	Object Displacement Objects manipulated to explore properties, including whole objects and their parts. Reaches for objects distanced or only partially visible.	Event/Discourse Organizes experience by performing action and attending to effects of own action with expectation something will occur.	Perceptual Primitive concepts of objects based on perceptual features (color, size, shape, sound), so can discriminate between objects.
Social	Self/Other Displacement Observes the presence and actions of people at a distance; interest in body parts and facial features.	Interactional Child uses schemes to control own level of input; participates in simple social games like peek-a-boo, pat-a-cake.	Functional Objects for primitive classes (preconcepts) such as instruments to shake and listen to, or grasp and squeeze.
Semiotic	Time/Space Displacement Reactive to immediately present sensory and proprioceptive stimuli; maintained for short time, reinitiated.	Locutionary Behaviors occur in response to stimuli, not purposefully to affect adult, but function to maintain adult interaction.	Convention Responds with recognizable behavior to action, people, or objects (smile, reach, pull, drop).
Sensory-Motor	Imitative Displacement Imitates other's behaviors if the behavior is already in child's repertoire.	Exocutionary Repeating patterns of verbal and nonverbal behaviors; sounds, actions, gestures.	Modality Variety of vowel sounds with marginal babbling caused by vocal tract closures.

Reprinted with permission from Norris, JA, and Hoffman, PR (1999). The SDS developmental model of integrated functioning, Baton Rouge, LA: EleMentory.

Situational Context

During the first months of life, external input directly impacting on the child was the primary source for initiation and maintenance of activation. With no representation of objects, people, or events existing within the internal network of connections, this unelaborated processing of input was all that could be conducted. But with formation of internal representations, units within the network begin to activate each other (Rumelhart & Mc-Clelland, 1986). That is, when sensory input activates units, these units spread their activation to internal units. Importantly, these internal units have only indirect connection to input units and to each other through layers of hidden units (see Fig. 1.7). The network thus creates patterns of activation separate from sensory input units. The network also includes a variety of connections between particular units at one level to particular units at another, allowing for context sensitivity in response of units at one level to those at another. This independence from sensory input enables the internal representation to interpret and maintain attention to the external object. It continues the activation even if the sensory input ceases, causing the child to continue to watch the object. Furthermore, existence of object representations forming within the overall event representation creates the possibility of initiating patterns of activation internally.

Existence of internal representations, concommitant with increasing motor skills, allows for a very different situational context to exist for the child. Objects that can be reached can be manipulated (Jens & Johnson, 1982; Lockman, 1986; Rose & Ruff, 1987). Schemas for objects are integrally connected to event representations for actions that govern these manipulations, allowing them to be repeated and reinitiated (Nelson, 1985). Furthermore, ability to activate subschemas enables the child to explore properties of the object and to discover part-to-whole relationships (Uzgiris, 1983). Socially, a greater interest in body parts and facial features is observed, as the child plays the "mine versus yours" game, touching, pulling hair, pulling off glasses, and in other ways manipulating the features of others. The child is beginning to discover an existence separate from other people, as these explorations form differential representations for self versus others (Mahler, Pine, & Bergman, 1975). These differential representations are forming both perceptually, or on the basis of physical differences, and functionally, based on differential roles within the event representation (i.e., Who gives the bath and who takes it) (Nelson, 1996). Representations also make it possible for objects that cannot be reached or manipulated to be observed (Piaget, 1954). Internal representations establish and maintain activation for the object or person, even when the actual input occurs at a greater physical distance from the child's sensory system. The changing situational context is thus characterized by longer attention

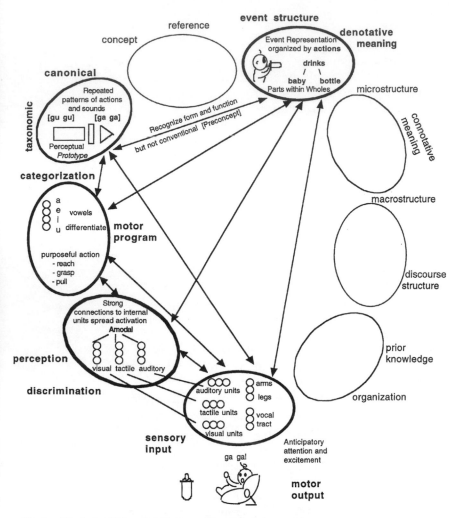

event structure

reference

concept

canonical

Event Representation organized by **actions**

denotative meaning

drinks
/   \
baby   bottle
Parts within Wholes

microstructure

connotative meaning

taxonomic

Repeated patterns of actions and sounds

[gu gu]   [ga ga]

Perceptual Prototype

Recognize form and function but not conventional [Preconcept]

categorization

a
e
i   vowels
u   differentiate

motor program

macrostructure

purposeful action
- reach
- grasp
- pull

Strong connections to internal units spread activation

Amodal

visual tactile auditory

discourse structure

perception

discrimination

auditory units

arms

legs

tactile units

vocal tract

visual units

prior knowledge

organization

sensory input

Anticipatory attention and excitement

ga ga!

motor output

Situational Context: Child reacts to familiar people or objects from a distance. (Contextualized-Decentered)

FIG. 1.7. Whole-to-part relationships form within event representation between 3 and 8 months. Emerging preconcepts of people and objects form from stable patterns of perceptual features and functional role within the event representation. The preconcepts are inseparably connected to the event representation through the unifying action, so cannot yet form a true concept. These internal structures allow for maintenance of attention to distanced objects and differentiated actions for objects within a familiar event. (Reprinted with permission from Norris, JA, and Hoffman, PR (1999). The SDS developmental model of integrated functioning, Baton Rouge, LA: EleMentory.)

to objects and people located at greater distances from the child, organized by developing representations of both the wholes and the parts for these entities (Moore & Dunham, 1995).

Discourse Context

Representations constructed by the child allow for an emerging ability to organize experience by differentially performing actions to objects and then attending to effects of these actions. The child's behavior is goal oriented, but established after the activity begins (no anticipation or true intention) (Lamb, 1981; Masur, 1983; Piaget, 1954). Event representations include an increasingly greater number of units coordinating action *schemes*. Event representations also provide a means for unifying touching, listening, and looking to allow for sustained attention to the object and consequently integration of new actions or states (i.e., effects of action) into patterns of connectivity. This expansion and extension across units rapidly builds complexity within internal representations. More complex event representations begin to form with roles for agents, actions, objects, and consequences for these experiences (Nelson, 1986, 1996). However, connections between performed actions and the object are much stronger than connections between observed actions of others and the object. This results in the child viewing himself as the cause of action and excluding the roles of others. Therefore, the concept of causality, or cause and effect, does not extend beyond the child as the agent (Piaget, 1952, 1960). In older children with limited development, the failure to watch their own actions for effects is prevalent, and the resulting lack of increasing complexity and purpose in their behavior is not surprising.

Representations constructed by the child for others and their roles within the event representation allows for the ability to differentially respond to people and their actions, as well as to attend to effects of these interactions (Harding, 1983; Mahler, Pine, & Bergman, 1975). The construction of differential roles within the event representation enables the child to be an active participant in simple social games such as peek-a-boo or pat-a-cake where the child can respond with recognizable behaviors such as smiles or body movements to adult actions (Ross & Lollis, 1987). As play continues, anticipatory reactions such as body wiggling or squealing may occur in response to the adult, which the adult interprets as a request to continue the game. Consequently, the child's actions unintentionally serve to control actions of others and to sustain the activity for a prolonged period (Harding, 1983; Snow, 1984). This repetition of the social game provides both time and repeated exposure needed to add complexity and connection strength to units mapping turn-taking, interactional strategies, communicative functions, and other aspects of social and pragmatic knowledge.

Semantic Context

The emergence of representational meaning can be observed at this stage of development. Sufficient patterns of connectivity exist for familiar objects and actions to allow them to form preconcepts. Preconcepts exist as stable patterns of perceptual features that form a prototype. These preconceptual representations are created on the basis of the intrinsic form and function of the object, such as recognizing that a ball is round (form) and it bounces (function), embedded within the sensory-motor events in which the object is experienced (pushing the ball) (Nelson, 1996). Thus, objects of a particular size, color, and shape begin to be discriminated as different from other objects because of their appearance within an event, even though the child does not yet have a concept of the object and its conventional use or function (Mervis, 1987). Rather, functional knowledge is limited to primitive classes of use, such as things that can be banged versus instruments to shake and listen to (Piaget, 1960). Consequently, familiar objects or objects that fit the prototype are responded to with recognizable and predictable behaviors, such as smiles, reaches, pulls, and drops (Roberts & Horowitz, 1986). One part of an event (the appearance of a bottle) functions as a signal for another event (eating) (Acredolo & Goodwyn, 1985).

Vocalizations at this stage also exhibit differentiated patterns of connectivity. Vocal behavior increasingly diversifies with new forms including more vowel-like sounds, and some marginal babbling in which vocal tract closures are imprecisely and irregularly alternated with vowel-like elements (Stark, 1979). Advances in growth and maturation of the motor system make these new forms of input possible. Squeals, growls, and trills also are produced. The integration of this input with existing representations results in their differential production in response to pleasurable and adverse stimuli (Bates, O'Connell, & Shore, 1987), indicating that the representations for these forms of vocal output are networked to preconcepts for objects and people that have formed in the internal representational network. Input from these stimuli readily spreads activation to units controlling these vocalizations.

Tyrone's Unorganized Response to Sound

Tyrone's cognitive development continued as expected. He manipulated objects, organized them by action schemes within event representations, and formed patterns of connectivity for the perceptual features related to an object's whole configuration and its parts. Some objects were differentiated into preconcepts, and Tyrone responded with anticipation to these objects and people. Socially, Tyrone watched people from a distance and established patterns of connectivity between people and objects they used.

When adults initiated games such as peek-a-boo he watched faces until his face was covered, and then reached, wiggled, and squealed when the blanket was removed from his face. But when his mother vocalized to him, Tyrone rarely vocalized back. Unlike other stimuli, patterns of connectivity for vocalizations had not begun to form differentiated schemas and were not becoming networked to preconceptual representations. Production of sound by an adult provided input to the system, but this input did not in turn activate internal units related to production of vowel sounds. These links between units had not been established during earlier months and so the system could not reproduce the sounds. Vocal reactions, when they did occur, continued to occur with a delay and were connected to reflexive responding rather than differentiated behavior. Reflexive responses in other aspects of Tyrone's behavior were becoming modified by experience, with strong interconnections forming with emerging complex representations. Connections with vocalizations were becoming increasingly diminished, and without excitation from other sources, weakening in strength and frequency of activation or occurrence. The weakest aspect of his development was becoming increasingly weaker.

A MEANS TO AN END: DEVELOPMENT FROM 7 TO 10 MONTHS

The first six months of development established internal representations for objects and people, their related actions, and part-to-whole relationships. Many of these integrated patterns of connectivity exist as event representations for frequently occurring experiences. The second 6 months of development focus on establishing relationships between objects that form paradigmatic groups, objects within the group sharing roles in unified sequences of actions to form event representations. Event sequences refine with emergence of scripts that define the event, including a beginning and ending, roles of actors, agents, recipients, and beneficiaries, and goals organized around the scripts (Barsalou, 1991). These complex event representations render the child more independent and adaptive to the physical and social environment, as shown in Table 1.6.

Situational Context

Greater displacement in thought is obtained as the child is able to maintain patterns of activation for an object schema while attending to effects of her own action on the object (Lamb, 1981; Masur, 1983). The event representation makes this possible. Within the event, the child maintains a role, such as the agent who performs an action, such as banging, on an

TABLE 1.6
Abilities Demonstrated between 7 and 10 Months of Age Across
the Cognitive, Social, Semiotic, and Sensory-Motor Domains Profiled
within the Situational-Discourse-Semantic Contexts of the
SDS:Development Model

	7–10 Months Level IIb		
	Situational Decentered Displacement	Discourse Collection Organization	Semantic Indication Reference
Cognitive	Object Displacement One object can be used to explore or manipulate a second object (i.e., means-ends behavior).	Event/Discourse Attention coordinated between two objects to maintain an event such as stacking, putting in.	Perceptual Recognizes objects by properties (things you roll, pull). Tracks until out of sight.
Social	Self/Other Displacement Uses other people to achieve personal purpose, such as raising hands up to request adult to lift up (i.e., means-ends behavior).	Interactional Uses behaviors to purposefully initate and terminate interaction with others; maintains own role.	Functional Differential actions applied to object according to the function of object (roll a car because it has wheels).
Semiotic	Time/Space Displacement Maintain interesting stimuli to achieve an outcome; visually tracks objects until not visible.	Locutionary Purposefully controls objects or people, but does not show or share objects with others (i.e., purpose but not intent).	Convention Culturally recognized gestures (wave, kiss, shake no); babbling-like language.
Sensory-Motor	Imitative Displacement Imitates unknown behaviors similar to ones in child's repertoire.	Exocutionary Well-formed patterns of movements including vocal syllables produced repetitively [dada], or repetitive banging.	Modality Vocal closures released into an open vocal tract such as [da] or [ba].

Reprinted with permission from Norris, JA, and Hoffman, PR (1999). The SDS developmental model of integrated functioning, Baton Rouge, LA: EleMentory.

42

object. Thus, within the event represention many schemas already exist for actions that formed strong patterns of connectivity during the first 6 months. Well-established representations enhance learning. Since actions can be spontaneously and automatically instantiated, new learning can focus on what can be accomplished by applying those actions. The focus of the child's attention is no longer on performing actions using his own body, but rather on effects of those actions on objects. From the general event representation, a script begins to form and generalize across events with similarities (see Fig. 1.8) (Nelson, 1996).

For example, banging a spoon and banging a block begin to form a pattern of connectivity that is separate from either event. Instead, a more abstract representation emerges comprised of a script such as "Child/self (agent) bangs (action)—(objects)." The scripts define roles and begin to increase predictability of experiences and afford the child a level of control (Barsalou, 1991). Thus, while events were largely under adult control during the first 6 months of life, they increasingly come under the child's control as he assumes a stronger participatory role (Brazelton & Tronick, 1980; Holdgrafer & Dunst, 1986).

Play and other experiences afford the child opportunities to apply many actions to the same objects, and to perform the same action with many objects (Piaget, 1954, 1960; Ross & Lollis, 1987). Patterns of connectivity across a wide variety of actions and objects are thus highly integrated. Focus on effects of actions on objects and interconnected patterns of connectivity across objects and actions allow for expansion of the event representation to include a series of actions and objects to accomplish one goal. The first action serves as a means to achieve the second action, or end. Early signs of this means-end behavior include pushing aside a barrier to obtain a blocked object. Near the end of this developmental stage strategies such as pulling on a blanket to obtain an object, requiring an understanding of tool usage (i.e., the instrument function within the event representation), are commonly used (Roberts & Horowitz, 1986; Uzgiris, 1983). The shared interconnections within events make such purposeful series of actions possible.

Similar displacement in thought is observed socially. The child increasingly understands herself to be different and separate from others because of respective roles within event representations. One way in which this is manifested is "stranger anxiety," indicating that the child recognizes that other people are distinct from oneself even when (or perhaps especially when) that person is in physical contact (Osofsky, 1987). Another manifestation is a social form of means-end behavior, such as raising hands up to indicate a desire to be picked up or held. This behavior is engaged in for its own effects, and not as a means to accomplish a different goal (i.e., the child signals to be picked up to be held, rather than picked up to reach a cookie on a table) until late in this stage (Holdgrafer & Dunst,

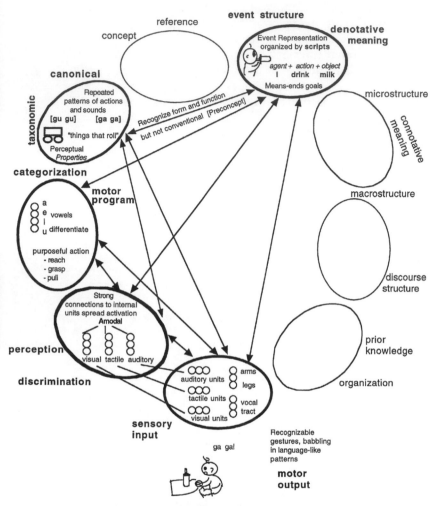

event structure

reference

concept

denotative meaning

Event Representation
organized by **scripts**

agent + action + object
I   drink   milk

Means-ends goals

canonical

taxonomic

Repeated
patterns of actions
and sounds
[gu gu]   [ga ga]

"things that roll"

Recognize form and function
but not conventional [Preconcept]

microstructure

connotative
meaning

Perceptual
Properties

categorization

**motor
program**

a
e vowels
i
u differentiate

macrostructure

purposeful action
- reach
- grasp
- pull

discourse
structure

Strong
connections to internal
units spread activation
Amodal

perception

visual tactile auditory

prior
knowledge

discrimination

auditory units   arms

legs

tactile units   vocal
tract

visual units

organization

**sensory
input**

ga ga!

Recognizable
gestures, babbling
in language-like
patterns

**motor
output**

Situational Context: Internal structures enable child to use objects and people (means) to achieve goals (ends).
(Contextualized-Decentered)

FIG. 1.8. Event representation is organized by scripts, rather than sensory-motor action beween 7 and 10 months. Child recognizes self and others as agents that cause actions to occur (i.e., roles). This allows the child to focus on the effects actions have on objects, an emerging form of problem solving that results in means-ends behavior. Goals are purposeful (Integration of action and communication as in signaling to be picked up) but not yet intentional (coordination of communication with people and objects, as in signaling to be picked up to reach an object). (Reprinted with permission from Norris, JA, and Hoffman, PR (1999). The SDS developmental model of integrated functioning, Baton Rouge, LA: EleMentory.)

44

1986). The appearance of means-ends indicates that patterns of connectivity are formed in which representations for objects, people, and events are connected like "roads across a landscape." This integration and complexity adds new and amazing flexibility to the system. If a direct action for obtaining or manipulating an object or person cannot be used, then an alternative route can be followed. The spontaneity of these means-ends actions, such as pulling on a bedspread the moment mother places her purse out of the child's reach indicates that the child can create and activate these alternative routes using existing connections without extensive learning. The connections established in the previous stage by attending to outcomes of actions have produced sufficient strengths to generalize to new situations, and the child anticipates which actions will result in the desired outcome (Acredolo & Goodwyn, 1985).

Discourse Context

Representations constructed by the child allow for an emerging ability to create and control the physical and social environment, rather than merely responding to the context that is present (Piaget, 1954). For the first time attention can be coordinated between two objects (Moore & Dunham, 1995). During this stage the child may try to maintain interesting stimuli using two objects, such as banging two hard objects together, or attempting to stack two blocks. The control means that the child is no longer dependent on others to initiate events, but can now initiate actions and maintain the activity for short durations (Mahler, Pine, & Bergman, 1975). The child's behavior thus becomes purposeful and directed toward achieving simple goals such as shaking a desired object, retrieving an object placed out of reach, or differentially banging one object while sucking on another. Communications produced at this stage are also social and purposeful (Holdgrafer & Dunst, 1986). That is, the child may vocalize in association with seeing a familiar object or person because of previously established connection weights between auditory, tactile, and visual information within a representation. A reach or vocalization may be produced for purposes of maintaining contact, being picked up, terminating interaction, or protesting an event. However, these communications are not intentional (Bates, Camaioni, & Volterra, 1975; Vedeler, 1987). At this stage, children do not have sufficient patterns of connectivity to understand that other people can help them achieve their goals. The purposeful communications reflect connections between the child and his goals with objects, but not the child, objects, and insights into potential actions of others to achieve those goals. Thus, a child may reach, pull, climb, cry, and try numerous other strategies to obtain an object, but cannot yet turn to another and directly point to the object of desire with the intent of having the adult retrieve it (Holdgrafer & Dunst, 1986).

Connections that exist between the child and others do allow the child to participate in social games that involve integration of actions with communications. For example, a game of pat-a-cake now can be maintained by a child who vocalizes whenever action stops (Ross & Lollis, 1987). Caregivers reinitiate the game when they hear the purposeful vocalization, interpreting it as an intentional command to play more (Adamson, 1995). These games not only reinforce the child's communications, but also model more conventional words and sounds that are appropriate in meaning and function to the context, such as "Play more" or "Do it again?" This social play and accompanying talk is particulary effective if the input provided by the parent matches or is slightly in advance of the child's current level of development, a concept Vygotsky (1962) refers to as interacting within the child's Zone of Proximal Development (ZPD).

The Zone of Proximal Development represents a range of input to the child that can be assimilated into existing representations while also maximally facilitating accommodations. In connectionist terms, the lower level of the zone represents patterns of connectivity already established. Input at this level activates existing patterns with minimal change to the system. The upper level of the zone represents new patterns of connectivity that can be established if the input provides enough information to facilitate forming connections between previously unlinked schemas, or reconfiguring patterns of connectivity within existing representations to form associated, new representions. Above the ZPD the child lacks critical representations, and so few new structures can be constructed. According to Vygotsky (1962), the process of collaboratively constructing new representations occurs through social mediation, where the adult acts as a mentor and engages the child in an activity at a level more difficult than the child can perform independently. The adult supports the child's participation by providing mediation, such as beginning an action and then letting the child complete it, telling the child the next step in a sequence that must be performed, pointing to some relevant bit of information needed to complete the task and talking about its function, or providing other similar support for learning. The adult in such interactions monitors how well the child is responding, and accordingly increases or decreases the amount of mediated support (Adamson, 1995).

This type of mediated support occurs as a natural part of parent-child interactions during language learning. Parents talk about objects or events that the child is already attending to, treat the child as a conversational participant even when the child is at a prelanguage stage of development, imitate the child's vocalizations and expand to model more conventional words or longer word combinations, extend the topic by adding information to a subject initiated by the child, use exaggerated intonation and stress to enable the child to attend to important aspects of language, slow their rate of speech production and repeat utterances to provide time to process information, and use words knowable to the child, such as pointing to objects while labeling and describing their actions or properties (Sachs, 1993; Snow, 1984). Each of these mediation strategies serves to activate patterns of connectivity that the child already has formed, provides input at a level that makes use of existing patterns of connectivity for sounds or meaning even if the specific word does not yet exist within the child's system, and provides simultaneous input from visual or other sensory sources that can help the child form relevant new patterns of connectivity for meaning and form of new words or syntactic structures.

Parents not attuned to their child's needs may not provide the appropriate level or type of social mediation needed to expand and refine the child's network of associated connections. The parent may fail to respond to the child's vocalizations, ignoring the child completely or attending to biological needs without responding socially to the child's purposeful behaviors. Or a parent may respond to the child, but be out of synchrony with the child's rate of processing information (Lojkasek, Goldberg, Marcovitch, & MacGregor, 1990). For example, the child may vocalize and the parent may imitate, but not until after the child's attention is directed elsewhere. Or the parent may provide input to the child that is well above his ZPD, and therefore is unusable to the child's system. For example, instead of imitating the child's vocalization, parents may talk in complete sentences using abstract words during their communicative turn (Mahoney & Powell, 1988). These types of responses may make it difficult for the child to form interconnected patterns, since the child lacks an internal representation for the input provided by the parent and has no structure to which information can be assimilated or compared.

When parents are responsive to initiations of children, the child's discovery that objects and people can be purposefully controlled provides both impetus and means to develop strategies to communicate these goals. It is not surprising that new developments emerge in the semantic context to facilitate this.

Semantic Context

More objects become meaningfully recognized during this stage, but based on the perceptual properties of the object and not the symbolic function (i.e., they remain preconcepts). For example, a child might roll a car or other wheeled object intermittently while exploring its parts, but without knowledge that cars are driven by people on a road. The perceptual property of the object, and not symbolic function, is responded to, resulting in no attempts to place people in the car or to drive along a road. This perceptually based familiarity results in other differentiated actions applied to recognized objects, such as pushing buttons versus pulling levers when presented with toys or objects (Nelson, 1986, 1996).

Patterns of connectivity existing within the system enable a child to re-activate sequences of action once they have begun, resulting in imitation of one's own behaviors. In addition, activation from input provided by actions of others is sufficient to result in activation of similar patterns existing within the system to produce imitation of other's behaviors (Kaye & Marcus, 1981; Stine & Bohannon, 1983). However, this imitation is restricted to unknown behaviors similar to one in the child's repertoire, meaning the basic patterns of connectivity must be in place for imitation to occur. Culturally recognized gestures, including points, reaches, pulling away, shaking no, smiling, kissing, hugging, waving, and eye contact toward a goal object emerge within routines through imitation during this stage (Holdgrafer & Dunst, 1986). These gestures are inseparable from the routine and its corresponding event representation in the same manner that objects and actions are part of the integrated event (Nelson, 1986, 1989). Parents provide prompts that serve as input, activating use of these gestures appropriately in social routines such as greeting, or playing social games such as peek-a-boo (Ross & Lollis, 1987).

Other behavioral imitations entered into internal representations through imitation of self and others include syllabic sound sequences such as [dadadada]. Early canonical babbling starts for most infants at 7–8 months of age and appears rather abruptly (Oller & Eilers, 1988). Evidence from anatomical, physiological, perceptual, and aerodynamic research suggests that the child's physical system is sufficiently mature to produce consonants at this time, and that perceptual categories for these sounds and their related oral gestures are well-formed schemata within the child's system (MacKain et al., 1983). Self-imitation of spontaneous productions and imitations of sounds produced by others both serve to strengthen connection weights between acoustic and production features for these sounds and to increase the frequency of their occurrence within a variety of contexts (Snow, 1989).

Tyrone's Failed Transition to Babbling

Tyrone's cognitive system is relatively unaffected by poor integration of auditory-vocal information into internal representations. His explorations with objects have resulted in event representations sufficiently complex to support means-end problem solving comparable to his peers, and he recognizes many objects by their perceptual properties. Socially, he can use means-end to signal his wants, and he can initiate and terminate interactions with others using nonverbal means. His event representations mark differential roles for agents, actions, and objects and his actions are appropriate to the properties of an object. Semiotically, nonverbal communications are produced, including waves, kisses, and head shaking, and he uses purposeful strategies to accomplish his goals.

Motorically, like his peers, Tyrone is capable of producing movements necessary for production of [ba] and [da] syllables (Stark, 1979), but even when these are spontaneously produced they are not integrated into well established patterns of vocalizations and syllable productions. Since syllables did not integrate with representations for social games, response to anticipated stimuli within event representations, preconcepts, or consequences of actions, the syllable is represented primarily as a perceptual entity, with no functional utility. To the child, the syllable is similar to a bird call: the internal representation recognizes it as familiar and associates it with its source, but the sound is not imitated or produced because it is not activated by connectivity to other representations. The schema for vocalizations continues to evolve in isolation, with few opportunities for increasing its connection strength for productive use. Development of the ability to produce a consonant does nothing to improve this status. The consonant by its nature has to be produced in the context of a vowel. Consequently, a spontaneously produced consonant will integrate with the vowel in the existing representation. But instead of the vowel connecting the consonant through its established connections to meaning and function, the vowel inhibits the consonant. Like other sounds, the emerging consonant is processed as nonadaptive background information. Rather than expanding into well-formed patterns of repetitive movements, or babbling, the sounds remain unrehearsed.

THE EMERGENCE OF RELATIONAL KNOWLEDGE: DEVELOPMENT FROM 10 TO 14 MONTHS

The ability to coordinate two objects and to use objects as a means to an end establishes the foundation for the next achievement in infant development, or the acquisition of relational knowledge. Relational knowledge refers to the use of objects for intentional functional purposes, such as the use of a spoon for eating, and meaningful use of objects in relationship with other objects in the same event or routine, such as a spoon used in relationship to a bowl. Emergence of relational knowledge begins near the child's first birthday, as profiled in Table 1.7.

Situational Context

Throughout the first year of development, knowledge is organized on the basis of event representations constructed from routines. During the

TABLE 1.7
Abilities Demonstrated between 10 and 14 Months of Age Across
the Cognitive, Social, Semiotic, and Sensory-Motor Domains Profiled
within the Situational-Discourse-Semantic Contexts of the
SDS:Development Model

	10–14 Months Level IIIa		
	Relational *Situational* *Relational* *Displacement*	*Descriptive List* *Discourse* *Descriptive List* *Organization*	*Labeling* *Semantic* *Labeling* *Reference*
Cognitive	Object Displacement Objects used in relationships (fork retrieves pancake) with appropriate use in routines. Uses objects and novel actions to experiment with objects to see what happens.	Event/Discourse Maintains extended attention to same event, but rapid change in action or focus. Anticipates next step of a familiar routine.	Perceptual Recognizes relationships between operating parts of wholes (knobs, levers, buttons, dials) and uses differentiated actions.
Social	Self/Other Displacement Recognizes things others can do (open a container). Returns frequently to adult for reassurance during distanced explorations.	Interactional Uses behaviors to intentionally initiate and terminate interaction with others; adult maintains conversation across several turns.	Functional Objects recognized for functional purposes (things you eat, drive). Imitate sound and action sequences and patterns.
Semiotic	Time/Space Displacement Words and response to objects highly contextualized to immediate environment; finds hidden objects.	Locutionary Communicative behavior produced with true intent and social purpose (reject, request object or action, or comment).	Convention Small vocabulary of single words, jargon as if talking; verbalizations supported by gestures; long strings of inflected sounds.
Sensory-Motor	Imitative Displacement Imitates unknown behaviors if the behavior is similar to one in child's repertoire.	Exocutionary Repeating patterns of verbal and nonverbal behaviors; sounds, actions, gestures.	Modality Variety of consonant CV and VC sounds, intonation changes; nonverbal, pulls, drops, bangs, reaches.

Reprinted with permission from Norris, JA, and Hoffman, PR (1999). The SDS developmental model of integrated functioning, Baton Rouge, LA: EleMentory.

second year, concepts and words must be abstracted from contexts that bind them. For this to occur, true concepts must form that are separate from the event representation (Nelson, 1996). This process began with formation of scripts within event representations including roles of people and objects specific to the event. Roles provide the basis for formation of more abstract categories (Barsalou, 1991). These early categories are referred to as slot-filler categories because they are composed of items that can fulfill the same roles, or fill the same slot, within the event representation (Lucariello & Rifkin, 1986). For example, items eaten at breakfast, such as bananas, cereal, or eggs, may be substituted for each other within a slot. The shared occurrence within the same role thus establishes patterns of connectivity between these items that bear little perceptual similarity to each other but yet are alike in function (see Fig. 1.9). These new concepts are different from primitive classes of perceptual preconcepts observed between 3 and 10 months. Patterns of connectivity that evolve from the slot-filler role create a level of representation that is based more on functional role than on perceptual appearance (Nelson, 1996). New patterns of connectivity between varied objects that fill the slot form a level of representation distanced from the event representation or the script from which the conceptual category evolved.

The conceptual structure that is beginning to form out of event representations is two dimensional. From the slot-filler categories, concepts form that are like each other on the basis of similarity of role or function. These are categories such as things you eat, wear, or ride on, as well as animals, vegetables, or buildings. This type of organization is referred to as paradigmatic (Nelson, 1996; Saussure, 1959/1915). Paradigmatic relationships can be seen as units of a particular level of the model, such as *mom dad sis* who can serve in the same functional slot at a higher level, for example, and can be persons who act to pick the child up. The other dimension of conceptual organization is related to the script, or relationships between agents, actions, and objects that unify the entities into a whole event. This type of organization is referred to as syntagmatic. Syntagmatic organization may be seen as organization imposed by units at one level upon those at a different level. For example, the eating routine's organization of a sequence of actions. Both the organization of integrated wholes and separation into conceptual categories or parts are critical to development of conceptual organization.

Manifestations of this emerging conceptual organization can be seen in cognitive characteristics of the situation at this stage of development. The child begins to use objects in appropriate relationships, such as using forks and spoons to eat, within familiar routines. Similarly, toys are played with according to expected actions, such as attempting to stack rings on a post, or placing pegs in a board (Fenson & Ramsey, 1980; Roth & Clark, 1987; Sachs,

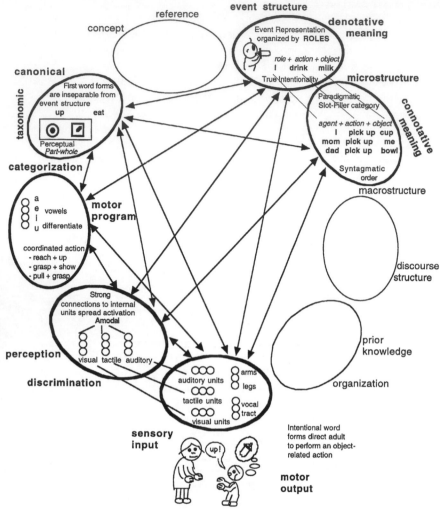

Situational Context: Internal structures enable child to use people to achieve goals (intention).
(Contextualized-Relational)

FIG. 1.9. Event representation is organized by roles between 10 and 14 months. Child can connect roles and actions of others to personal roles and actions, so understands that adult's action can be used to accomplish child's goal (signaling to be picked up to reach an object). Preconcepts become structured by the script to form slot-filler categories of objects that can function within the same role (paradigmatic organization of the event representation). Sequence of actions imposed by adult orders roles in the event, thus imposing syntagmatic organization in the microstructure. Sound patterns merge with event representation to result in word forms that refer to the event structure but not individual concepts. (Reprinted with permission from Norris, JA, and Hoffman, PR (1999). The SDS developmental model of integrated functioning, Baton Rouge, LA: EleMentory.)

1984). Socially, the child begins to understand roles of others within the event. The child may hold out a container, recognizing that the adult can open it (Bates, Camaioni, & Volterra, 1975; Chapman, 1981; Seibert, Hogan, & Mundy, 1982). Object permanence also is observed as the child can find hidden objects. To accomplish this, the child must maintain relationships within the whole event, recognizing that someone must have moved or altered the location of the object before it can be expected to be somewhere different (Nelson, 1996). Relationships present within the event structure and the ability to form slot-filler categories also enable the child to imitate unknown behaviors if they are similar to one in the child's repertoire (Holdgrafer & Dunst, 1986; Piaget, 1954). While the child is continuing to construct knowledge about her own roles within events, actions are increasingly influenced by an active awareness of the roles and impact of others. Understanding the roles of others provides motivation to influence those roles to accomplish one's own goals (Mahler, Pine, & Bergman, 1975).

Discourse Context

To act intentionally, one must know that behaviors of others can be controlled. Therefore, expansion of the event representation to incorporate a script with roles and functional relationships enables the emergence of true intentionality. Existence of roles associated with actions and outcomes different than one's own results is necessary to understanding that other people can help achieve goals (Lewis, 1987; Nelson, 1996). The event representations must include patterns of connectivity between roles and actions of others as well as roles and actions of the child in relationship to objects. Construction of an event representation capable of coordinating roles of the child and adult provides a new means of problem solving and adapting to the environment.

The expanded event representation also results in maintenence of extended attention to the same event, but with a rapid change in action or focus (Kaye & Marcus, 1981). This suggests that despite coordination of dual roles within the event representation, temporal and causal connections present in adult event representations are not established in the child's conceptual structure (Nelson, 1996). Rather, actions and objects are organized by association, with input from one object or action spreading activation to the higher level routine that links that action or object to others in the routine. For example, the child may attend to the food and dishes present on a highchair tray for an extended period, alternately spooning food, banging on the tray, eating bites with fingers and other event-related actions. The event representation lacks a tool for establishing relationships between these action sequences, and so they occur in random order with no overall goal or sequence.

Similarly, the expanded event representations enable the child to become interested in toys that have a variety of knobs, buttons, and levers that can be manipulated with no regard to sequence (Fenson & Ramsey, 1980; Roth & Clark, 1987; Sachs, 1984). Once the lever scheme has been activated, it can be repeated and cause the child to intentionally pull it again. That is, the end of the lever pulling script (i.e., seeing a window open on a toy) is interconnected with the beginning of the script (i.e., grabbing the lever) and so activation of the script becomes self-perpetuating and results in extended attention to the event if there is a rapid change in action or focus and no temporal sequence is required. Toys that require a temporal sequence for success cannot be manipulated. However, in highly familiar contexts of routine action sequences, beginnings of temporal sequences can be observed (Nelson, 1985, 1986). When adults impose temporal order on the routine, the child is able to participate and anticipate actions before they occur, indicating connections marking temporal relationships are forming. This is observed in behaviors such as holding out hands to be wiped at the end of the eating event. Cues provided by the adult, such as saying "Time to get cleaned up," or moving toward the sink provide input that is recognized as part of the event representation when performed in that context (Nelson, 1985; Vygotsky, 1962). That input is sufficient to activate the relevant action sequence even before the action has begun.

Semantic Context

The elaborated event representation also allows for emergence of first word forms (Snow, Perlmann, & Nathan, 1987). These emergent word forms are different from the adult form, representing the entire event rather than a specific concept. For example, "eat" holistically represents the entire eating event, and not the action of eating. The word enters the event representation in the same manner as other elements of the event, through sensory input occurring simultaneously with sights, sounds, touches, and other perceptions received through the sensory system. Multimodal experiences, such as parental talk during nursing, bathing, or dressing provide opportunities for units activated for speech production to interconnect with the sensory input provided by visual, auditory, and tactile input related to speech production, and also to actions and agents occurring in concert. With repeated similar experiences, strong connection weights form among vocalization, touch, and visual image. The schema that develops associates components of the event, so that eventually the activation of part of the sequence spreads activation to other parts of the event representation. That is, appearance of a familiar object or person spreads activation to units for sounds and words associated with the event representation. The child consequently produces the word in context, and the adult imparts a contextually appropriate meaning on the utterance (Snow, Perlmann, & Nathan, 1987). Thus, the adult treats the word with far greater specificity in meaning and intent than was actually allowed by the embedded nature of the word within the whole event. Intentional communication requires both context and nonverbal support to establish reference, since words are not yet specific and conventional (Grieve & Hoogenraad, 1979; Stoel-Gammon & Cooper, 1984).

Production of word forms may occur as naming, where activation of the event representation activates production of the word. In many cases, the name is spoken spontaneously, with no intent to influence behavior of others, as a rehearsal or practice mechanism (MacNamara, 1982). In other cases, names are produced to establish joint attention or focus with an adult, with no expected resultant action or outcome (i.e., the informing function) (Halliday, 1975). Much of the child's talk during this second year involves naming, a behavior that externalizes the child's developing symbol and provides adults an opportunity to expand or modify the child's word form and its meaning. This process of sharing through labeling builds the child's vocabulary and establishes the foundation for more complex communications later (Moore & Dunham, 1995; Snow, 1987). But naming also serves intentional communication purposes with expected actions or outcomes. These intentional communications can appear in nonverbal forms, such as points or other gestures, but most typically they are achieved by accompanying words and vocalizations with gestures that clarify the meaning and intent of the communication.

For example, the word "eat" may generate representation of the whole event when spoken by others in the relevant context. In the course of the eating routine, parents refer to the event, as in "Time to eat" or "Eat your food." They also behave as if the child is saying "eat" whenever the child vocalizes in this context, but in particular if the sounds produced by the child approximate the word. Patterns of connectivity for the sound and motor production of the word are networked to the schema for "eat" in the same manner as actions, smells, and objects are part of the schema. The word is not a symbol at this stage, but rather part of the sensory information occurring during eating and consequently part of the overall event representation. When the word is later uttered by the parent in the context of the kitchen, it activates the event representation for eating and the child performs the next action in the event sequence, that is, crawling to the highchair. Hearing the word propagated intentional action in the child. Thus, the child might appear to comprehend the meaning of the word while in fact having only a nonspecific understanding of the meaning. Since the meaning is tied to the event representation, the word is not generalized but rather can only be used in the specific contexts where learning originally occurred.

The child also produces the word intentionally. A child spotting a favorite food commonly encountered within the eating routine might utter the word "eat" accompanied by a reaching gesture while looking at the adult (Chapman, 1981; Seibert, Hogan, & Mundy, 1982). The sight of the food activated patterns of connectivity to the event representation for eating and consequently to the word form, which was then produced. Any response by the parent, including denying food or providing it, will strengthen the pattern of connectivity between that specific word form and that specific event, but not for conventional meaning of the word. Uttering the word affects behavior of the intended listener, even if the desired outcome was not achieved.

Tyrone's Nonverbal Event Representation

While the normally developing child is in the process of making an important transition into representational meaning, Tyrone lacks the tools for this transition. The event representation is forming slot-filler categories, providing a means for concepts to separate from the event representation and form concepts independent of the routine event or event representation. But acoustic patterns and motor sequences that associate word forms with these concepts are not developing as part of this preconceptual structure. When concepts separate, they will do so without patterns of connectivity integrating them with words. The concepts will have only a nonverbal composition.

Tyrone's representations also lack prerequisite social attachments of word forms to intentional communication. Tyrone's event representations are developing normally in most respects to this point in development. Like other children, much of the event representation has formed through interactions with people and objects using all sensory modalities (Rose, Gottfried, & Bridger, 1983). The auditory mode was in many respects redundant and somewhat secondary to others, such as vision and touch (Piaget, 1954; Uzgiris, 1983). That is, hearing a word could not create a meaningful representation for an object, since the word would have to refer to meaning within Tyrone's network to do so. Rather, words map onto concepts constructed through object manipulation or observation. Tyrone has had normal experiences in these sources of input and has constructed fairly typical representations. His integration of visual and tactile information within social interactions has resulted in formation of a gestural system that works well at this stage of development to intentionally control behaviors of others. Since words are nonspecific and can only refer to the event representation, pointing and reaching work just as well. Both are bound to the immediate context of the here and now, and both require the context to interpret meaning and intent. Tyrone hasn't noticed that he needs sounds or words for communicative purposes.

But Tyrone's representations, with their failure to incorporate acoustic and motoric patterns for speech, will soon prove to be inadequate to support advances in communication and learning.

EXPRESSING REPRESENTED MEANING: DEVELOPMENT FROM 14 TO 18 MONTHS

Formation of slot-filler categories results in formation of presemantic concepts, or concepts that exist in the world of events or activities. They are presemantic, meaning concepts cannot yet be created from lexical meanings of words, independent of an experience (Bruner, 1983; Grieve & Hoogenraad, 1979; Vygotsky, 1962). Words map onto these already formed concepts and are used within events as they occur. These words establish presymbolic reference, where meaning is recognized in the "here and now" context of an ongoing activity (see Table 1.8). Inclusion of language as an integral part of events begins to change the structure of the event representation and leads to ongoing changes in representational structure and organization that continues throughout childhood (Nelson, 1996).

Situational Context

As patterns of connectivity for words integrate into event representations, the nature of the representation begins to change. Language used by adults helps to make important parts of the event salient and serves to mark and move the event forward (Nelson, 1986, 1996). Thus, temporal and causal connections between constituent actions that were lacking begin to form. For example, each time a bowl is placed on the tray of the highchair and a spoon is used to retrieve food from the bowl, connection weights between units representing these objects strengthen. Subschema comprised of smaller events within the whole begin to evolve. Parents assist in formation of subschema through the process of parsing. Parsing occurs as adults establish joint attention for an object within a routine by performing actions while talking about salient features of the object or event (Nelson, 1985). The adult might stop the child from grabbing food from the bowl, holding up the spoon while saying "Use your spoon," and then assisting the child to retrieve food with the spoon. This attention helps the child momentarily isolate the object, creating a slot in the emerging script for that item while simultaneously integrating it with other elements of the subschema. In connectionist terms, this momentary focus increases connection weights

TABLE 1.8

Abilities Demonstrated between 14 and 18 Months of Age Across
the Cognitive, Social, Semiotic, and Sensory-Motor Domains Profiled
within the Situational-Discourse-Semantic Contexts of the
SDS: Development Model

	14–18 Months *Level IIIb*		
	Situational *Relational* *Displacement*	*Discourse* *Descriptive List* *Organization*	*Semantic* *Labeling* *Reference*
Cognitive	Object Displacement Uses familiar objects appropriately independently of actual routines; pictures recognized as depicting objects or animals, but not actions.	Event/Discourse Uses sequence of actions with related objects to accomplish a goal (stack rings on post). Watches actions within ongoing event.	Perceptual Manipulates perceptual obects and parts (open door to put something in; put objects in containers).
Social	Self/Other Displacement Talks during event to share the experience ("car go" "up" "no more"). Anticipates response of others; understands other's mental states.	Interactional Shares responsibility for the communication, maintaining interaction for several turns. Coordinates object & adult.	Functional Know body part functions; pretend & self-help action. Recognizes attributes of animals and other people (actions, sounds).
Semiotic	Time/Space Displacement Presymbolic reference; meaning is recognized in here and now context ("cup" can mean "I want" or "drink," etc.), Familiar objects looked/asked for if expected in a context (ask for cup).	Locutionary True intention to greet; request a game, object, or action; show off, gain attention; acknowledge express feelings; protect self or self-interests.	Convention MLU 1.0; Many semantic relations (agent, action, object) conventional word mixed with jargon; uses gestures in combination.
Sensory-Motor	Imitative Displacement Spontaneous imitation of actions and words produced in a familiar context. Imitates global actions, such as scribbling to imitate coloring or writing.	Exocutionary Sounds and intonation are language-like, with strings of sounds that resemble sentences. Cluster reduction, unstressed syllable deletion.	Modality Words produced are usually one, sometimes two, syllables, with a few sounds (usually b, p, m) predominating. Devoicing.

Reprinted with permission from Norris, JA, and Hoffman, PR (1999). The SDS developmental model of integrated functioning, Baton Rouge, LA: EleMentory.

for features of the spoon, and between the spoon in relationship to the food and the bowl, thus establishing the represention for the spoon as a pattern of connectivity that is part of the whole and one that can be activated as a subunit with activation independent of the whole (see Fig. 1.10).

This independence results in new behaviors such as use of familiar objects appropriately independent of the actual routine (Piaget, 1962; Wolf & Gardner, 1979). A child encountering a spoon on the floor in the hallway will pretend to eat with it, even though no actual food, bowls, highchairs, or other elements of the routine are present. Similarly, the child begins to recognize pictures of familiar objects encountered in books even when not depicted within a routine or other ordinary context of occurrence.

Use of language by adults to establish attention to a specific object creates a momentary isolation of connectivity that also serves to enhance language development. The object becomes associated with the word "spoon" because of the co-occurrence of the action and the talk, whereby both sources of simultaneous input form interconnected patterns of activation. The isolation strengthens patterns of connectivity between the spoon and the word "spoon" specifically. In so doing, the word forms stronger patterns of connectivity with the concept of the spoon, and weaker connections to the event representation as a whole. A growing vocabulary of presymbolic words thus emerges that represent different aspects of the event, such as the agent performing the action, the object receiving the action, and the action designating the relationship (Tomasello & Farrar, 1984). These words map onto the slot-filler concepts that have already formed within the context of the event representation. The patterns of connectivity for the sound patterns received spread activation to units involved in speech production, resulting in spontaneous imitation of words. The adult in turn accepts and frequently repeats the child's speech approximations, interpreting them as meaningful in context and consequenting them with action or attention.

This cycle of shared input and output assures the child's entry into speech. The child's use of the word in a known context, whether spontaneously produced or in imitation, externalizes it (i.e., "spoon"). The adult's expansion of the utterance to convey the interpreted meaning (i.e., "That's your spoon"), or extension to include new aspects of the event (i.e., "Now eat with your spoon") strengthens and adds complexity to existing patterns of connectivity. Recursive interactions continue to increase the complexity of language patterns networked within the event representation and enable an increasing number of semantic relations to be expressed. The event representation thus provides a supportive context for language to form (Snow, Perlmann, & Nathan, 1987). At this stage the conceptual system is not independent of language, but rather the two evolve interdependently with achievements in each supporting developments in the other. That is, without language many aspects of the event could not be

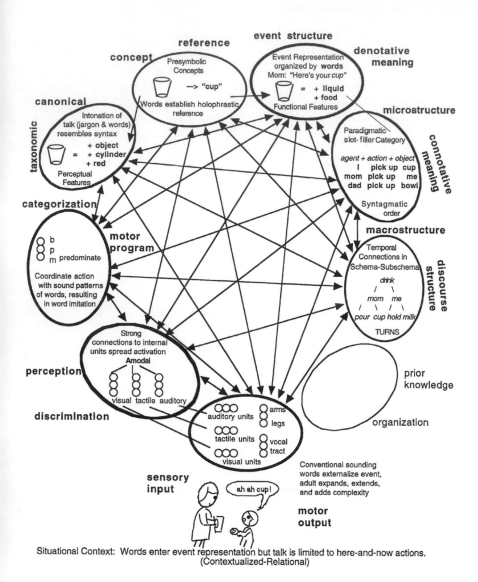

reference

concept

Presymbolic Concepts

—> "cup"

Words establish holophrastic reference

canonical

Intonation of talk (jargon & words) resembles syntax

= + object
+ cylinder
+ red

Perceptual Features

taxonomic

event structure

Event Representation organized by **words**
Mom: "Here's your *cup*"

= + liquid
+ food

Functional Features

denotative meaning

microstructure

Paradigmatic slot- filler Category

agent + action + object

I	pick up	cup
mom	pick up	me
dad	pick up	bowl

Syntagmatic order

connotative meaning

categorization

motor program

b
p
m predominate

Coordinate action with sound patterns of words, resulting in word imitation

macrostructure

Temporal Connections in Schema-Subschema

drink
/ \
mom me
/ \ / \
pour cup hold milk

TURNS

discourse structure

perception

Strong connections to internal units spread activation

Amodal

visual tactile auditory

prior knowledge

discrimination

auditory units
tactile units
visual units

arms
legs
vocal tract

organization

sensory input

ah ah cup!

Conventional sounding words externalize event, adult expands, extends, and adds complexity

motor output

Situational Context: Words enter event representation but talk is limited to here-and-now actions. (Contextualized-Relational)

FIG. 1.10. Event representation is organized by words as adult uses words to isolate or "parse" a concept from the event from 14 to 18 months of age. Parsing forms presemantic concepts, or concepts that must be created within an ongoing experience. Once formed, words map onto the concepts so connections of words to concepts are stronger than connections to the whole event. Child's use of word (reference) externalizes concept, where adult expands and extends it. This creates a cycle: growth in concepts leads to words, external words expand and extend concept. (Reprinted with permission from Norris, JA, and Hoffman, PR (1999). The SDS developmental model of integrated functioning, Baton Rouge, LA: EleMentory.)

shared. Sharing helps the child form conventional concepts, and concepts provide a representational structure that supports interpretation of the word with less and less contextual support (Nelson, 1996).

Words that emerge during this period are not used only to label, although labeling is a function engaged in with high frequency. Rather, the single word is used to mark the entire relationship between the agent, action, and object of the event (Bloom, 1970; Miller, 1981). The meaning of these utterances is dependent on the context for interpretation. Thus, "cup" spoken while holding the cup could mean "See my cup," "Put milk in my cup," or "You take this cup." The utterance refers to the interconnected network of cognitive, social, semiotic, and sensory-motor knowledge that operates to enable functional communication. The focus on agents, actions, objects, states, locations, and other semantic relations is demonstrated in perceptual and functional actions the child engages in during this time. It is an emphasis on the relationship between objects with other objects, objects and their parts, people and objects, and changing states of objects within meaningful events that motivates the child, and not single objects. These relationships are the subject of much of the child's talk, even if only one word is used to express it.

Socially, talk during an event facilitates sharing the experience. Nonverbal participation in an event provides a forum for the child to construct a personal model or representation of what happens. The addition of language enables sharing and comparison of the experience with others (Bloom, 1993). Language is the primary medium for making select aspects of an event salient ("Oh, oh, it spilled"), for extending the event to include future actions ("We need to get a sponge and clean it up"), and for expressing feelings ("That's so silly" versus "That makes me so mad"). Language thus provides a window into the minds of others and helps to orient the child to social and cultural interpretations of events. Without language, many aspects of social and cultural knowledge cannot be entered into the child's mental representations (Nelson, 1996).

Discourse Context

Discourse organization at this stage is highly collaborative, with the adult asking questions, providing prompts, expanding and extending the child's ideas, and providing opportunities for turns to occur (Baker & Nelson, 1984). This results in the maintenance of interaction across several turns with shared responsibility for communication. Once again the event structure with its roles and relationships makes this possible. The child has a script for the conversational event and expects the adult to fulfill the role of acknowledging, answering, asking, or informing (Snow, Perlmann, & Nathan, 1987). This expectation primes the network to maintain activation of the existing representation and to integrate new information into the schema, building overlapping patterns of connectivity that result in a primitive topic maintenance.

This shared maintenance and responsibility for communication within an event provides opportunities for temporal sequences to form between actions, consequences, states, and new actions. Adults mark these sequences using language ("Let's hit the peg."; "Oh oh, you missed it, let's try again."; "I'll hold it while you hit.") Parent talk serves to organize the event through time, integrating short action sequences into extended event sequences that the child's representational system cannot yet independently support (Nelson, 1996). At the same time, patterns of connectivity for language that integrates the events through time begin to enter into the child's network. It will be several months before the time markers enter the child's verbalizations, but intonation patterns in the child's jargon resemble syntax, including temporal terms. Nonverbally at this stage, the child uses a series of actions with related objects to accomplish a goal, indicating that sequence and duration are forming conceptually within the event representation (Piaget, 1952, 1954). The prelinguistic system that is forming will support later language learning, particularly syntax. The integration of the two types of information about the event and its organization (i.e., experience and language) are interdependent and reciprocal, each fostering development in the other and each enabling the child to function productively and generatively (Bruner, 1983; Nelson, 1996; Vygotsky, 1962).

Semantic Context

A small vocabulary of words appears during this stage, expressing a range of semantic relations and pragmatic functions (Halliday, 1975; Miller, 1981). The word "truck" produced in a different context can be a request (Give me the truck), protest ("Don't take my truck"), statement ("I have the truck"), or question ("Where did the truck go?"). For this to occur, the word must refer to the entire relationship. When asking "Where did the truck go?" the child must mentally construct the truck in relationship to a specific location to recognize that it is gone. Referring to the object in context serves to activate a similar representation in the listener. The word externalizes the thought, the externalized thought is shared and expanded. The shared meaning then enters into the child's knowledge representation (Nelson, 1985).

Learning words is possible because of the occurrence of the word in a context. An unfamiliar word can mean anything, but the child assumes that language is relevant to the context. By understanding the context through the event representation and interpreting the speaker's intention through the roles and relationships within the representation, a meaning can be extracted (Nelson, 1996). All clues to meaning, including points and gestures, facial expressions, and intonation provide simultaneous input to the network. Each source of input provides salient information, activating patterns of connectivity for specific perceptual and functional features that are likely to be associated with the unfamiliar words. The meaning assigned is partial and ambiguous, lacking depth and allowing for potential incorrect information. The word thus has little flexibility or power to generalize to a broad range of contexts or uses (Bloom, 1970). But once the category is established, future uses of the word or experiences with the concept add refinement and clarity, building a flexible meaning that captures different interpretations in varying contexts. For many words, it may be years before the full adult use of the word is achieved. However, the ability to use words to establish reference marks the transition to symbolic language (Bates, O'Connell, & Shore, 1987; Clark, 1983, 1993).

Tyrone's Different Learning System

Up to this level of development, Tyrone has appeared to have a fairly normal learning system, with the exception of an inability to integrate acoustic and productive aspects of speech into his developing representations. In many ways, the lack of integration of speech information appeared to be of little consequence. Tyrone progressed through the developmental sequence, interacting in socially appropriate ways, acquiring routines and self-help skills at a rate comparable to peers, playing with toys in the same manner as his age-mates, and communicating as effectively as others using nonverbal means. He formed concepts that separated from the event representation, recognized objects outside of their typical context of use, and used objects contextually in functionally appropriate ways. He explored objects, learning about their part-to-whole relationships and manipulated buttons and levers to achieve anticipated outcomes as competently as other toddlers.

But Tyrone is going to find "keeping up" increasingly more difficult and in a short while, impossible. The period of presymbolic learning is nearing an end in normal development, and further advances require a symbolic tool for distancing thought from experience. Already the network has begun to construct this new way of thinking, as concepts separate from the event representation and take the words with them. Children begin to expect words to refer to something specific within the context, and not to the event representation as a whole. They listen to the words spoken by others and use all available clues to assign a meaning to the word. This contextual mapping of words to concepts results in the rapid acquisition of words that the child can understand and use. The occurrence of unknown words causes the child to seek meaning, a strategy for learning new concepts not available to Tyrone. The imitation of words heard provides opportunities for adults to expand and extend the utterance, establishing the foundation for syntax and linking the event representation through relationships that may not be evident nonverbally. Tyrone will lack access to this learning also.

The acoustic information that appeared to be redundant and secondary to other sources of input during prelinguistic development is suddenly critical to further advances in learning. Without this input, or comparable input though a medium such as manual sign, Tyrone's learning will remain grounded in experience while his peers go on to decontextualized, culturally mediated learning.

THE EMERGENCE OF SYMBOLIC LANGUAGE: DEVELOPMENT FROM 19 TO 26 MONTHS

Symbolic representation, including emergence of true words, comes out near the child's second birthday. Evidence of this symbolic ability is observed both verbally and nonverbally, as thought begins to separate from the ongoing event. Thought can now use the event representation and other forms of mental representation to create what could be rather than what is (Piaget, 1954; Vygotsky, 1962). In Piagetian terms, the system is reaching a new equilibration, or a qualitative change in the manner in which the system functions (see Table 1.9).

Situational Context

Separation of concepts and language away from the immediate context of an event means that they have to be represented within the system in a new way. Connections between concepts, words, and their meaning can no longer be part of the event representation in which they were learned (Nelson, 1996). This happens as a consequence of both external experiences that provide input to the system, and the internal structure of the system that is designed to assimilate new information into existing representational structures and to generate accommodations that modify patterns of connectivity. External experiences are characterized by redundancy, meaning that the same objects are used to perform similar actions in new contexts, and different objects are used to perform similar actions in old contexts (Nelson, 1985, 1986). For example, in the context of the eating routine, the child's shirt may come under focus if something is spilled, or if sleeves are getting into the food, or the child wipes her mouth on the shirt.

TABLE 1.9
Abilities Demonstrated between 19 and 26 Months of Age Across the Cognitive, Social, Semiotic, and Sensory-Motor-Domains Profiled within the Situational-Discourse-Semantic Contexts of the SDS: Development Model

	19–26 Months Level IV (Corresponding to Brown's Stage I)		
	Situational Symbolic Displacement	Discourse Sequential Organization	Semantic Descriptive Reference
gnitive	**Object Displacement** Performs pretend actions with own body, but requires lifesize props. Talks about own action, comments on changes within ongoing event. Meaning unclear outside of context.	**Event/Discourse** Short, isolated schema combined in temporal sequence, including short series of self-help and pretend for familiar actions (feed doll and put to bed).	**Perceptual** Perceptual actions including puts objects in container, builds towers, shapes in form boards. Adj + N such as "big block," determiners this/that prepositions in/on in two-word phrase.
ial	**Self/Other Displacement** Actively watches others in play but does not participate. Concept of self as individual, differentiates things belonging to self versus others.	**Interactional** Engages in short verbal dialog exchanging information by asking & answering questions. Cooperates with adult in shared activites (dressing, reading).	**Functional** Associates objects with people who use them (put baby in bed). Uses most familiar objects appropriately. Possessives by word order (mommy shoe), pronouns I/mine, mainverbs.
iiotic	**Time/Space Displacement** Symbolic reference to objects/needs that are not in the immediate vicinity; talks about whatever draws attention in the immediate environment. Can refer to objects or persons not present within very familiar context.	**Locutionary** Informative function emerges (sharing information about nonpresent objects. Where go? Puppy gone.). Follows and gives simple requests within familiar events (no eat, two truck).	**Convention** MLU 1.01–1.99; at least 250 unique syntactic types of two-word combinations that express objects, actions, characteristics, states, locations, roles. Word order & intonation whquestion; What that? That me?
sory-Motor	**Imitative Displacement** Imitation of novel action or word sequences and patterns not already in child's repertoire. Verges on imitating vertical line with crayon or pencil.	**Exocutionary** Begins to climb, jump, run, throw; navigates sequences (up and down stairs with one hand and held). CVCV and VCVC syllable shapes and clusters appear, but cluster reduction, weak syllable and final consonant deletion, metathesis.	**Modality** Initial consonants /b/t/k/g/m/n/h /w/f/s/; final /p/t/k/n/r/s/. Phonetically appropriate /p/b/t/d/k/g/m/n /ng/h/w/. Gestures accompany words and communicate much of the meaning. Scribbling for pleasure, not representation, emphasis on circles.

Reprinted with permission from Norris, JA, and Hoffman, PR (1999). The SDS developmental model of
grated functioning, Baton Rouge, LA: EleMentory.

The caregiver is likely to focus attention on the action and condition of the shirt, using language to describe the circumstance ("Oh, oh, we spilled milk on your *shirt*"; "Let's pull your sleeves up so we don't get your *shirt* dirty"). Connections are established between the shirt, the word, and the context of the eating routine. But the shirt also is encountered and focused on in the dressing routine, as the caregiver asks "What *shirt* do you want to wear?" while viewing a drawer with folded shirts, and "Let's put your *shirt* on," while pulling one over the child's head.

The use of the word "shirt" in context specifies which of the potential objects needs to be considered. The word thus serves to isolate, or parse, the object from the whole while it is the focus of attention. The word "shirt" used in two different contexts to refer to the same object means that the object and the word used to refer to it cannot belong to either event exclusively. The mental representation of the concept of a shirt, as well as the word used to refer to it, can be activated through input from the eating routine, but also the dressing routine, the bathing routine, the shopping routine, and many other routine and incidental experiences. The shirt soon develops a pattern of connectivity that is linked to all of these events, like the complex root system of a tree (see Fig. 1.11). This complex pattern of connectivity for shirt, with each context contributing both overlapping and different elements of meaning results in the status of the representation of shirt as a separate concept. This new representational power is manifested in many ways, such as the emerging ability to perform pretend actions outside of an actual event, if life-sized props are available. Thus, the child encountering a cup will pretend to drink even when no other contextual cues for the event are available (Fenson & Ramsey, 1980).

Separation of words from the event occurs at the same time that concepts separate. The parsing of the concept that occurs is accompanied by language as the adult refers verbally to the concept (Nelson, 1996). The simultaneity of occurrence results in strong patterns of connectivity forming between the word and the corresponding concept. Thus, at this stage of development the language is not independent of the concept, although both are becoming independent of the event representation. This distancing of the concept and word from the event representation allows for words to begin to substitute for absent objects in the child's thought and verbal reference. Activation of any part of the complex network to which the concept is integrated, such as feeling hunger, can activate an associated concept and word(s) (i.e., "Want cookie"). Producing the word in context can recreate absent objects or scenes. Thus, words begin to create the shared context or situation symbolically (Brown, 1973; Bruner, 1983; Vygotsky, 1962).

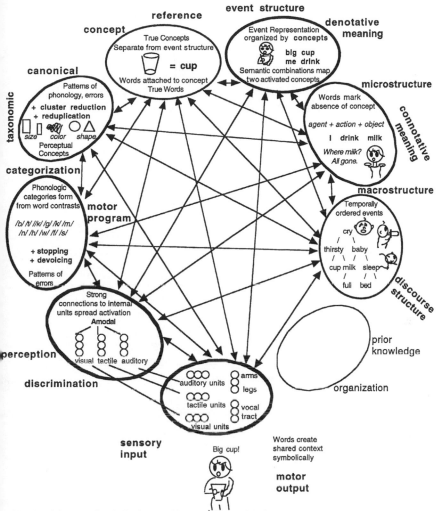

Situational Context: Symbolic play with lifesize props; words refer to objects that are part of action.
(Contextualized-Symbolic)

FIG. 1.11. Concepts and associated words separate from event structure between 19 and 26 months, creating true concepts and true words. Words still attached to concepts so cannot create past or future, but can refer to absent objects through connections to the microstructure script. Two concepts can be activated at once, resulting in two-word utterances that are semantic rather than syntactic. Properties also separate from the concept to form new perceptual concepts, referred to with words of color, size, or shape. Sound repertoire large and rapidly refining, resulting in patterns of correct productions and errors (phonological processes). (Reprinted with permission from Norris, JA, and Hoffman, PR (1999). The SDS developmental model of integrated functioning, Baton Rouge, LA: EleMentory.)

67

Discourse Context

While the process of parsing results in parts separating from the whole, this is only one developing property of the connectionist network. At the same time, syntagmatic development, or expanding interconnections of the parts continues to integrate into elaborated wholes. The shared responsibility for moving events forward, including prompts provided by parents to perform the next step in a routine or to anticipate the next change in an event, all serve to provide input that forms patterns of connectivity between subevents (Snow, Perlmann, & Nathan, 1987; Nelson, 1996). The strength of these patterns of connectivity is sufficient at this stage to activate a series of short, isolated schema that are combined in temporal sequence to form a primitive, but topically related event in both self-help and play (Piaget, 1954). That is, activation of one subevent spreads input to the next subevent networked within the same event representation. A child will feed a doll, then brush its hair, and then put it to bed. No causal links between the event are present, and the child does not have adult understanding of why a baby needs to be fed before bedtime. In the child's representational system, connections enable the sequence to occur. Language marks the event, referring to salient objects, people, or action, including those that are expected but not present (e.g., "Where cup?" "Puppy all-gone"). But the language is part of the concept, and therefore can't represent the event in communication or cognition, so that only topics supported by objects can be referred to using words (Nelson, 1996).

Semantic Context

In the same manner that concepts separate from the event representation, properties of objects, such as color, size, number, or status, begin to separate from concepts (Nelson, 1986). Using our tree analogy, branches of conceptual units of connectivity begin to sprout from conceptual branches, which themselves have separated from the tree trunk (i.e., event representation) and the sensory input, or root system. For example, during the dressing routine the caregiver may say, "Let's put on your *red* shirt." In the same event, references to other objects characterized by their color might also occur, as in "Here are your *red* socks," "Your pants are *red*, too," or "Is this *red*?". The property of being red cannot belong to any one object in the event, but forms an existence as connected to but separate from any object or any representation of an object. *Red* also occurs in the context of many other events, such as eating ("These strawberries are *red*"), bathing ("Do you want a *red* or a blue towel?"), riding in the car ("We have to stop at the *red* light"), or playing ("Let's build a red house"). The ability to form concepts becomes increasingly distanced from the perception (Blank, Rose, & Berlin, 1978).

Words for properties, such as *red, broken, big,* or *two* begin to be imitated and spontaneously used in familiar contexts (Brown, 1973). The representational system in which interconnecting branches of connectivity are simultaneously activated allows for two concepts to be activated at the same time. When two concepts are activated (i.e., "big" and "block") corresponding words are also activated because of the inseparable bond between the word and the concept. Therefore, the child produces two-word combinations at this stage that express intended relationships between objects, actions, characteristics, states, locations, and roles (Bloom, 1970). Flexibility of the network, like a giant tree with thousands of branches, is demonstrated by appearance of at least 250 unique syntactic types expressing as many different kinds of semantic and pragmatic functions (Miller, 1981). These two-word combinations are indicative of how the network simultaneously activates parts (i.e., words that refer to separate concepts) and patterns of connections between them (i.e., the meaningful utterance), like two sides of a coin that always exist in an interdependent relationship.

While gestures still support the meaning of the words, the sound repertoire incorporated into the network is large and rapidly refining. From this stage of development forward, children add approximately 4 to 10 vocabulary words daily (Mehrabian, 1970). The auditory and productive aspects of phonology and speech are organizing according to the same principles as all other aspects of the connectionist network. That is, words are not produced as a series of isolated phonemes, but rather as integrated combinations of sounds with no boundaries between words in connected speech (Locke, 1993). Thus, at each moment of processing, all of the sounds that are in the acoustic stream are simultaneously providing input to the system and establishing patterns of connectivity for those sound patterns as a whole. At the same time, the patterns for individual phonemes within that stream are also activated because of the acoustic and perceptual categories that are part of the structure of the hearing mechanism.

In the same manner that concepts encountered within many events parse from the whole event representation, phonemes encountered within many different words parse from the whole representation to form separate phonemic structures for individual sounds. This network of connectivity between all of the words that share phonemes results in patterns of correct productions across words, as well as patterns of error. That is, a child might consistently substitute the /t/ phoneme for /s/ in all or most phonetic contexts. At the same time, patterns of connectivity differ in connection weights for each word linked to a concept, so that productions that differ from the typical pattern are equally possible. Across time, repeated input from adult productions results in reweighting and reconfiguring of the patterns within the system. This reweighting results in continuous progress within the child's system toward phonological organization and productions that match the input received from adults.

Tyrone's Communicative Frustration

Tyrone will start to notice the lack of ability to process and/or use language during this stage, resulting in numerous episodes of frustration. Like his peers, Tyrone is establishing a new, qualitatively different system of representation. Concepts are parsing away from the event representation because of their co-occurrence in many different contexts and routines, but not as efficiently, because of the difficulty in processing language clues. As they separate, there are no words to accompany the concepts, since the acoustic and production representations never formed. Similarly, Tyrone has been forming syntagmatic connections between agents, actions, and objects within the event routine, and has formulated slot-filler categories within the script for specifying these relationships. Consequently, Tyrone is able to think in semantic relationships and can differentiate conceptually between noticing that his shirt is dirty versus wanting to wear his red shirt, but without language he has no means of easily communicating this information to others. With no symbol for externalizing thought, the thought cannot be shared. Tyrone's earlier strategies of pointing or gesturing require the participant to interpret his meaning and intent. But as his ideas become distant from the immediate context, and his thoughts form specific relationships between specific concepts, these nonverbal means become increasingly ineffective. Tyrone resorts to tantrums, crying, or abandoning the interaction when he cannot make his wants and ideas known.

FORMING NEW CONCEPTS USING WORDS: DEVELOPMENT FROM 25 TO 30 MONTHS

Language development through the second year occurs as words map onto concepts that are created through their existence within an event representation (Clark, 1993; Nelson, 1996). Language helps the concept separate from the event representation but the language and conceptual system are not independent. The prelinguistic mental representations must support language development. But at age two, the language accompanying events begins to lingusitically form mental representations that are not first part of the conceptual system, but instead first part of the linguistic system (Nelson, 1996). The ability to linguistically form mental representations changes the potential of the system to learn, as the child can now exchange memory with others (Table 1.10).

TABLE 1.10

Abilities Demonstrated between 25 and 30 Months of Age Across the
Cognitive, Social, Semiotic, and Sensory-Motor Domains Profiled within
the Situational-Discourse-Semantic Contexts of the
SDS: Development Model

	25–30 Months Level V		
	Situational *Pre-op Logical* *Displacement*	*Discourse* *Reactive Causal* *Organization*	*Semantic* *Attributive* *Reference*
gnitive	Object Displacement Attends to abstract symbols that suggest real objects (peg people, miniatures, drawing of head only). Language refers to own actions and consequences on status of others ("I feed baby. Baby all done.").	Event/Discourse Three or more related action sequences are embedded within longer episodes of action with some temporal and causal links (get food, pour into pan, cook on stove, serve). Talks about action.	Perceptual Objects matched & sorted by one abstract perceptual property (color, texture, size, shape). Comments on properties and location. Includes copula but no tense (I is big). Adj in object position (I want red truck).
ial	Self/Other Displacement Plays near others using same toys or materials and talks about actions or need from own perspective but not coordinated with the role of others within the interaction.	Interactional Maintains extended verbal dialog when adult responds contingent to child's topic. Asks questions but may not wait for answers. Peer interactions prevalent.	Functional Asks, watches, and experiments to discover function of unfamiliar object or event. Relates two things to the same action (Want milk and cookie). Pronouns me, my, it.
niotic	Time/Space Displacement Language used to recreate familiar objects or events in another time and location ("I drink juice" while pretending to pour juice); follow pictured actions across time in a storybook.	Locutionary Interactions with peers involve requests, commands, protests, declarations, or comments about own actions. Tantrums and negativism common. Aware of consequences, react "Oh-oh!".	Convention MLU 2.00–2.49; use of morphemes to specify same semantic relations previously expressed in word order. A/the specify general versus specific, "my" possessive, main verb tenseing, "no" precedes verb, use "and".
sory- Motor	Imitative Displacement Imitates functional actions with new or familiar objects in a role other than child's own (tries to open door with keys, cooks).	Exocutionary Sequences of behaviors used to assert power, regulate others. Morphological markers add to syllable shape. Final clusters appear/ps/ts/.	Modality Initial consonants /p/b/t/d/k/g/m/n/h/w /j/l/f/s/; final /p/t/d/k/m/ n/ng/r/f/s/sh/ch/. Phonetically appropriate: /p/b/t/d/k/g/m/n/ng/ h/w/j/f/. Communication less reliant on gestures.

Reprinted with permission from Norris, JA, and Hoffman, PR (1999). The SDS developmental model of inte-
ted functioning, Baton Rouge, LA: EleMentory.

Situational Context

From early infancy, one role that parents serve is to attempt to orient the child to the symbolic world. Parents present toys and encourage their child to look and interact, engage in storybook reading by pointing to pictures while naming and talking about the object, and provide opportunities to watch television and videotaped programs with muppets, cartoon characters, or people who sing and dance (Snow, 1983, 1984). These toys, illustrations, and visual images are different from an actual object used within a routine to accomplish goals. They are external representations of objects and events for which the child constructs an internal representation. To understand toys and pictures, the child must generate representations for these symbolic representations and associate them with representations of actual objects (Piaget, 1954). The event representation provides a structure for accomplishing this generalization (see Fig. 1.12).

Input from the sensory-motor system enables a child to construct a mental representation of a toy or a picture just like any other object encountered in the environment. This representation would construct a pattern of connectivity for the perceptual and functional features inherent to the object, including its size, shape, color, sound, and action. But the direct sensory input would not provide the child direct experience with the object in a routine or event that is needed to construct an understanding of how people use the objects, a condition necessary for symbolic play. The child must impart roles of real objects and real people within the event representation to miniatures and two-dimensional drawings. At least three sources of input are available for establishing connections between the representation of the symbolic object with those of the real object (and therefore an access route to the event representation). First, there are direct models that others provide using toys in routine contexts. Initially with lifesize toys, and gradually with smaller representations, adults model driving cars, feeding dolls, and placing figures in castles and doll houses. Connection weights for using a cup to drink share features with using a cup to give a drink to the doll. The event representation enables the doll to take on the same role in the slot-filler category as the child. The child is then able to attribute the same actions and characteristics to the doll that they learned in their own role as the recipient of the drink. By using the event representation, the network can produce an inference regarding roles and actions of the doll. Use of this strategy for forming new patterns connecting information within the child's network occurs frequently, as the child is observed imitating a range of functional actions with new and familiar objects in a role other than the child's own. The child's representation of self as a concept enables the child to function in a slot-filler category originally held by a parent or older sibling, and so the

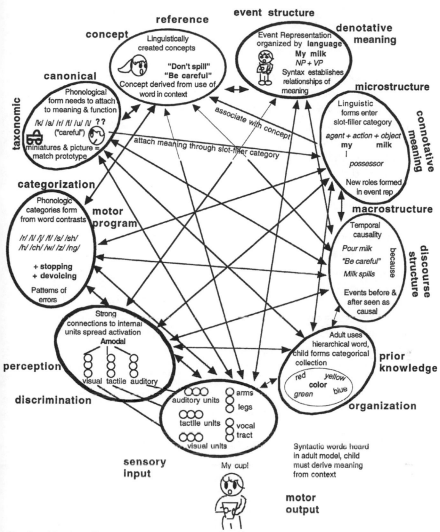

Situational Context: Plays with miniatures, interpretation of pictures as symbols representing real objects. (Contextualized-Symbolic)

FIG. 1.12. Symbols begin to be created and used as internal representations between 25 and 30 months. Pictures and miniatures perceptually are matched to the closest existing prototype, and enter the associated slot-filler category. The symbol then has the same association to the concept as the real object. Similarly, syntactic words perceptually enter the network and then are assigned a slot-filler category according to context of use (from the familiar "I drink milk" the word "my" in "my milk" enters the role of agent). Different function of the word creates a new kind of role, "possessor." Thus language creates new concepts of time, casuality, role, and so forth for linguistically created words that do not name objects or actions. (Reprinted with permission from Norris, JA, and Hoffman, PR (1999). The SDS developmental model of integrated functioning, Baton Rouge, LA: EleMentory.)

child begins to role play (pretend to cook dinner, or pretend to wash the car).

A second source of generalization is the perceptual similarity of the toy to the actual object. Because the representation of the actual object (i.e., a cup) has begun to form a concept separate from the event representation, and many different cups have contributed to the formation of the separated representation, the concept is not like any of the actual cups encountered (Fenson & Ramsey, 1980; Piaget, 1954). Connection weights for features most commonly encountered through experiences with cups form a prototype, or an idealized interpretation of what constitutes a cup (Clark, 1993). But experiences have also provided many connections to features that are unique to a certain cup, or only found among a subset of cups, or specific to certain uses of cups, or characteristic of certain people. Thus, wide variation in perceptual and functional features will still activate the concept of cup as the most probable interpretation of an object compared to other possible interpretations.

The context in which the object is embedded will determine which conceptual category existing within the system best fits the object (Clark, 1983, 1993). In a connectionist network, concepts can easily be viewed as fluid, with no rigid boundaries or features that must be present to activate the concept. Rather, the concept that has the greatest input from all sources within the context will be retrieved as the correct interpretation. Thus, a miniature cup that bears some perceptual similarity to an actual cup is likely to be interpreted as a cup because nothing else in the child's experience has greater similarity to the small object and consequently the strongest pattern of activation within the system will be the representation of a cup. Once activated, connections between the concept and the event representation from which it parsed will be activated, thus enabling the child to use the toy in the same slot-filler roles as the real object (Norris & Hoffman, 1994).

A final source of generalization is the use of language when playing with the toy (or looking at the picture). In addition to adults modeling actions with the toy, they also talk about actions as they occur. Words used by the adult are inseparable from the concept, and thus serve to activate the correct conceptual category for the child. Activation of the conceptual category provides connections to the event representation, or an interpretation of what to do with the toy. This use of language serves to communicate representations (i.e., the adult's interpretation of what the toy represents is shared with the child through the use of the word) so that the child learns how others interpret unfamiliar objects without direct experience. Language begins to function as a means for the child to become aware of cultural knowledge while simultaneously distancing learning from sensory-motor experience (Nelson, 1996).

Discourse Context

Increasing knowledge of the roles of self and others within event representations acquired through experience and through language used to talk
about the event enables greater complexity to form (Nelson, 1996; Piaget,
1960). Increased complexity serves to unify the event into a cohesive whole.
For example, in the role of an agent performing an action on an object, the
child establishes the temporal relationship between the initiating action
(for example, picking up a cup and drinking) and the consequence (the
cup is empty). Repeated experiences not only form temporal connections,
but also causal ones as the child learns that drinking a little does not empty
the cup but drinking a lot does. When the event does not go according to
the script, a deviation results in a focus on causality. For example, picking
up a cup that slips and falls empties it, resulting in the same consequence
but a different action immediately preceding it in time. Causality at this
stage has strong temporal links, with interpretations that immediately preceding actions caused the consequence. Children report that they got hurt
because they fell rather than they tripped over a toy, or that the milk is
all gone because it spilled rather than they didn't hold the cup tightly
(Piaget & Garcia, 1974). The unexpected event (i.e., falling or spilling) becomes inserted temporally into the script and connections between it and
the consequence are more salient than the actual cause.

This temporally and causally linked sequence is observable in the child's
play and accompanying talk (Piaget & Garcia, 1974; Vygotsky, 1962). The
child now performs three or more related temporal-causal sequences (i.e.,
a subevent), which are embedded in longer episodes of play with the same
toys. For example, in a play kitchen the child might remove food from
the cupboard and pour it into a pan, cook it on the stove, and say "it's
hot." The learned temporal connection between the stove and the hot food
establishes the causal link without a true understanding of the causality.
Language used by adults is an important source of causal understanding.
Within routine and pretend events, adults mark the causal relationships
using language during the ongoing event ("I have to cook it first," "Be careful, its hot"). These comments contain words such as "first" and "careful"
that are not part of the concrete experience of the event or routine. These
words do not map onto already formed concepts. Their meaning is not
knowable through direct action. Instead, language accompanying events
begins to lingusitically form mental representations that are not first part
of the conceptual system, but instead first part of the linguistic system
(Nelson, 1996). These undefined words set up patterns of connectivity
for the sound sequences that are not attached to concepts. The context
must be used to derive some meaning. Context is the immediate temporal
sequence of action and consequence, linked by the unknown word, from

which an emerging concept of causality must form. The ability to linguistically form mental representations is a critical feature of the network that makes abstract language development, including syntactic forms for time, causality, status, or cohesion possible (Brown, 1973).

Semantic Context

Abstract concepts that parsed from more concrete concepts, including size, shape, color, or number, a few months earlier continue to expand in number and complexity. At this stage, sufficient conceptual organization exists for the child to match and sort by one of these perceptual properties, such as color or size (Davidson, 1983; Piaget, 1952, 1954). This organization is derived from the slot-filler categories of events. For example, in the dressing routine the child is asked to find a red shirt on one day and a blue shirt the next. The child must determine what is salient about the shirts that makes one red and one blue from possibilities including sleeve length, material, logos, or collar style. The occurrence of the color word in other event representations, such as the red (or blue) ball or cup or towel eliminates most of the possibilities and establishes the strongest patterns of connectivity to perception of color. The shared role within these slot-filler categories results in the set of colors forming a subcategory of items as uniquely related. One source of input that unites this set is the use of an hierarchical word "color" by the adult. Unlike the words red or blue that were an inherent aspect of the real object, the word "color" is an abstraction that has no corresponding object to which it can refer. It is derived by using language to form a linguistic representation that is meaningful by its patterns of connectivity to the set of individual colors. This is not to imply that two-year-old children have the heirarchical organization of adults. Rather, children have a collection of concepts that are included within the overall label "color."

Formation of linguistic representations makes the emergence of syntax and morphology possible within an event representation (Nelson, 1996). In conversations with children, adults provide input to the child at a level only slightly in advance of the length and complexity of the child's utterances (Adamson, 1995; Sachs, 1993; Snow, 1984). In so doing, most of the words activate concepts already established within the child's network. But other words are produced by the adult, including grammatical markers for time, and cohesive markers such as pronouns and articles, that do not activate conceptual representations. The input received from these words thus establishes the phonological representation which then must be connected to features of meaning and function. Part of this might be accomplished through interconnections between language, concepts, slot-filler categories, and event representations. For example, at this stage the possessive "my" appears to communicate the semantic relationship previously expressed in word order (Brown, 1973), as in "Tyrone cup." The adult, during interaction with the child, produces the utterance "No, that's my cup" as the child reaches for a coffee mug. The relationship observable in the event is between the mother and the cup, but the word "mommy" was not uttered; instead the unknown word "my." So both "my" and "mommy" are slot fillers for the event representation, leading the child to infer that "mommy" and "my" were substitutable terms. But other experiences, where daddy and big brother and grandfathers are each referred to as "my" require a reinterpretation of the meaning and function of the word. The best fit is the concept that had formed and was expressed through the word combination to mark possession. This relationship can only be discovered through many occurrences in a context where the speaker consistently referred to ownership or possession.

The grammatical morpheme begins to form increasing patterns of connectivity to the abstract slot-filler category "possessor" but only when in the speaker's role. This information was previously marked in conversation by referring to the person, a fairly concrete one-to-one mapping strategy (Clark, 1993). This works receptively, where the possessive "my" refers to other people in the role of owning. Expressively, the word must also develop patterns of connectivity that limit its use so that "my" is used only when the speaker is in the role of possessor within the event representation. For this to occur the network must be complex and well integrated.

Tyrone's Limited Learning System

By this stage, Tyrone has developed concepts for most everyday objects encountered in routines and other direct experiences. Attention begins to focus on toys and pictures, as well as objects used by adults and other people in the environment. Tyrone has nonverbal sources of input to discover the representational nature of these objects, just as do his normally developing peers. He can learn through models provided by others, or through associations based on perceptual similarity to the actual object. But the most efficient channel for learning, or the use of words to share interpretations of the object, is not available to Tyrone. Concepts that are not easily modeled and that are not perceptual, such as finding out that a storybook character was "listening," are not accessible to Tyrone (Vygotsky, 1967).

Similarly, Tyrone's development within the discourse context is increasingly affected by failure of language to develop. Talk, both by adults and by the child, serves to move an event forward. The use of temporal and causal terms makes the temporal relationships explicit (Nelson, 1996). In a nonverbal experience, Tyrone can represent that a series of actions occurred in a temporal order, and that a consequence occurred following an action. But without language to share interpretations of the event, Tyrone cannot access the reasons why (i.e., "I have to cook it first"). Furthermore, use of these words in context creates concepts through linguistic representations that only later acquire meaning. These concepts cannot be learned by Tyrone and their absence will limit future development. Semantically, Tyrone may be able to organize concepts into collections and thus be able to sort and match characteristics such as color or size. But with no access to the label to refer to this collection as a whole, Tyrone has no method for referring to it or for integrating it into other representations. Tyrone's semantic learning will increasingly be limited to personal experience, while peers are learning scientific and cultural knowledge imparted via words.

EMERGENCE OF TIME AND ABSTRACTION: DEVELOPMENT FROM 31 TO 34 MONTHS

Increasing complexity of event representations, incorporation of abstract concepts into event representations, and separation of concepts away from event representations, as well as their recombination into collections, all lead to greater symbolic abilities. Nonverbally, the child can reenact and invent events both directly and indirectly experienced. But language adds the potential of freeing thought from experience (Vygotsky, 1962). Emergence of this is seen during this stage as language provides a tool for greater displacement of thought from the here-and-now (see Table 1.11).

Situational Context

Beginning in this stage, the past, or an event that the child did experience at a sensory-motor level, is remembered and can be talked about at a later time and location (Bates, Benigni, Bretherton, Camaioni, & Volterra, 1979). Memory can be constructed nonverbally in the same manner that other events are constructed. That is, input from sensory modalities simultaneously activates patterns of connectivity that form connection weights between them. The complexity of the experience would result in a chaotic memory of what happened unless it is organized within an existing script or event structure (Nelson, 1996). Thus, specifics of the memory enter slot-filler categories, and any remarkable or unexpected action within the experience is integrated into the general event structure as a subevent. The represented event is thus not an exact copy of the actual event, but is rather an integration of the experience with the event structure. Merging new experience with established event structure provides for sufficiently strong connection weights to be capable of reactivating the memory at a later time. The memory, at least for a time, can be remembered as the specific event.

TABLE 1.11

Abilities Demonstrated between 31 and 34 Months of Age Across
the Cognitive, Social, Semiotic, and Sensory-Motor Domains Profiled
within the Situational-Discourse-Semantic Contexts of the
SDS: Development Model

	31–34 Months Level Vb		
	Situational Pre-op Logical Displacement	Discourse Reactive Causal Organization	Semantic Attributive Reference
gnitive	Object Displacement Establishes context from words with minimal reliance on actual objects or people (plays with few props; follows action in pictures; reports events that already occurred with emerging use of past tense, future can/will).	Event/Discourse Elaborated action sequences with details, causality, outcomes (baby cries and so feed, burp, wrap in blanket, rock to sleep). Discourse connected by cause; but, so, or, if: time; before, after.	Perceptual Can substitute objects if perceptual similarity (pen used for baby). Parts within wholes (Open my car door). Elaborated NP subject & object with attributes (number, color, texture, size), differential negative forms.
ial	Self/Other Displacement Stays near others in same activity but not social; language to others focuses on own actions and needs. Talks to characters during play ("Eat your food") followed by action.	Interactional Maintains an extended topic with adult scaffolding to increase sentence length and length of story; discourse devices used (cohesive use of the, you).	Functional Play themes and representations show cultural and world knowledge. The role of others taken in play that are less often experienced (doctor). Pronouns: gender (he/she his/her), number (we/them) sub/obj confused
miotic	Time/Space Displacement Recreates experiences occurring at great distances in time and space from original event; talks about future actions if in immediate time frame ("I will get my car").	Locutionary Refers to own intention and the probability that future action will change present state, or implies change has occurred (It can break; it broked).	Convention MLU 2.50–2.99; 1,000 words, many simple complete five-word sentences with elaborated NP + VP. Tense-ed, modal can, will, won't; negative inserted; conjunc clauses; why, who?
sory- Motor	Imitative Displacement Imitates actions for world events (zoo, dance), reenactments of events infrequently experienced. Draws lines, circles on imitation; scribbles have definite lines and forms.	Exocutionary Planned actions (walk back-ward, jumps down, forward, tip-toe, stand one foot). Initial clusters /fw/ bw/kw/tr/sp/st/sn/sl/. Final clusters /ps/ts/ns/nch/nk/.	Modality Initial consonant /p/b/t/d/k/g/m/n/w/ r/l/j/f/s/sh/h/ch/. Final /p/t/k/b/g/m/ n/ng/r/f/s/sh/v/z/ch/. Appropriate: /p/b/t/d/ k/g/m/n/ng/h/w/j/f/. Gestures merely embellish or emphasize meaning of words.

Reprinted with permission from Norris, JA, and Hoffman, PR (1999). The SDS developmental model of
egrated functioning, Baton Rouge, LA: EleMentory.

Its specific features also integrate into slot-filler categories of the general event representation (see Fig. 1.13).

Talk that occurs during actual experience also serves to organize and interpret it (Bruner, 1983). Parents use words to mark temporal and causal connections between actions (i.e., "Let's brush all of that sand off of your hands so it doesn't get on your cookie" spoken as the transition between wiping the sand and handing the cookie). Words signal important information to attend to, partition the event into subevents, and form mental representations that are merged into ongoing experience (Nelson, 1996). Language in this role serves to internally construct and represent the event. When remembering and recalling the event, both the words and the event representation are sources for reactivating patterns of connectivity, thereby recreating the event in memory or play. In play, the child is still a part of the ongoing activity, so the self is not separated from the here-and-now. To accomplish this separation, a symbolic tool such as language is required.

Within the connectionist network, integration of language with event and concept representations makes sharing and retaining memories possible for personal and social purposes. Parents talk during an event, moving it forward and marking important elements. When parents don't talk during the event, the memory may be similar, but ways of talking about it later are less elaborated and specific (Tessler & Nelson, 1994). Later, shared events provide opportunities to help children talk about the remembered event at a displaced time and different location. Adults ask questions, prompt the child to remember a significant action sequence, model words that the child can use to communicate information to others, and in other ways collaboratively construct remembered events in linguistic form with the child (Nelson, 1996). Input from the adult's questions or prompts activates concepts the child cannot independently activate. This process of collaboratively retelling adds connection strength to weakly connected units with each recounting, so that over time the child can tell longer sections with more details and fewer prompts. Verbal recounting is decontextualized, meaning that there is no input from the environment that maintains or activates the action sequences. As a result, internal symbols must generate the activation.

The event representation begins to not only recall an experienced event, but also to generate an action sequence in words immediately before it occurs, as in "I will drink some milk." As children begin to form linguistic representations for abstract concepts such as time, they can use these terms in context of a familiar event (Nelson, 1996). Activation of the representation creates knowledge that milk can be drunk before the action of drinking the milk occurs. The preceding event, seeing the milk, spreads activation to the next action in the script and to the word marking the transition between actions in the event sequence. This simultaneous activation

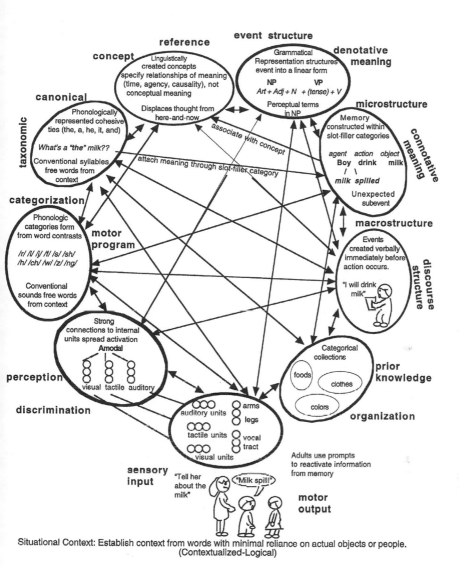

FIG. 1.13. Language frees thought from experience, resulting in displacement of thought from here-and-now between 31 and 34 months. Linguistic forms continue to enter through perceptual representation and attach meaning through slot-filler categories and event sequences. The event structure changes from one organized by concepts to one organized by the linear structure of grammer. Memories also enter into slot-filler categories of the event representation, and thus can be reactivated internally by external prompts, so that simple past events can be recounted. The immediate future can be created in words before the action occurs. (Reprinted with permission from Norris, JA, and Hoffman, PR (1999). The SDS developmental model of integrated functioning, Baton Rouge, LA: EleMentory.)

81

enables language to be uttered before the motor scheme for drinking is instantiated. The first step toward the symbolic future has been taken.

Discourse Context

Event representations continue to elaborate with a greater number of linguistically created concepts establishing links that form transitions between events. This is seen in elaborated action sequences produced with details, including causality and outcomes. Many of the actions are accompanied by language with words such as "but," "so," "if," "before," or "after" included (Brown, 1973). This occurs as the event representation is increasingly represented linguistically and consequently becomes less and less dependent on the ongoing event (Nelson, 1996).

The early event structure could only construct patterns of connectivity for occurrences present in the ongoing event. But as the same routine was repeated through multiple experiences, different items that fit within the same role in the event representation began to form a category of represented concepts within the slot filler category. The language used to refer to these concepts parsed from the event because it was part of the structure of the concept. Increasingly, any concept that could be enacted within the event could also be referred to using words, so that by this stage the words could represent the objects. In other words, what was originally learned in the context of the event representation now separates from it, and becomes the source of input that recreates the event representation using linguistic symbols.

Ability to maintain a topic through a series of action sequences begins to be manifested verbally as well as in play, especially when the adult provides assistance through prompts and questions to continue to talk about a topic. The adult uses her ability to connect ideas across a series of sentences to provide a scaffold for the child to learn these linguistic strategies (Bruner, 1983; Dore, 1986; Rondal, 1980; Wilkinson & Rembold, 1982). In the adult models and prompts, linguistic devices are used to maintain cohesive discourse, including pronouns, articles "a/the," and temporal terms such as "before" and "after" (Brown, 1973). These terms indicate clues to meaning, such as a referent that is either being introduced for the first time (e.g., There is *a* cat) or that the speaker is continuing to refer to the same entity (e.g., *The* cat is sleeping). Occurrence of these unknown words uttered between words with known meanings results in formation of a linguistically created event representation. At first the child begins to use words based on construction of the phonological sequence within the representation with very little meaning attached. In other words, cohesive ties are grammatically produced rather than semantically specified (Nelson, 1996). Presence of the category will result in patterns of connectivity for meaning forming from contexts of use. In these contexts, adults expand, extend, ask for clarification, or repair the child's utterance to conform to conventional use of these terms.

Semantic Context

Concepts of size, shape, color, and so forth that had parsed away from basic-level concepts appear linguistically in elaborated noun phrases (Brown, 1973). Words continue to be part of the conceptual structure but use of the linguistic symbol removes conceptual structure further from the event representation from which it formed. Words restructure the multidimensional event into linear form as syntax is used to express the information linguistically. The structure of organization is influenced by both the event representation and the emerging grammatical representation (Nelson, 1996).

Grammatical representation emerged from the event representation in the same process as concepts emerged. The event representation provides a context in which linguistically created mental representations can form, initially according to patterns of connectivity for the phonemic structures heard. As these phonemic structures appear repetitively in the context of sentences, patterns of connectivity for the word as a unit strengthen, and the word parses away from the whole in the same manner that other concepts separate. However, since little meaning can be assigned to these linguistic representations they are different from concept-based representations. Unlike concrete concepts, linguistic concepts begin to form strong patterns of connectivity between conceptual representational structures according to the manner in which they are used to unify these slot-filler categories. Thus, patterns of connectivity are primarily created from phonemic input (as opposed to the multisensory input of other concepts) and patterns of connectivitity that develop are primarily linguistic, serving as strategies for interconnecting slot-filler categories in a linear arrangement (as opposed to the multidimensional arrangement of thought). The linear order specifies how ideas are to be considered in relation to each other (Tomasello & Farrar, 1984). The meaning is relational, Indicating clues to meaning such as agency, possession, action, or state rather than conceptual meaning.

Once constructed, the grammatical representation can serve as a tool for organizing thought. The linear order provides a reliable tool for keeping thoughts straight (Nelson, 1996). It also provides a tool for ordering events in a sequence different from the actual event or from the event representation. This property adds new flexibility to the system to recreate an old event in a new way (Bruner, 1986). This new grammatical representational structure develops rapidly, and, during this stage, forms such as elaborated noun phrase order, pronouns that refer to gender, verb tense, and modal verbs indicating potential future action all begin to appear (Brown, 1973). Formulation of linguistic mental representations based on phonemic structures serves to further refine the phonological representations. The range of conventionally produced phonemes increases as well as the syllabic structure of words, resulting in minimal dependence on context or gesture for listeners to interpret the intended word (Locke, 1993).

Tyrone's Emerging Phonemic System

The lack of a tool such as language to acquire and refer to new concepts and to share meanings with others results in increasing frustration, or disequilibrium in Piagetian (1954) terms. Internal disequilibrium is generally resolved by seeking new input from the environment. For example, when trying to communicate that he wants to wear his red shirt (as opposed to the blue one mom has selected), Tyrone may point to his shirt, push away the blue shirt, or run and grab the red shirt. Interpreting his actions, mom might say "Oh, you want your *red shirt*." Tyrone's motivation to communicate the information was high, and he observed the environment for any indication that his message was being interpreted. The words provided one such indication, and they were simultaneously spoken in reference to acquisition of the desired object. The disequilibrium activated patterns of connectivity resulting in focused attention, an active search for contextually relevant input, extended duration of attention, and integration of unknown information into the network in an active search for a solution.

This focused attention on processing new information provides the opportunity for acoustic signals that were ignored in infancy to be attended to and integrated into the child's network of representations. In other words, Tyrone is now strongly motivated to attend to the auditory signal because his system lacks a representational mechanism for externalizing thought and for recombining concepts internally. Attention results in enhanced activation of this acoustic information, integrating input with weak patterns of connectivity that have been constructed for speech but have not become embedded within event or conceptual representations. That is, through nearly three years of exposure to speech, Tyrone does have many patterns of connectivity established, but they have only weak connection strengths, and have formed without integration into conceptual structures and, as a result, have never developed into speech.

Tyrone's new focus on speech results in fairly rapid formation of patterns of connectivity for phonemes and for sentence intonation and syllable shape. Although the level of his apparent development is like that of an infant, the status of his learning is very unlike an infant. Tyrone has already constructed a representational network of concepts and event representations; he already knows how to initiate, take turns, and terminate conversational interactions nonverbally; he uses nonverbal representations of actual objects in play, and he has developed the physical structures and motor coordination necessary for speech production. These accomplishments provide Tyrone with a network of internal representations to which accoustic signals can simultaneously assimilate on many levels throughtout the network. If Tyrone can process acoustic signals with enhanced attention and focus, then he should progress to the use of words in far less time than that required of an infant.

In his current development, Tyrone cannot access linguistic representations acquired by his peers. His development now has severe limitations since he can no longer construct the same concepts or elaborate the structure of event representations with the same complexity as his peers. With no symbolic representations for past and future, he cannot simultaneously incorporate two time periods into his thought, one created and maintained through activation of linguistic representations and the other through activation of present context. He has no tool for thinking about what he will do independent of what is occurring. And he has no ability to access meaning and function of grammatical forms and constructions. Their absence will prevent later development of a linguistic representational ability separate from conceptual structure of thought.

EMERGENCE OF EXTENDED DISCOURSE: DEVELOPMENT FROM 35 TO 40 MONTHS

In just a few short months the representational network changes from one in which a single word is used to refer to an inseparable event representation to one in which linguistic representations create imaginary events (Bruner, 1986). Grammatical and discourse representations provide a linguistic means for moving agents and actions across a series of related events to create stories and elaborated play sequences (Wolf & Gardner, 1979). This is made possible by the emerging complexity of the linguistic representation (see Table 1.12).

Situational Context

Development of the event representation began with the child constructing a representation of his own actions in relationship to objects and people within daily routines. As patterns of connectivity became elaborated across the slots of the event representation, sufficient connection weights for roles of others enabled the child to function in those roles in play, or to refer to those roles in language when props or other artifacts of the

TABLE 1.12
Abilities Demonstrated between 35 and 40 Months of Age Across
the Cognitive, Social, Semiotic, and Sensory-Motor Domains Profiled
within the Situational-Discourse-Semantic Contexts of the
SDS: Development Model

	35–40 Months Level VI		
	Situational Decontext-Egocentered Displacement	Discourse Abbreviated Plan Organization	Semantic Interpretative Reference
Cognitive	Object Displacement Language decontextualizes and can be used to recount a personal experience; predicts future events in real or imaginary situations based on present evidence although logic may be faulty). Words support objects or toys in play.	Event/Discourse Elaborated sequences of plot-related events, but sequence is not well planned or goal oriented; talks about aspects of event throughout and coordinates ideas in space, perspective, or time across sentences.	Perceptual Interest in perceptual properties of objects is strong. Uses words that interpret distinctions (big-fat-tall versus little-thin-short). Interest in shapes, size, counting. Uses blocks to make buildings or vehicles. Adj used in elaborated phrases (one little dog).
Social	Self/Other Displacement Plays with others in same activity but no coordinated goal (each paint) (associative). Talks about past and future possible acts (I'm gonna paint Barnie).	Interactional Takes turns with adults and peers in conversation; can give reports on personal events as a near monologue. Takes other's perspective (I versus you).	Functional Language used for functioning within many social roles; switch role talking to and for doll in same event. Words interpret desires, feelings, thoughts (I know, think, wish).
Semiotic	Time/Space Displacement Language refers to things that are possible and future actions that could happen independent of actual experience. Demonstrations used to support meaning.	Locutionary A variety of utterances are used to report, entertain, show off, and regulate the actions of others. Embeds subordinate clauses to ordinate ideas.	Convention MLU 3.00–3.99; adult-like talk: three to seven word sentences include complex structures. Auxiliary verbs present but may have errors, used in neg. and questions. Past modals (would); combine two clauses, embedding.
Sensory-Motor	Imitative Displacement Imitates roles of others, producing dialogue consistent with less familiar and unexperienced roles (policeman, space traveler). New vocabulary learned without direct participation.	Exocutionary Bilateral coordination (rides trike, alternates feet upstairs) Walks backward, sideways, on tip toes, marches. Invents spellings with syllables.	Modality Decontextualized language requires greater phonemic accuracy: /p/b/t/d/ k/g/m/n/ng/h/w/j/ r/l/f/s/ occurs appropriately. Gestures represent action ("Like this" [demonstrates]).

Reprinted with permission from Norris, JA, and Hoffman, PR (1999). The SDS developmental model of integrated functioning, Baton Rouge, LA: EleMentory.

event representation were present. As concepts separated from the event representation, still greater displacement was possible, and the child participated in events created from infrequently experienced events, such as pretending to be a doctor or a store clerk (Vygotsky, 1978). The result of this expansion in complexity of representational structures is a network of thousands of interrelated events and conceptual representations.

The interrelated nature of the network makes generalization from any one conceptual structure to another and the association of a new representation to established ones possible. This ability to acquire meaning or function through association with existing conceptual structures allows for new creativity and generativity within the network (Rumelhart & McClelland, 1986). At this stage the child is able to observe unexperienced roles and behaviors of figures such as police officers or astronauts, or even animals such as kangaroos, and imitate their actions (Sachs, 1984; Stambak & Sinclair, 1993). The child uses event representations similar to existing ones and is able to use slot-filler categories to modify the representation to accommodate new information (see Fig. 1.14). This ability to generalize begins to free the child from learning through direct experience (Piaget, 1954, 1960). Instead, personal observations of others' actions, even when viewed on television or at a distance, can provide input that can be interpreted and reconstructed in the internal event representation.

Development and separation of language from the event representation adds further flexibility to the system. Since words and their concepts are connected to, but parsed from, the myriad of event representations from which they evolved, they can easily be activated by new contexts of use (Nelson, 1985, 1996). Dialogue produced by superheros, police officers, and other observed agents thus can be interpreted in context. The dialogue "We have to catch him," spoken as a villain is running will activate connections between familiar words and the relationships between them, while simultaneously activating concepts of the superheros and the villain in the chasing event. These two sources of input and information allow the observed event to be interpreted. The child further uses known words to interpret unknown meanings, as in the dialogue "It's time to power-up," spoken while pressing buttons that appear to provide immediate strength and energy. The words "It's time to" activate well-established associations with meaning, having been heard within routines since early infancy (It's time to ... go to bed, eat dinner, go to day care, take a bath). The expected meaning for the unknown word "power-up" is predicted to be an action that changes the current activity, activated by the semantic relationships maintained between these words (Dollaghan, 1985; Stoel-Gammon & Cooper, 1984).

Merging linguistic expectations with visual input establishes patterns of strong connectivity between the action of pressing the button and the

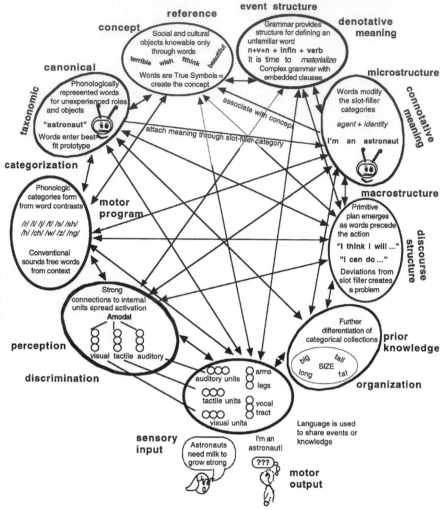

Situational Context: Language establishes context independent of people or objects for personal events.
(Decontextualized-Egocentered)

FIG. 1.14. By 35 to 40 months, the interrelated network makes possible generalization from any one conceptual structure to another, and association of new information with established structures. The resulting creativity and generativity of the network makes play in unexperienced roles, like an astronaut, possible. Language begins to decontextualize, or be used independently of an actual experience, such as talking about what will happen later. Words are true symbols, creating concepts that cannot be seen such as "wish," "think," or "know." Grammar helps establish the meaning of unfamiliar words. Primitive planning is seen in personal narratives, reflected in words such as "can" or "will." (Reprinted with permission from Norris, JA, and Hoffman, PR (1999). The SDS developmental model of integrated functioning, Baton Rouge, LA: EleMentory.)

words "power-up." When the child is imitating the scene and spontaneous running begins, connectivity to the powering-up event would elicit use of that dialogue and imitation of the action. So at this stage of learning, words support objects and create possible future actions before they happen. Children also begin to use this language independently of the actual experience, as in saying "I'm gonna power-up" while riding in the car.

Discourse Context

Discourse context is increasingly represented in language. Discourse includes organization of conversational interchanges, such as turn-taking, topic maintenance, and methods for initiating and terminating an interaction. Discourse also includes organization of factual, expository, or procedural information for sharing, termed transactional discourse by Britton (1982), and organization of events that convey culturally signifiant messages, often in the form of stories, called narrative discourse (Bruner, 1986). Discourse of all genres develops as a product of cognitive and social/cultural input provided through linguistic forms (Blum-Kulka & Snow, 1992; Bruner, 1983). That is, during procedures such as making cookies with a child, or examining a butterfly, or telling a fairy tell, language serves as the primary medium for exchanging information. Information becomes increasingly less individual and experience-based and more cultural and learning-based (Norris & Hoffman, 1993; Vygotsky, 1962). For example, while looking at the butterfly, the adult might label it as an insect and show that it has six legs. Discourse requires the cognitive, social, and linguistic capacity to hold in mind a representation of a complex reality formulated in language (Nelson, 1996). Without this ability, children appear distractible and unwilling to listen, and disengage from conversations rapidly unless they are maintained by others.

Narrative discourse, unlike conversation, is often conducted as a monologue. Instead of taking turns and sharing responsibility for interchange, one speaker must organize and present a coherent telling of an event. Temporal organization is basic to a narrative (Bruner, 1986). Temporal organization emerged earlier in the context of an event representation where linguistic representations established categories for interpreting time. Narratives emerge as events deviate from the expected or typical event representation. The deviation impels the narrative to emerge to first describe, and in later development to resolve the noted difference (Feldman, 1989). In the typical, or canonical event, breakfast might ensue as pouring cereal and milk, eating the cereal with a spoon, and putting the dirty dishes in the sink. A deviation in this temporal sequence, such as having no clean spoons and attempting to eat the cereal with a fork constitutes a difference that is problematic.

To share the event later, language is needed to communicate the story. While the sequence of actions could be enacted in play (and in fact elaborated sequences of plot-related events are observed in play), social and cultural aspects of the story can only be expressed in words (Nelson, 1989, 1996). Reactions to the attempt to use the fork ("That was so funny" versus "That was so frustrating") can only be shared using language. These social aspects are learned in the context of the event, as the adult looks at the smiling child and says "That's so funny," or to the frustrated child and says "It makes you feel mad when it doesn't work." Even when the story is enacted in play, there is often ongoing talk about aspects of the event that coordinate ideas across time and specify feelings, reactions, and problems. Much that occurs in symbolic play could not be created without the use of language (Stambak & Sinclair, 1993).

Events that have the strongest patterns of connectivity are those that are personally experienced and familiar, closely following the canonical script of a routine event. With this level of internal representation and reliable activation of patterns of connectivity a child at this stage can report on a personal event that contains a problem as a near monologue. The recounting may contain a primitive plan or intention ("I think I can break it. And I stepped on it. And it broked"). Other types of story telling will require prompts and scaffolded support provided by adults collaborating with the child to recount the experience (Bruner, 1983). However, independence from the actual event and from the scaffolded support of others is beginning to emerge.

Semantic Context

Components in the event representation allowed for formation of slot-filler categories, or collections of items that could fulfull that role within the event. Over time, an increasing number of items formed patterns of connectivity to the event slot. Some of these were similar in perception and performed the same function within the event, such as colors (i.e., Find your *color* shirt), in which case they formed strong patterns of connectivity between them. These words form a subcategory within the larger collection, particularly if the subcategory had been identified with a name (e.g., color). During this stage, further differentiation among members of a category is seen as children begin to specify distinctions with words, as in big, little, fat, tall, thin short, and so forth. Emergence of these terms suggests that children are able to attend to one aspect or dimension of bigness (or smallness) such as height or girth, and refer to that dimension independently of the overall whole, as when calling a very short but heavy person "fat" (Blank, Rose, & Berlin, 1978).

Distinctions within the subcategory remain as collections rather than hierarchies (hierarchies are not usually constructed before five years of age). The child does not understand that fat is opposite of thin, or tall opposite of short, and that both are dimensions of the superordinate category of big versus small. Rather, they are relatively independent concepts that refer to the salient dimension within a context. Adults who label superordinate categories (i.e., "What size do you want?") create a linguistic representation to which children must attach meaning and in so doing begin to form hierarchical structure (Nelson, 1996). Naming establishes categories and shapes categories to have the meanings maintained by the shared culture. Meanings for categories that form independently of language may be different from those in the culture.

Discourse provides a context for children to learn that others may think differently from them and to begin to acquire cultural thought. Language is required for this to occur. During an event, adults model what is in their thinking by using language to talk about it, as in "I think your shoes are in here" or "I know what to do." They encourage children to talk about their thoughts, asking questions such as "What do you think is in here?" or commenting on the child's behavior as in "You know you're not supposed to be up there." By this stage, children have interpreted these linguistic representations and begin to generate their own comments using words such as I know, think, or wish (Abbeduto & Rosenberg, 1985). These linguistically created concepts represent the transition into true symbols.

Many connections are present for establishing relationships for words, so that the mean length of utterance (MLU) is three to four words but sentences of up to seven words are commonly produced (Miller, 1981; Miller & Chapman, 1981). Sentences include complex structures, such as elaborated noun phrases containing a quantifier and an adjective (One little dog) as well as auxiliaries and modals in the verb phrase. Just as the event representation may be embedded by a deviation from the canonical structure, sentences may have an embedded clause inserted into the canonical structure. Hierarchies are beginning to form in both the conceptual and the linguistic system.

Tyrone's Profile of Language Delay

Studies of late talkers have repeatedly shown that by three years of age, many children spontaneously begin to use language, even without intervention. However, the profile of language is characterized by vocabulary that is within the lower limits of average, but delayed significantly in syntactic and morphological development (Paul, 1993; Paul, Spangle-Looney, & Dahm, 1991; Rescorla, Roberts, & Dahlsgaard, 1997; Rescorla & Schwartz, 1990). Tyrone is beginning to fit this profile. Recall that up until two years of age, acoustic information was redundant to other sources of input and was not the primary source of forming event representations and concepts. Those structures within Tyrone's network were relatively normal. Conceptual development at two years of age could continue to progress typically, as concepts parsed away from event representations. The difference was the lack of integration of words with concepts and the foundation that words would establish for later development. Presence of language allows for concepts to recombine in new ways, independent of the event representations as adults label collections of subcategories, or refer to abstractions using words. Tyrone's current development is limited to attaching words to slot-filler categories, or those that evolved nonverbally from the event representation. He cannot acquire higher level lexical representations until he has sufficient vocabulary attached to concepts, to begin to recombine them into more abstract collections.

Syntactic development is delayed to a far greater extent because while conceptual development (and therefore the conceptual structure for words to map onto) could continue without language, relational meanings could not be expressed. Tyrone required word forms to begin to express semantic relationships, and semantic relationships were needed to provide a frame for syntactic forms to emerge. Linguistic representations requiring facility with acousitic and phonological forms must be present for syntactic markers to evolve from the event representation. So while the representational structure was present to support vocabulary acquisition, no similar structures were constructed to support syntactic development. Tyrone's system is qualitatively different from normal and will continue to limit the transition toward symbolic language and thought.

REPRESENTING MEANING IN SYMBOLIC LANGUAGE: DEVELOPMENT FROM 41 TO 48 MONTHS

The presymbolic child learns through direct experience, creating event representations and conceptual structures through sensory-motor interactions with the environment. Talk is embedded within the internal representations for the event. That is, connection weights representing words are activated in the same manner as other components of the event structure. The words and the event are inseparable. But as concepts and corresponding words separate from the event representation and words separate and form a grammatical representation, language itself becomes symbolic, independent of the concepts or the event representation. Representational ability begins to change from experience-based to language-based (Piaget, 1960; Vygotsky, 1962, 1978). These changes are profiled in Table 1.13.

TABLE 1.13

Abilities Demonstrated between 41 and 48 Months of Age Across the Cognitive, Social, Semiotic, and Sensory-Motor Domains Profiled within the Situational-Discourse-Semantic Contexts of the SDS: Development Model

	41–48 Months Level VII		
	Situational Decontextualized Displacement	Discourse Abbreviated Plan Organization	Semantic Interpretative Reference
nitive	Object Displacement Language decontextualizes and can be used to recount an event observed but not personally or directly experienced. Recounting understood by others who have some knowledge of the event.	Event/Discourse Elaborated sequences of plot related events, with embedded episodes of plans, cause, end. Overall does not focus on a problem and plan to solve it, but some actions include a plan.	Perceptual Draws pictures to represent objects or events. Categorizes by same/different, dimensions (animals, red things). Perceptually based logic (more because its taller). Complex noun modifiers (four big blue cars).
al	Self/Other Displacement Cooperates with adults to achieve goals (bake cookies, simple chores). Takes on reciprocal roles in shared play, talking to and for characters. Assigns roles to other children acts out roles using puppets.	Interactional Begins to adjust length of discourse to conform to the social context and participant expectations. Asks questions to find out how and why things are done or occur.	Functional Greater focus on future events and can infer possible actions (He might find a space man). Express facts, rules, beliefs, attitudes, emotions: focuses on function words (It isn't on, I need to go, because I couldn't).
iotic	Time/Space Displacement Language establishes the context by setting the scene and specifying the subjects and objects of an event, but often assumes shared information that listener may not have. Refers to possible and future actions. Emerging separate thought versus action (I know, . . .).	Locutionary Begins to differentiate between recountings of actual events versus fictional stories or fantasy. Reasoning emerges, resulting from integration of reporting, predicting, and projecting. Tease, warn, convey humor.	Convention MLU 4.0–4.49. Many compound and complex sentences, coordinating and subordinating clauses to relate complex events. Vocabulary surpasses 1,500 words. Most verbs correctly inflected, contracted auxiliaries and negatives, gerunds.
ory- otor	Imitative Displacement Imitates complex actions and verbal expressions. Imitates pretend actions performed by superheros and other fanciful figures. Uses imitation to draw complex figures.	Exocutionary Emerging maturity in locomotion including arm swing; runs smoothly, throws, & catches. Uses many polysyllabic words (impossible, everywhere); may have syllable simplifications.	Modality Adult-like grasp (pincer). Begins to perform self-help actions (button, laces, brush teeth). Phonemically appropriate /p/b/t/d/k/g/m/n/ng /h/w/j/r/l/f/s/z/sh/ch/ in most word positions. Errors: /v/dz/. Begins to recognize letters, pretend writing.

Reprinted with permission from Norris, JA, and Hoffman, PR (1999). The SDS developmental model of grated functioning, Baton Rouge, LA: EleMentory.

Situational Context

Play during the previous stage evolved to enable the child to observe un-experienced roles and behaviors of others, such as astronauts or police, and to replicate their actions in play. The child also could use the dialogue of these characters in the context of play, and often independently of it. Increasingly, linguistic representations form that allow for abstract concepts to be constructed through collaborative interactions with others. That is, the grammatical context in which words are produced begin to provide as many clues to meaning as the event context. The growing independence of language from experience results in symbolic representations of knowledge, generated using language symbols. One result of this is the ability to recount an observed or unexperienced event in language, without support of context or props (Bruner, 1983; Westby, 1985). People, places, and time frames specified in language become the situational context, while actual objects and people present in the physical environment become irrelevant to the shared meaning (Nelson, 1989; Norris & Hoffman, 1993). When recounting a trip to the beach, the kitchen provides little of relevance to support the talk. At this stage, the child's recounting lacks clarity and cohesion, and so is best understood by others who have some knowledge of the event. But the shared topic is linguistically created using symbolic representations of the event, and thus is completely decontextualized language.

Language is a system of both internal mental representation and external linguistic representation. Internally, linguistic symbols serve as the means for constructing new knowledge and establishing relationships of meaning and function according to linguistic structures (see Fig. 1.15). This property of language serves to organize thought according to consistent and reliable relationships expressed grammatically. Structural properties of language in turn permit more complex logical and theoretical thought than is possible through other semiotic forms (Nelson, 1996). Externally, language provides a means of sharing knowledge and perceptions, such as a recounting a previously experienced beach event. In addition, language provides a means for cultural knowledge to enter into the child's mental representations. The child's thought becomes mediated by cultural ways of thinking and speaking, so that the child's concepts and beliefs become conventional, or more like those expressed by others. The result is individuality balanced with, or determined by, sociality.

This process occurs as the input from the adult's language serves as a source of input to the child. The child is able to use this linguistic input because of internal linguistic representations that have been constructed for words and grammar within the child's network. Exchange of linguistic meaning was not possible until the child could interpret relationships of meaning using the word order principles of language, and had a large

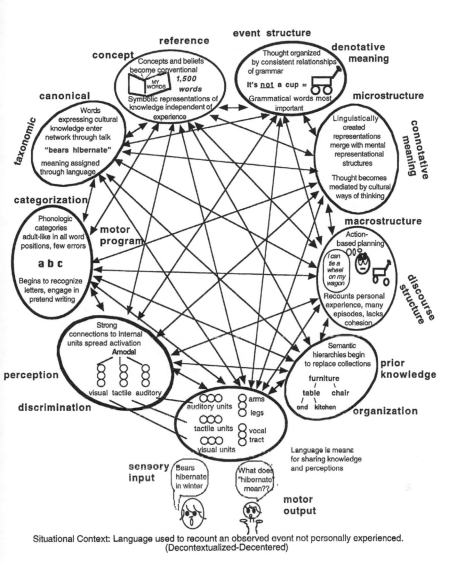

Situational Context: Language used to recount an observed event not personally experienced.
(Decontextualized-Decentered)

FIG. 1.15. Representational ability changes from experience-based to language-based between 41 and 48 months of age. Abstract concepts form through collaborative construction with others, including questions and explanations. Talk creates symbolic representation of knowledge independent of experience, or true language. For the first time, new knowledge can be constructed internally within the network from words and grammar. Externally, language allows for a means for cultural knowledge to enter the event representation, so child's concepts and beliefs become more conventional. Phonological forms are nearly adult-like. Semantic hierarchies begin to form, although it will be many years before the semantic hierarchy is well developed and integrated. (Reprinted with permission from Norris, JA, and Hoffman, PR (1999). The SDS developmental model of integrated functioning, Baton Rouge, LA: EleMentory.)

lexicon. By the fourth birthday children have a sufficiently complex linguistic representation to interpret another's knowledge in context and to use language as the input source to enter parts into their own mental representations (Donald, 1991; Nelson, 1996). That is, learning through verbal explanation is possible without an accompanying direct experience. The linguistically created representation merges with the child's mental representation as a single, inseparable representation because of direct connections that remain between the event representation and language. Language does not yet create an independent event representation formed from linguistic symbols. For this to occur, language must be organized semantically, that is, separate from the event and comprised of its own linguistic hierarchies (Nelson, 1985, 1986). This achievement is not reached until after seven years of age, recognized by Piaget (1954) as concrete operational thought.

Discourse Context

The emerging logic of the cognitive system, now mediated by symbolic language, allows for the appearance of planning in the context of play, art, and self-help routines. Plans do not yet focus on an overall problem and a plan to solve it, but rather action plans such as how to get wheels to stick on a cardboard box car. In play, many episodes are embedded within the sequence of plot-related events so that play developing the same theme may be long in duration with some episodes including action based plans. Similarly, mediated logic is observed in emergent reasoning abilities, and children begin to look for the cause of an event and not just the consequence.

Emerging reasoning ability and linguistic ability to exchange personal and cultural knowledge leads to questions regarding how and why things are done or occur. At earlier stages, children use "why" as a means of socially participating in discourse, but do not listen for or expect an answer. The meaning of the "why" question to the younger child is primarily pragmatic. At this stage, the meaning of the "why" question becomes semantic as well, as the child uses this as a strategy to obtain information from others that can help to add clarity to ambiguous concepts or to linguistically created representations lacking meaning (Miller, 1981). This tool adds new power to learning, as the child does not have to discover information fortuitously through sensory-motor exploration, but instead can ask for information and receive an immediate answer. The power of this expectation is experienced by adults whose four-year-old repeatedly demands to know "why" upon receiving the answer "I don't know."

The ability to engage in extended discourse, deliver monologues, observe turn-taking and other conversational rules, structure information using conventional grammar, and perform a wide range of communicative functions using language results in a four-year-old with many adult-like discourse skills (Applebee, 1978; Dore, 1986).

Semantic Context

The network at this stage has constructed over 1,500 words that refer to concepts within the child's conceptual structure (Dollaghan, 1985; Stoel-Gammon & Cooper, 1984). Words and concepts are still integrated, although the relationship is flexible and beginning to separate. This occurs as semantic hierarchies in language form to replace collections of presymbolic conceptual categories. Through language, adults provide insights into the manner in which culture imposes categories (Gelman & Coley, 1991; Gelman & Markman, 1986). The foundation for these is constructed through slot-filler categories derived from the event representation. From these, children organize elements into basic collections such as foods, colors, animals, books, and so forth. Categories are assigned a label (i.e., "food" or "animals") and the label is linguistic, naming the category and not the concept derived from the event structure.

These linguistic labels then can be recombined to form greater abstractions (Nelson, 1986, 1996). For example, the category "animals" can be recombined with "hunters" to create the concept of "predators." Relevant features from the first concept form new patterns of connectivity with relevant features from the second concept to form a new concept, different from both. Similarly, the category of "animals" can be recombined with "food" to create the concept of "prey." "Predators," "prey," and "life" can be recombined to form the concept "survival" and so forth. In this manner, hierarchical inclusion begins to form. Only rudimentary beginnings of this hierarchical organization is observed at this stage, as children begin to categorize by basic level categories, such as "tables" or "chairs." More superordinate categories such as "tools" or "furniture" are not understood. Collections remain the primary strategy for organizing concepts (Nelson & Nelson, 1990).

Emerging hierarchical organization within the network is also observed in linguistic representations. Many compound and complex sentences are produced. Children at this stage produce coordinating and subordinating clauses, such as "The kitty ran, and we couldn't find it" or "I think we gotta put a bandaid on it." Superordinate terms such as "and" or "if" function to recombine propositions of two separate sentences, resulting in a different meaning than either utterance produced independently (Miller, 1981).

The hierarchical links in grammar become more informative to the meaning of the utterance than the vocabulary words. For example, in the sentence "It is not a chair" the important feature is the word "not."

This superordinate term changes the meaning from the concept of a chair to any possible concept except a chair (Blank, Rose, & Berlin, 1978). A child's ability to inhibit activation to the concept of "chair" based on its grammatical relationship to the word "not," provides the network a strategy for producing an inference based on what is not, rather than what is. It will be several years before a true hierarchy based on semantic organization of concepts and syntactic organization of relationships is complete (Nelson, 1996). However, the four-year-old child has constructed important patterns of connectivity at many levels of representation that form the foundation for this later development.

Tyrone's Future Language Learning

Tyrone is beginning to construct language as a representational system, but at a delayed rate compared to his peers. Syntactic advances are slower to be achieved than vocabulary acquisitions, even after word order strategies emerge. Phonological representations are also delayed, resulting in limited intelligibility. Is it likely that Tyrone will "catch-up" in language?

The more advanced representational language becomes, the more dependent it is on rapid processing of acoustic input. Abstract meanings are dependent on processing syntactic relationships, requiring linguistic representations to create and process information. Acoustic input must rapidly activate and form networks of relational meanings between words in multiply embedded sentences, and across boundaries of sentences present in discourse. Many studies suggest that a qualitative difference in processing the acoustic signal results in life-long differences in learning for many children. Strominger and Bashir (1977) reported that the children they studied as preschoolers had residual deficits at school-age, with written language problems most prevalent. Similar long-term difficulties have been identified in other populations of children with delayed preschool language development (Aram & Nation, 1980).

Studies of school-age children with language and learning disabilities have revealed language difficulties across all aspects of language, from phonology through connected discourse and social-pragmatic abilities (Gibbs & Cooper, 1989). These range from subtle differences in phonemic awareness (Kamhi, Catts, Mauer, Apel, & Gentry, 1988) to problems with phonological rules, poor word retrieval (Denckla & Rudel, 1976), and difficulty with morphological inflections and derivations (Wiig & Semel, 1980), comprehension and production delays in syntax (Donahue, Pearl, & Bryan, 1982), limited vocabulary development, and difficulty with metalinguistic analysis of language (Van Kleeck, 1994). All aspects of discourse also have been found to be problematic, including generating narratives (Roth & Spekman, 1986), maintaining text cohesion (Liles, 1985), conversational competence (Donahue, 1984), and social-pragmatic abilities with peers and adults (Donahue, 1994; Dorval, McKinney, & Feagans, 1982).

IMPLICATIONS FOR INTERVENTION

Connectionist principles, structured around a multidimensional model such as the Situational-Discourse-Semantic Development model can be used to guide intervention. This process begins with an observational assessment of the child's performance in routines, play, social games, conversation, and other contexts of learning and functioning. Each observation is used to determine characteristics of the situation, including a comparison of response to objects versus people. If, for example the child responds to objects at a higher level than to people, lack of integration of patterns of connectivity for social knowledge within the event representation is implicated. This is a common profile for children with autism or other pervasive developmental disabilities. In this case, the level of interaction would need to be lowered so that input from social sources could be integrated into the event representation.

For example, the child might sort objects by perceptual properties such as color or shape, indicating that connections are forming for slot-filler categories related to objects and their attributes, but ignore talk about the activity and turn the body or walk away as the adult attempts to interact. This means that the child cannot yet include people in interactions with objects, and has not constructed their role in the event script. Other people do not have a place in the child's well-structured representation and so they are rejected. The language is not useful or meaningful because words cannot refer to the role of others within the event representation, and so words cannot serve as a means to an end, or to insert new knowledge into the event representation.

The level at which the child can include people needs to be found and the event representation constructed beginning at that level. To do this, patterns of connectivity might have to be introduced into the event representation at a very basic level. It may be necessary to reduce the level of input to Level I (0–1 month), where people are responded to only when touching or very near the child and only unintentional reflexive movements are produced, which the adult interprets as meaningful. Intervention would then consist of repeated short cycles of interaction, where the child would produce an unintentional behavior (i.e., a random hand movement), the adult would impute meaning as if the child initiated an interaction, and the adult would respond by touching the child by playing a simple game (i.e., pat-a-cake) or chewing on the child's fingers with an object, such as a puppet. This interaction cycle would establish patterns of connectivity between the child's action, the adult role, and the consequences to the child. Once patterns of connectivity were incorporated for the adult's role, intervention would build toward gradually more complex social interactions, using the continuum of the SDS:D scale to guide steps in the process. When social interactions between people become intentional, objects can be introduced by responding to the child's intentional communication as if it was a request for a "turn" playing with the object. The adult would then talk about the child's actions as joint focus on the object was established, to establish patterns of connectivity between words and the slot-filler categories, as well as between words and the means-ends role of talk to the adult and consequences within the event representation.

Similarly, if Tyrone had not started spontaneously acquiring words, interactions might need to begin at Level I, providing him an opportunity to link acoustic signals to events. For example, the adult might begin with vocalizations such as giggles elicited by a tickle, causing a variety of interesting consequences to occur contingent to production of sound (i.e., blowing bubbles, putting a sticker in a book, or a social game such as a finger play). The interaction would abruptly end, followed by an invitation for Tyrone to reinitiate, such as "Let's do that again." The adult would wait briefly for a vocalization, and if none was produced a giggle would be elicited. The goal of the interactions is to help Tyrone make the discovery that his voice controls actions of the adult and to establish patterns of connectivity between sound production and actions of the event representation.

Children who manifest poor organization for the discourse context are having difficulty formulating event representations. Often these children have characteristics of Attention Deficit Hyperactivity Disorder (ADHD) and are distracted by images and sounds, flitting between objects and toys without interacting long enough to form organized action sequences (Norris & Hoffman, 1996). In this case, the adult needs to structure the discourse, continuing to point out several things on a page instead of allowing the page to be turned, and providing the child with a series of objects that can be used to form an action sequence. This mediated interaction allows patterns of connectivity to develop for discourse, including linguistic forms that structure and create cohesion across the linear order of sequences. For example, the adult provides the child with a pot, and as the child turns to leave, the adult says "That's right, you do need to cook the hot dog" and directs the child to put it in the pot. As the child begins to disengage, the adult models touching the pan, saying "Ow! That's hot!" and before the child can leave, the adult begins to unwrap a band-aid to place on the "owie." Initially 6 seconds of attention can be extended to 30 seconds, and then a minute, and finally several minutes playing short action sequences using the same sets of toys as the child forms event representations to guide these sequences.

As the child's interest increases, the adult can model and ask for language that can be used to structure and to parse concepts within the event representation, as in "Be careful, don't touch the pot. Now you tell me" (spoken while reaching toward the pot). Any word approximations or imitations are expanded to be a few words more complex than the child's utterance, and then extended to include a related idea.

In all interactions, situational-discourse-semantic principles are followed. Situationally, the adult must establish a level of input that maximizes successful learning. Once the learning situation is selected, the adult must work to increase discourse complexity, including expanding duration of the event and imparting control of interactions to the child. Semantically, the adult must accept the communications produced by the child, even if these lack conventionality and intent. These communications then can be enhanced using strategies such as modeling, expansion, and extension.

Understanding how the complex system of language forms from the initial reflexive responses of infancy, through progressively more elaborated event representations can enable interventionists to understand how and why atypical profiles of development can occur. These theoretical models can then be used to guide the sequence and process of effective intervention.

CONCLUSIONS

Human learning, particularly language development is so multidimensional and complex that we may never understand all of the principles involved or the mechanism for constructing the system. Machines, such as connectionist computers, may never be able to replicate even a small part of this complex process. Theoretical models based on connectionist networks provide a means for imagining how such a complex and integrated representational system might form in human learning. Connectionist models provide a way of envisioning what happens at a cellular level to produce the equivalent of an assimilation or accommodation if connection weights between units are translated as the transfer of activation between cells. The re-creation of patterns of connectivity each time a concept is instantiated allows for a unique pattern of activation for each context of use. This property accounts for subtle variations in meaning in different contexts. Similarly, patterns of connectivity that can be activated provide a model for understanding how event representations and concepts can form in overlapping whole-to-part relationships with gradual displacement from the original event.

This chapter profiles how a multidimensional model such as the SDS:D model can merge with a connectionist perspective to integrate a range of sometimes apparently conflicting research. It demonstrates, for example, how language can function both as part of the conceptual structure and be separate from it. It provides a beginning point for discussion of the integrated relationship between language and cognitive, social, and sensory-motor achievements. Many details of this combined model are incomplete and speculative. But the combined perspectives show how language can be both interdependent and independent of cognition as lower levels of connectivity are used to support increasingly higher levels of displacement and abstraction using the same structures and the same mechanism for constructing representations. It also demonstrates how many aspects of development can initially form normally, despite delays or deficits in one or more other areas, and how learning differences ultimately place limits on higher level functioning.

Future research will provide advances in connectionist models that will integrate multisensory input while simultaneously forming subpatterns of modality specific structures. Each advance will help us understand more about how collaborative construction of internal representations take place and how they function. The role of the input of other people, providing expansions, extensions, and excisions just above the level of those patterns of connectivity already established, will enable us to better understand what is needed to facilitate change. The journey into this understanding has just begun, and our tools for replicating this process in a machine are primitive compared to the human mind of the infant. Nonetheless, the model of connectionism provides us with a means for imagining how construction of internal structures can take place, functioning with sufficient consistency to allow for conventional cultural meaning, while at the same time offering flexibility to capture nuances of meaning in infinitely differing contexts. The potential of connectionism to integrate a wide range of processes and structures within a multidimensional model needed to achieve this goal makes it one of the exciting theoretical challenges of the future.

REFERENCES

Abbeduto, L., & Rosenberg, S. (1985). Children's knowledge of the presuppositions of *know* and other cognitive verbs. *Journal of Child Language, 12*, 621–641.

Acredolo, L., & Goodwin, S. (1985). Symbolic gesturing in language development. *Human Development, 28*, 40–49.

Adamson, L. B. (1995). *Communication development during infancy*. Madison, WI: Brown & Benchmark Publishers.

Applebee, A. N. (1978). A child's concept of story: Ages 2–17. Chicago: University of Chicago Press.

Aram, D. M., & Nation, J. E. (1980). Preschool language disorders and subsequent language and academic difficulties. *Journal of Communication Disorders, 13*, 159–170.

Baker, N., & Nelson, K. (1984). Recasting and related conversational techniques for triggering syntactic advances by young children. *First Language, 5*, 3–22.

Barsalou, L. W. (1991). Deriving categories to achieve goals. In G. H. Bower (Ed.), *The psychology of learning and motivation: Advances in research and theory* (vol. 27, pp. 1–64). New York: Academic.

Bates, E., Benigni, L., Bretherton, I., Camaioni, L., & Volterra, V. (1979). *The emergence of symbols: Cognition and communication in infancy*. New York: Academic Press.

Bates, E., Camaioni, L., & Volterra, V. (1975). The acquisition of performatives prior to speech. *Merrill-Palmer Quarterly, 21*, 205–224.

Bates, E., O'Connell, B., & Shore, C. (1987). Language and communication in infancy. In J. D. Osofsky (Ed.), *Handbook of infant development* (pp. 149–203). New York: John Wiley & Sons.

Blank, M., Rose, S. & Berlin, L. (1978). *The language of learning: The preschool years*. New York: Grune & Stratton.

Bloom, L. (1970). *Language development: Form and function of emerging grammars*. Cambridge: MIT Press.

Bloom, L. (1993). *The transition from infancy to language: Acquiring the power of expression*. New York: Cambridge University Press.

Blum-Kulka, S., & Snow, C. (1992). Developing autonomy for tellers, tales, and telling in family narrative events. *Journal of Narrative and Life History, 2*, 187–218.

Brazelton, T. B., & Tronick, E. (1980). Preverbal communication between mothers and infants. In D. Olson (Ed.), *Social foundations of language and thought* (pp. 299–315). New York: Norton.

Britton, J. (1982). Writing to learn and learning to write. In G. M. Pradl (Ed.), *Prospect and retrospect: Selected essays of James Britton* (pp. 94–111). Montclair, NJ: Boynton/Cook.

Brown, R. (1973). *A first language: The early stages*. Cambridge, MA: Harvard University Press.

Bruner, J. (1983). *Child's talk: Learning to use language*. New York: Norton.

Bruner, J. S. (1986). *Actual minds, possible worlds*. Cambridge, MA: Harvard University Press.

Chapman, R. S. (1981). Exploring children's communicative intents In J Miller (Ed), *Assessing language production in children* (pp. 111–138). Austin, TX: PRO ED.

Charon, J. M. (1992). *Symbolic interactionism: An introduction, an interpretation, an integration* (4th edition). Englewood Cliffs, NJ: Prentice Hall.

Clark, A. (1993). *Associative engines: Connectionism, concepts, and representational change*. Cambridge, MA: MIT Press.

Clark, E. V. (1973). What's in a word? On the child's acquisition of semantics in his first language. In T. E. Moore (Ed.), *Cognitive development and the acquisition of language* (pp. 65–110). New York: Academic Press.

Clark, E. V. (1983). Meaning and concepts. In J. H. Flavell & E. M. Markman (Eds.) *Handbook of Child Psychology, Vol. 3: Cognitive development* (General editor, P. H. Mussen (pp. 787–840). New York: John Wiley and Sons.

Clark, E. V. (1993). *The lexicon in acquisition*. New York: Cambridge University Press.

Davidson, A. (1983). *Maths and me*. Auckland, New Zealand: Shortland Publications.

Denckla, M. B., & Rudel, R. (1976). Naming of object-drawings by dyslexic and other learning disabled children. *Brain Language, 3*, 1–15.

Dollaghan, C. A. (1985). Child meets word: "Fast mapping" in preschool children. *Journal of Speech and Hearing Research, 28*, 449–454.

Donahue, M. L. (1984). Learning disabled children's conversational competence: An attempt to activate the inactive listener. *Applied Psycholinguistics, 5*, 21–35.

Donahue, M. L. (1994). Differences in classroom discourse styles of students with learning disabilities. In D. N. Ripich, & N. C. Creaghead (Eds.), *School discourse problems* (2nd ed.). San Diego: Singular Press.

Donahue, M. L., Pearl, R., & Bryan, T. (1982). Learning disabled children's syntactic proficiency on a communicative task. *Journal of Speech and Hearing Disorders, 47,* 397–403.

Donald, M. (1991). *Origins of the modern mind: Three stages in the evolution of culture and cognition.* Cambridge, MA: Harvard University Press.

Dore, J. (1986). The development of conversational competence. In R. S. Schiefelbusch (Ed.), *Language competence: Assessment and intervention* (pp. 3–60). San Diego: College Hill.

Dorval, B., McKinney, J. D., & Feagans, L. (1982). Teachers' interactions with learning disabled children and average achievers. *Journal of Pediatric Psychology, 17,* 317–330.

Elkind, D. (1974). *A sympathetic understanding of the child.* Boston: Allyn & Bacon.

Feldman, C. F. (1989). Monologue as a problem-solving narrative. In K. Nelson (Ed.), *Narratives from the crib* (pp. 98–122). Cambridge, MA: Harvard University Press.

Fenson, L., & Ramsey, D. (1980). Decentration and integration of the child's play in the second year. *Child Development, 51,* 171–178.

Field, T. M., Woodson, R., Greenberg, R., & Cohen, D. (1982). Discrimination and imitation of facial expressions by neonates. *Science, 218,* 179–181.

Fogel, A., Diamond, G. R., Langhorst, B. H., & Demos, V. (1982). Affective and cognitive aspects of the 2-month-old's participation in the face-to-face interaction with the mother. In E. Z. Tronick (Ed.), *Social interchange in infancy: Affect, condition, and communication* (pp. 37–58). Baltimore: University Park Press.

Gelman, S. A., & Coley, J. D. (1991). Language and categorization: The acquisition of natural kinds of terms. In S. A. Gelman & J. P. Byrnes (Eds.), *Perspectives on language and thought: interreations in development* (pp. 146–196). Cambridge, MA: Cambridge University Press.

Gelman, S. A., & Markman, E. M. (1986). Categories and indiction in young children. *Cognition, 23,* 183–209).

Gibbs, D., & Cooper, E. (1989). Prevalence of communication disorders in students with learning disabilities. *Journal of Learning Disabilities, 22,* 60–63.

Gibson, E. J. (1969). *Principles of perceptual learning and development.* New York: Appleton-Century Crofts.

Goscheke, T., & Koppelberg, D. (1991). The concept of representation and the representation of concepts in connectionist models. In W. Ramsey, S. P. Stich, & D. E. Rumelhart (Eds.), *Philosophy and connectionist theory* (pp. 129–162). Hillsdale, NJ: Lawrence Erlbaum Associates.

Grieve, R., & Hoogenraad, R. (1979). First words. In P. Fletcher & M. Garman (Eds.), *Language acquisition: Studies in first language development* (pp. 93–104). New York: Cambridge University Press.

Halliday, M. A. K. (1975). *Learning how to mean: Explorations in the development of language.* New York: Elsevier-North Holland.

Harding, C. G. (1983). Setting the stage for language acquisition: Communication development in the first year. In R. Golinkoff (Ed.), *The transition from prelinguistic to linguistic communication* (pp. 93–104). Hillsdalle, NJ: Erlbaum.

Holdgrafer, G., & Dunst, C. J. (1986). Communicative competence: From research to practice. *Topics in Early Childhood Special Education, 6,* 1–22.

Jens, K., & Johnson, N. (1982). Affective development: A window to cognition in young handicapped children. *Topics in Early Childhood Special Education, 2,* 17–24.

Kamhi, A., Catts, H., Mauer, D., Apel, K., & Gentry, B. (1988). Phonological and spatial processing abilities in language and reading-impaired children. *Journal of Learning Disabilities, 53,* 316–327.

Kaye, K., & Marcus, J. (1981). Infant imitation: The sensory-motor agenda. *Developmental Psychology, 17,* 258–265.

Lamb, M. (1981). The development of the expectancies in the first year of life. In M. Lamb & L. Sherrod (Eds.), *Infant social cognition* (pp. 155–175). Hillsdale, NJ: Erlbaum.

Lewis, M. (1987). Social developpment in infancy and early childhood. In J. D. Osofsky (Ed.), *Handbook of infant development* (pp. 419–493). New York: John Wiley & Sons.

Lewkowicz, D. J. (1994). Development of intersensory perception in human infants. In D. J. Lewkowicz & R. Lickliter (Eds.), *The development of intersensory perception* (pp. 165–204). Hillsdale, NJ: Lawrence Erlbaum Associates.

Liles, B. (1985). Cohesion in the narrative of normal and language-disordered children. *Journal of Speech and Hearing Research, 28,* 123–133.

Locke, J. L. (1993). *The child's path to spoken language.* Cambridge, MA: Harvard University Press.

Lockman, J. J. (1986). Perceptuomotor coordination in sighted infants: Implications for visually impaired children. *Topics in Early Childhood Special Education, 6,* 23–36.

Lojkasek, M., Goldberg, S., Marcovitch, S., & MacGregor, D. (1990). Influences on maternal responsiveness to developmentally delayed preschoolers. *Journal of Early Intervention, 14,* 260–273.

Lucariello, J., & Rifkin, A. (1986). Event representations as the basis for categorical knowledge. In K. Nelson (Ed.), *Event knowledge: Structure and function of development* (pp. 189–204). Hillsdale, NJ: Erlbaum.

MacKain, K., Studdert-Kennedy, M., Spieker, S., & Stern, D. (1983). Infant inter modal speech perception is a left-hemisphere function. *Science, 219,* 1347–1349.

MacNamara, J. (1982). *Names for things.* Cambridge, MA: MIT Press.

Mahler, M. S., Pine, F., & Bergman, A. (1975). *The psychological birth of the human infant.* New York: Basic Books.

Mahoney, G., & Powell, A. (1988). Modifying parent-child interaction: Enhancing the development of handicapped children. *Journal of Special Education, 22*(1), 82–96.

Massaro, D. W. (1987). *Speech perception by ear and eye: A paradigm for psychological inquiry.* Hillsdale, NJ: Lawrence Erlbaum Associates.

Masur, E. (1983). Gestural development, dual-directional signaling, and the transition to words. *Journal of Psycholinguistic Research, 12,* 93–110.

McClelland, J. L., & Rumelhart, D. E. (1986). *Parallel distributed processing: Explorations in the microstructure of cognition: Volume 2: Psycholinguistic and biologic models.* Cambridge, Mass: MIT Press.

Mehrabian, A. (1970). Measures of vocabulary and grammatical skills for children up to age six. *Developmental Psychology, 2,* 439–446.

Meltzoff, A. N., & Kuhl, P. K. (1989). Infants, perception of faces and speech sounds; Challenges to developmental theory. In P. R. Zelazo & R. G. Barr (Eds.), *Challenges to developmental paradigms* (pp. 67–91), Hillsdale, NJ: Erlbaum.

Meltzoff, A. N., & Moore, M. K. (1983). Newborn infants imitate adult facial gestures. *Child Development, 54,* 702–709.

Mervis, C. B. (1987). Child-basic object categories and early lexical development. In U. Neisser (Ed.), *Concepts and conceptual development: Ecological and intellectual factors in categorization* (pp. 201–233). New York: Cambridge University Press.

Miller, J. F. (1981). *Assessing language production in children.* Baltimore: University Park Press.

Miller, J. F., & Chapman, R. S. (1981). The relation between age and mean length of utterance in morphemes. *Journal of Speech and Hearing Research, 24,* 154–161.

Moore, C., & Dunham, P. J. (1995). *Joint attention: Its origins and role in development.* Hillsdale, NJ: Lawrence Erlbaum Associates.

Morehead, D. M., & Morehead, A. E. (1974). From Signal to Sign: A Piagetian view of thought and language during the first two years. In R. Schiefelbusch & L. Lloyd (Eds.), *Language perspectives: Acquisition, retardation, and intervention* (pp. 153–191). Baltimore: University Park Press.

Muma, J. (1978). *Language handbook.* Englewood Cliffs, NJ: Prentice Hall.

Murray, L., & Trevarthen, C. (1986). The infant's role in mother-infant communication. *Journal of Child Language, 13,* 15–31.

Nelson, K. (1985). *Making sense: The acquisition of shared meaning.* New York: Academic Press.

Nelson, K. (1986). *Event knowledge: Structure and function in development.* Hillsdale, NJ: Lawrence Erlbaum.

Nelson, K. (1989). *Narratives from the crib.* Cambridge, MA: Harvard University Press.

Nelson, K. (1996). *Language in cognitive development: Emergence of the mediated mind.* New York: Cambridge University Press.

Nelson, K., & Nelson, A. J. (1990). Category production in response to script and category cues by kindergarten and second grade children. *Journal of Applied Developmental Psychology, 11,* 431–446.

Norris, J. A. (1991). Providing developmentally appropriate intervention to infants and young children with handicaps. *Topics in Early Childhood Special Education, 11*(1), 21–35.

Norris, J. A. (1992). Assessment of infants and toddlers in naturalistic contexts. In W. A. Secord & J. S. Damico (Eds.), *Best practices in school speech-language patholog: Descriptive/nonstandardized language assessment* (pp. 21–32). San Antonio, TX: The Psychological Corporation.

Norris, J. A. (1995). Extending language norms for school-age children: Is it pragmatic? *Language, Speech & Hearing Services in Schools, 26,* 342–352.

Norris, J. A., & Damico, J. S. (1990). Whole language in theory and practice: Implications for language intervention. *Language, Speech & Hearing Services in Schools, 21,* 201–210.

Norris, J. A., & Hoffman, P. R. (1993). *Whole language intervention for school-age children.* San Diego, CA: Singular Publishing Group.

Norris, J. A., & Hoffman, P. R. (1994). Whole Language and representational theories: Helping children to build a network of associations. *Journal of Childhood Communication Disorders, 16,* 5–12.

Norris, J. A., & Hoffman, P. (1996). Attaining, sustaining, and focusing attention: Intervention for children with ADHD. *Seminars in Speech and Language, 17,* 59–71.

Norris, J. A., & Hoffman, P. R. (1997). The SDS:Development Model of integrated functioning. (Unpublished assessment scale) by J. A. Norris & P. R. Hoffman Baton Rouge, Louisiana.

Oller, D. K., and Eilers, R. E. (1988). The role of audition in infant babbling. *Child Development, 59,* 441–449.

Osofsky, J. D. (1987). *Handbook of infant development.* New York: John Wiley & Sons.

Paul, R. (1993). Patterns of development in late talkers: Preschool years. *Journal of Childhood Communication Disorders, 15,* 7–14.

Paul, R., Spangle-Looney, S., & Dahm, P. S. (1991). Communication and socialization skills at ages 2 and 3 in "late talking" young children. *Journal of Speech and Hearing Research, 34,* 858–865.

Piaget, J. (1952). *The origins of intelligence.* New York: International Universities Press.

Piaget , J. (1954). *The construction of reality in the child.* New York: Basic Books.

Piaget, J. (1960). *The child's conception of physical causality.* Paterson, NJ: Littlefield, Adams.

Piaget, J., & Garcia, R. (1974). *Understanding causality.* New York: Norton.

Ramey, C. T., Beckman-Bell, P., & Gowen, J. W. (1980). Infant characteristics and infant-caregiver interactions. In J. J. Gallagher (Ed.), *New directions for exceptional children: Parents and families of handicapped children* (pp. 59–84). San Francisco: Jossey-Bass.

Rescorla, L., Roberts, J., & Dahlsgaard, K. (1997). Late-Talkers at 2: Outcome at 3. *Journal of Speech, Language, and Hearing Research, 40,* 556–566.

Rescorla, L., & Schwartz, E. (1990). Outcome of toddlers with expressive language delay. *Applied Psycholinguistics, 11,* 393–407.

Roberts, K., & Horowitz, F. (1986). Basic level categorization in seven- and nine-month-old infants. *Journal of Child Language, 13,* 191–208.

Rondal, J. (1980). Fathers' and mothers' speech in early language development. *Journal of Child Language, 7,* 353–369.

Ross, H. S., & Lollis, S. P. (1987). Communication within infant social games. *Developmental Psychology, 23,* 241–248.

Rosch, E. (1978). Principles of categorization. In E. Rosch & B. Lloyd (Eds.), *Cognition and categorization.* Hillsdale, NJ: Erlbaum.

Rose, S. A., Gottfried, A. W., & Bridger, W. H. (1983). Infants' cross-modal transfer from solid objects to their graphic representations. *Child Development, 54,* 686–694.

Rose, S. A., & Ruff, H. A. (1987). Cross-modal abilities in human infants. In J. D. Osofsky (Ed.), *Handbook of infant development* (2nd ed., pp. 318–362). New York: Wiley.

Roth, F., & Clark, D. (1987). Symbolic play and social participation abilities of language-impaired and normally developing children. *Journal of Speech and Hearing Disorders, 52,* 17–29.

Roth, F., & Spekman, N. (1986). Narrative discourse: Spontaneously generated stories of learning-disabled and normally achieving students. *Journal of Speech and Hearing Disorders, 51,* 8–23.

Rumelhart, D. E. (1980). Schemata: The building blocks of cognition. In R. J. Spiro, B. C. Bruce, & W. F. Brewer (Eds.), *Theoretical issues in reading comprehension: Perspectives from cognitive psychology, linguistics, artificial intelligence, and education.* Hillsdale, NJ: Lawrence Erlbaum.

Rumelhart, D. E., & McClelland, J. L. (1986). *Parallel distributed processing: Explorations in the microstructure of cognition: Volume 1: Foundations.* Cambridge, MA: MIT Press.

Sachs, J. (1984). Children's play and communicative development. In R. L. Schiefelbusch & J. Pickar (Eds.), *The acquisition of communicative competence* (pp. 109–140). Baltimore: University Park Press.

Sachs, J. (1993). The emergence of intentional communication. In J. Berko Gleason (Ed.), *The development of language.* New York: Macmillan.

Sander, L. W. (1969). The longitudinal course of early mother–child interaction: Cross case comparison in a sample of mother-child pairs. In B. M. Foss (Ed.), *Determinants of infant behavior.* London: Methuen.

Sander, L. W. (1977). The regulation of exchange in the infant–caregiver system and some aspects of the context-content relationship. In M. Lewis & L. Rosenblum (Eds.), *Interaction, conversation and the development of language* (pp. 133–156). New York: Academic Press.

Saussure, F. D. (1959/1915). *Course in genreal linguistics.* New York: The Philosophical Library, Inc.

Schaffer, H. R. (1977). *Studies in mother-infant interaction.* New York: Academic Press.

Schaffer, H. R. (1984). *The child's entry into a social world.* London: Academic Press.

Scoville, R. (1984). Development of the intention to communicate: The eye of the beholder. In L. Feagans, C. Garvey, & R. Golnkoff (Eds.), *The origins and growth of communication* (pp. 109–122). Norwood, NJ: Ablex.

Seibert, J. M., Hogan, A. E., & Mundy, P. C. (1982). Assessing interactional competencies: The early social-communication scales. *Infant Mental Health Journal, 3,* 244–258.

Seidenberg, M. S., & McClelland, J. L. (1989). A distributed, developmental model of word recognition and naming. *Psychological Review, 96*(4), 523–568.

Small, S. L. (1994). Connectionist networks and language disorders. *Journal of Communication Disorders, 27,* 305–323.

Snow, C. E. (1983). Literacy and language: Relationships during the preschool years. *Harvard Educational Review, 53,* 165–189.

Snow, C. E. (1984). Parent-child interaction and the development of communicative ability. In R. L. Schiefelbusch & J. Pickar (Eds.), *The acquisition of communicative competence* (pp. 69–108). Baltimore: University Park Press.

Snow, C. (1987). Relevance of the notion of a critical period to language acquisition. In M. H. Bornstein (Ed.), *Sensitive periods in development: Inter disciplinary perspectives.* Hillsdale, NJ: Erlbaum.

Snow, C. E. (1989). Imitativeness: A trait or a skill? In G. E. Speidel & K. E. Nelson (Eds.), *The many faces of imitation in language learning.* New York: Springer-Verlag.

Snow, C. E., Perlmann, R., & Nathan, D. (1987). Why routines are different; Toward a multiple-factors model of the relation between input and language acquisition. In L. Galda (Ed.), *Children's language* (pp. 65–97). Hillsdale, NJ: Erlbaum.

Stambak, M., & Sinclair, H. (1993). *Pretend play among 3-year-olds.* Hillsdale, NJ: Lawrence Erlbaum Associates.

Stark, R. (1979). Prespeech segmental feature development. In P. Fletcher & M. Garman (Eds.), *Language acquisition* (pp. 15–32). New York: Cambridge University Press.

Stern, D. N. (1985). *The interpersonal world of the infant: A view from psychoanalysis and developmental psychology.* New York: Basic Books.

Stine, E. L., & Bohannon, J. N. (1983). Imitation, interactions and acquisition. *Journal of Child Language, 10*, 589–604.

Stoel-Gammon, C., & Cooper, J. (1984). Patterns of early lexical and phonological development. *Journal of Child Language, 11*, 247–271.

Strombinger, A. Z., & Bashir, A. S. (1977). *A nine-year follow-up of language-delayed children.* Paper presented at the annual convention of the American Speech-Language-Hearing Association, Chicago.

Tallal, P., Miller, S. L., Bedi, G., Byma, G., Wang, X., Nagarajan, S. S., Schreiner, C., Jenkins, W. M., & Merzenich, M. M. (1996). Language comprehension in language-learning impaired children improved with acoustically modified speech. *Science, 271*, 81–84.

Tessler, M., & Nelson, K. (1994). Making memories: The influence of joint encoding on later recall. *Consciousness and Cognition, 3*, 307–326.

Tomasello, M., & Farrar, M. (1984). Cognitive bases of lexical development: Object permanence and relational words. *Journal of Child Language, 11*, 477–493.

Tronick, E. Z. (1982). *Social interchange in infancy: Affect, cognition, and communication.* Baltimore: University Park Press.

Uzgiris, I. C. (1983). Organization of sensorimotor intelligence. In M. Lewis (Ed.), *Origins of intelligence* (2nd ed.) (pp. 135–189). New York: Plenum.

Uzgiris, I. C., & Hunt, J. (1975). *Assessment in infancy: Ordinal scale of psychological development.* Urbana: University of Illinois Press.

van Gelder, T. (1991). What is the "D" in "PDP"? A survey of the concept of distribution. In W. Ramsey, S. P. Stich, & D. E. Rumelhart (Eds.), *Philosophy and connectionist theory* (pp. 33–60). Hillsdale, NJ: Lawrence Erlbaum Associates.

Van Kleeck, A. (1994). Metalinguistic development. In G. Wallach & K. Butler (Eds.), *Language learning disabilities in school-age children and adolescents* (pp. 53–98). New York: Merrill.

Vedeler, D. (1987). Infant intentionality and the attribution of intentions to infants. *Human Development, 30*, 1–17.

Vihman, M. M. (1999). Phonological development: *The origins of language in the child.* Cambridge, MA: Basel Blackwell.

Vygotsky, L. S. (1962). *Thought and language.* Cambridge, MA: MIT Press.

Vygotsky, L. S. (1967). Play and its role in the mental development of the child. *Soviet Psychology, 5*, 6–18.

Vygotsky, L. S. (1978). *Mind in society.* Cambridge, MA: MIT Press.

Westby, C. E. (1985). Learning to talk—talking to learn: Oral-literate language differences. In C. Simon (Ed.), *Communication skills for classroom success: Therapy methodologies* (pp. 181–218). San Diego, CA: College Hill Press.

Wiig, E., & Semel, E. (1980). *Language assessment and intervention for the learning disabled*. Columbus, OH: Charles E. Merrill.

Wilkinson, L., & Rembold, K. (1982). Parents, and peers' communication to toddlers. *Journal of Speech and Hearing Research, 24*, 383–388.

Wolf, D., & Gardner, H. (1979). Style and sequence in symbolic play. In M. Franklin & N. Smith (Eds.), *Early symbolization* (pp. 117–138). Hillsdale, NJ: Erlbaum.

Wolff, P. (1969). The natural history of crying and other vocalizations in early infancy. In B. Foss (Ed.), *Determinants of infant behavior*. London: Methuen.

Wolff, P. H. (1987). *The development of behavioral states and the expression of emotions in early infancy*. Chicago: University of Chicago Press.

2

Dynamic Systems Theory: Application to Language Development and Acquired Aphasia

Sarah S. Christman
The University of Oklahoma Health Sciences Center

Modern connectionism has had such an impact on cognitive psychology and the behavioral neurosciences that it is difficult to consider certain aspects of human behavior without invoking connectionistic principles or adopting its phraseology. Although levels of behavioral description may vary from the neuroanatomical to the metaphorical, it is not uncommon to find disparate brain and language functions characterized by the same connectionistic terminology (e.g., both operating from "distributed networks" driven by simultaneously "activating" forces that, when lesioned, produce errors of "excessive excitation" or "inadequate inhibition" [cf. Dell, 1988; Kertesz, 1991; Mesulam, 1990]). Part of the popularity of the interactive activation (IA) and parallel distributed processing (PDP) models that inform these characterizations (McClelland & Rumelhart, 1981, 1986; Rumelhart & McClelland, 1986) lies in the apparent surface validity of an inferred neurocognitive (brain-language) interface. Indeed, as Habib and Demonet (1996, p. 226) have noted, "no-one now would think of neural substrate (sic) of cognitive functions other than in terms of multiply interconnected, large-scale networks subserving distributed processing of function" (Mesulam, 1990)."

Converging evidence from many disciplines suggests that the fundamental structures of IA/PDP models may actually be neurologically realizable for complex cognitive functions such as attention, memory, and language (cf. Chase & Tallal, 1990; Cohen, Servan-Schreiber, & McClelland, 1992; Edelman, 1993; Friston, Tononi, Reeke, Sporns, & Edelman, 1994; Goldman-Rakic, 1988a, 1988b; Jacobs & Grainger, 1992; Kertesz, 1991;

Mesulam, 1990; Parks et al., 1991; Stemberger, Elman, & Haden, 1985; Sutherland, 1986), though see Siegel (1992) for a cautionary note. Isomorphism between the "lower-level" physiological and the "higher-level" conceptual aspects of information processing have been strongly supported for simple linear PDP models (Smolensky, 1986). In these systems, mathematical entities such as "units" or "connections" can be simultaneously mapped onto local biological (e.g., neurons, synaptic contacts) and psychological (e.g., concepts, conceptual interrelations) phenomena. Isomorphism is less directly established within complex non-linear PDP models, however, because mappings must be made from the collective output of single units to groups of neurons or to networks of concepts (Smolensky, 1986). There is an appealing symmetry to modeling interdependent systems as working in analogous ways and subject to comparable constraints. Perhaps because the connectionistic perspective lends itself so easily to biological description, it has become the dominant theoretical force in cognitive neuroscience (Small, 1994).

Of course, the popularity of a dominant theory often attenuates as new ideas evolve. The tenets of connectionism have quite usefully framed the search and shaped the interpretation of what might be the neurocognition of language and have informed our understanding of normal and disordered cognitive processing. "If it isn't broken, why fix it?" paraphrases a popular saying and asks a legitimate question about the subject of this chapter. Given connectionism's diverse utility and power, is dynamic systems (or "chaos") theory nevertheless emerging to supplant it as the new worldview in the study of brain and language?

There is a relatively small but rapidly growing body of literature characterizing various biological systems as dynamic and deterministically chaotic (i.e., self-organizing, locally unpredictable but globally stable) (cf. Babloyantz, Salazar, & Nicolis, 1985; Basar, 1990; Duke & Pritchard, 1991; Frank et al., 1990; Kelso, 1995; Mandell, 1985; Parks et al., 1991; Pritchard & Duke, 1995; Skarda & Freeman, 1987). While connectionistic and dynamic (chaotic) models are not incompatible, the latter subsumes many elements of the former and represents a significant paradigm shift in scientific thought. If connectionism is like watching a good movie in a theatre then chaos is like watching it while wearing 3-D glasses: Things may not be as they have previously seemed.

The conventional use of the word "chaotic" usually connotes negative events whose random and ungovernable characteristics are considered threatening unless and until they are brought under external control. As an example, if a physician pronounced his patient's heart, nervous, or intellectual functions to be in a chaotic state, there would surely follow an immediate call for a cure—unless chaos were understood to be the desirable index of health that some researchers have claimed it to be (Allman, 1993). Some sense of this persepective shift might be gained by considering the following fundamental and oxymoronic tenet of the theory: Normal biological, physical, and mental complex systems generate a beneficial and uniquely configured stable turbulence that continually self-organizes in response to changing environmental conditions. The emergent nature of chaos is not unlike that ascribed to connectionistic systems (or others capable of internal change), which are able to self-modulate (or "learn") simply by virtue of being active (Hebb, 1949; Mesulam, 1990).

Chaotic systems differ in that their constant random background activity keeps them continually ready to phase-shift into and out of new situationally adaptive patterns of activity to which they have been attracted (Pritchard & Duke, 1995). Because change is accomplished at local rather than global levels of processing, all functional creativity and flexibility generated through internal flux can exist without cost or compromise to overall system identity. It is an interesting paradox that in this context, chaos is a desirable condition essential for many normal human functions and, by extrapolation, abnormality can be understood as a loss of chaos with consequent reduction in the flexibility that this state provides.

While it is yet too early to evaluate the ultimate contributions of chaos theory to the communication sciences, it is not too soon to become acquainted with its relevant theoretical principles or informed about the ways in which these are being applied to the study of speech, language, and hearing. The first two sections of this chapter review the basic elements of connectionism and chaos theory, exploring their points of intersection and reviewing interwoven applications of both to the study of speech and language. The third section proposes the paradoxical construct that aphasia is a chaos-reduced condition and suggests a dynamic systems perspective from which the aphasias might be viewed. Finally, the last section considers the merits of chaos theory as a complement to connectionism, especially in view of common criticisms of the latter, and poses questions for future research. Discussion throughout highlights the neurobiological aspects of the chaos/connectionism interface.

I. ELEMENTS OF DYNAMIC SYSTEMS THEORY: CONNECTIONS AMIDST CHAOS

This section identifies the major attributes of normal connectionistic and chaotic systems, highlighting the architectural and functional elements of both that suggest their conceptual linkage to neural and mental levels of processing.

Architecture

Although some have flatly asserted that, "The properties of the units and connections in many PDP models correspond to the basic properties of neural circuitry" (Parks et al., 1991, p. 209), the homologous mappings among (PDP/neural) nodes/neurons, connectionistic pathways/neural circuits, and activation/action potentials are incomplete for many cognitive functions. Nevertheless, Mesulam (1990) asserts that multifocal neural networks possess internal architectures remarkably like those that characterize PDP models: They are comprised of cytoarchitectonically local circuits or nodes (analogous to PDP "units") that are linked together into functionally overlapping and widely distributed large-scale networks (just as PDP units are linked by activation pathways into distributed networks). Mesulam identifies Wernicke's area in the temporoparietal junction and Broca's area in the frontal operculum, together with their connections, as the localizable neurology important for purposeful speech repetition and essential for coordination of the wider language network.

Several important structural elements of biological chaotic systems will be immediately familiar to students of connectionism: Both are configured with layers of nodes having branching pathways linked to larger/smaller layers of more grossly/finely organized nodes and branchings, which in turn are linked—ad infinitum. Functionally, pathways in both kinds of systems are traversed flexibly and often bidirectionally and operations are crucially dependent on both internal feed-forward and feedback mechanisms (Hao, Vandewalle, & Tan, 1994). Branching pathways in chaotic systems, however, are recursively reiterative so that each progressively smaller substrate preserves the often complex configuration of the whole (Allman, 1993).

In very complex systems (neurological or cardiovascular, for example) internal pattern may be difficult to discern and an observer's gestalt impression (of structure and/or function) may appear to be one of great irregularity and unpredictability. Nevertheless, there exists, in chaotic systems, an orderly organizational framework, often described as fractal, that possesses a self-similar structural regularity at all levels of scale, which serves as the scaffolding on which flexible behavioral determinism is built. It is important to understand that the regularity within chaotic systems is not found in specific instances (i.e., "tokens") of structure or function but rather in the constraints that determine the internally repeating (fractal) nature of the system (though the nature of those constraints is an underexplored area of study) (McClelland & Rumelhart, 1986). The presence of fractal chaos at every level of function undoubtedly helps such systems to balance exquisitely between total entropy (disorder) and rigid periodicity: Such systems can shift states freely at local levels of processing but do so within the context of coherent overall structure and function. Fractal systems are stable enough to process and store information efficiently and yet flexible enough to transmit it easily (Waldrop, 1992).

Scale invariance is found across diverse biological domains. It is, for example, a quality of the structure of neural pathways, blood vessels, and bronchial tubes (Gleick, 1987) and is characteristic of the behavior of noncoding DNA and heartbeat sequences (Peng et al., 1994). Structural or behavioral scale invariance in fractal-like entities is essentially the product of internal computational algorithms that are "smart" enough to define the constraints on internally repeating processes without having to specify the parameters for creation of each instance of a behavior or shape. Thus, fractal biological systems can direct, by structural constraint (perhaps coded in DNA), the progressive arborization of neurons, blood vessels, and bronchial tubes without needing to store the discrete instructions for the formation of each and every branching structure. Likewise, they can specify, by constraint, repeating behavioral patterns (whether firings of action potentials, contractions of muscles, or perhaps the construction of syllables) at progressively more global levels of activity without having to repeat anew the instructions for the performance of each and every instance of behavior.

Fractal structure enables tremendous amounts of surface area to be enclosed in incredibly small spaces, as with the cerebral cortex in the skull, the lungs in the thorax, or even DNA in cells (Allman, 1993). As a point of interest, fractal DNA seems to be a phenomenon that appears with increasing frequency as species complexity increases along an evolutionary hierarchy (as in from "bacteria to fruit flies to mammals," Allman, 1993, p. 85). It may represent an evolutionary adaptation that serves flexible complex organisms by permitting the encoding of maximal genetic information while also providing for resistance to damage through scalar redundancy (Allman, 1993). Although Gould (1996) argues against evolution with intent, he and others have suggested that it is a process that seems to favor variety and the survival of complex structured systems rather than the converse.

Although it remains unclear just why a trend toward complexity prevails, perhaps hierarchical fractal "building block" designs facilitate system learning (see the Nonlinearity section following) and economize the effort of adaptive change. As Waldrop (1992) suggests, once the genetic codes for useful structural shapes or behavioral constraints have become biologically instantiated, they can be reshuffled to yield innumerable organismic permutations. In this way, small changes in code organization, which will be reflected across all levels of system operation, can create immediate quantal alterations in organism structure and function. This postulated mechanism for adaptation in complex systems echoes Lieberman's (1984) functional branch point theory of evolution: small spontaneous reactions to environmental conditions may trigger "avalanches of novelty" wherein some variations are extinguished but others are amplifed and stabilized until the next evolutionary leap occurs. Stabilization has been conceptualized as instantiation of fractal feedback loops not present in previously extant structures (Waldrop, 1992). It is interesting that evolution might provide a macroscopic perspective from which to view the establishment and behavior of chaotic dynamic systems.

To summarize, chaotic systems possess an outwardly irregular, seemingly disorganized appearance that is actually constrained internally with a regular self-similar architecture (Gleick, 1987). Local flexibility within the context of redundant, overarching functional constraints is a key behavioral characteristic of these systems that is explored in more detail in the sections following. Having noted the importance of fractal structure to chaotic systems, Calvin's (1996, p. 35) disclaimer on this subject should be noted: "That the same principle is seen at several levels does not . . . mean that it constitutes a level-spanning *mechanism*; an analogy does not a mechanism make." He suggests that the search for neuro-behavioral mechanisms is best conducted within the firing patterns of cerebral cortex circuitry, at a level of neural organization well above that of cellular chemistry, but below that of perception and planning, and certainly well below that of species evolution. Calvin rightly asks us to look beyond fractal structure for the answers to why and how chaotic systems change, and at least for the "how" aspects of these issues, we will need to address additional concepts related to deterministic self-organization (such as sensitivity to initial conditions and phase shift attractors) before a clear picture will emerge. Further, questions about the nature of fractal scale-insensitive system constraints are especially intriguing and are somewhat related to the concept of attractor states. In that context, they will be revisited in subsequent sections of this chapter.

Nonlinearity

The most intriguing characteristic of connectionistic and chaotic systems is the emergent quality of their behavior, as if the act of processing in and of itself contributes to the outcome of system computations. This is the essence of *nonlinearity*: The nature of a system's behavior in a given instance depends precisely on those internal and/or external environmental conditions facing it at the moment processing is initiated. As processing progresses, inherent feedback mechanisms naturally alter a system's internal states, so that at any point in time a dynamic system will be somewhat different than it was just moments ago and will therefore face temporally evolving sets of initial conditions (Hao et al., 1994). Through feedback devices, a system has some control over its immediate internal configuration even if it cannot always influence the outside forces that impinge upon it. Critically dependent on feedback, initial conditions, and internal constraints (fractal structure), nonlinear dynamic systems have the capacity to "learn," "self-organize," and "morph" at high speed (Gleick, 1987; Kelso, 1995).

As mentioned above, within the fractal architecture of chaotic dynamic systems, there is a certain degree of order masquerading as randomness (Gleick, 1987). Systems that combine fractal structure and function can handle cascades of (neural/activation) activity across self-similar levels of structure in a manner that might appear in particular instances to be irregular and unpredictable, but that actually, upon examination, turn out to be extremely ordered as a whole. Arising from structure, this cascading function is what, in part, permits the speed and flexibility of computation seen in all manner of parallel and distributed dynamic systems. According to Mesulam (1990), the operational adaptability of neurocognitive systems arises from inherent architectural and functional redundancies: Individual local neural circuits, each participating in several functionally related larger networks, provide multiple routes for cognitive processing. Overlapping neural networks can

> sustain parallel distributed processing in the sense that... major cortical components can communicate not only directly but also through the mediation of several other parallel pathways, allowing for a rapid and multidimensional sampling of a very extensive informational landscape. The network can thus solve a computational problem (such as expressing a thought) by simultaneously (and iteratively) considering many permutations, boundary conditions, and goals. (Mesulam, 1990, p. 605)

It is this ability to simultaneously manipulate various types of information that permits the kind of behavioral diversity found in parallel, distributed, dynamic information processors. Furthermore, it is a property of such systems that they become more efficient as the number of constraints (i.e., "boundary conditions") on processing are increased, unlike serial processors, which slow down as constraints and conditions are added (Mesulam, 1990).

In a paper describing the likely neurocognitive networks for attention, memory, and language (in human and rhesus monkey brains), Mesulam (1990) suggests that the parallel and distributed nature of cognitive processing can be understood within the context of a nervous system massively parallel and distributed in form and function. However, he issued the disclaimer that not all the elements of "parallel distributed processing" described by McClelland, Rumelhart, and Hinton (1986) can be found in biological "wetware." Mesulam emphasizes that local cortical circuits not only perform regional computations, but also, critically, serve as focal points for the convergence of information from more distant areas of distributed functional networks (see also Damasio, 1989). Recognizing the inadequacies of pinpoint cognition, he emphasizes that language is not found in these major cortical nodes per se (though they are essential for normal processing); rather, he suggests that language emerges as a quality of the operation of concatenated hierarchies of networks. This view is consistent with that of Small (1994) who suggests that, in a PDP system, the processing units, the patterns of activation weights among their connections, and the manner in which weights are computed, will collectively determine the behavior of the model as it might operate for language.

A characteristic shared by both neural and artificial PDP systems is the summative way in which neurons/units seem to acquire "strength." Although artificial and biological neural systems operate in a fundamentally parallel fashion, seriality can be found in the micromechanics of both unit activation and neural excitation. PDP unit connections acquire activation "weight" in an additive fashion (Small, 1994) just as postsynaptic neurons develop action potentials from the temporal and/or spatial summation of impinging presynaptic stimuli (Kandel, Schwartz, & Jessell, 1991). Although all behavior is time-dependent, necessarily unfolding in a sequence, Mesulam (1990) emphasizes that cognitive products are not achieved in a fundamentally additive way (e.g., by summing the outputs of serialized processing stages) but rather arise from the simultaneous activity of core network components engaging simultaneously and in concert to yield mentation. The brain, after all, is a massively parallel system at all levels of function, including the molecular (Rambidi, 1993). Even though some elements of its function may arise from serial processing at some level, this does not compromise the emergent, nonlinear nature of its processing.

McKenna, McMullen, and Shlesinger (1994, p. 587) have noted that the brain is "a dynamic system that is non-linear at multiple levels of analysis" (see also Calvin, 1996; Rossler & Rossler, 1994) and suggest that:

> the emerging capability to record the spatiotemporal dynamics of neural activity by voltage-sensitive dye and electrode arrays, provides opportunities for observing the population dynamics of neural ensembles within a dynamic systems context. New developments in the experimental physics of complex systems, such as the control of chaotic systems, selection of attractors, attractor swiching, and transient states, can be a source of powerful new tools and insights into the dynamics of neural systems. (p. 587)

It seems that chaos theory is motivating a new generation of neuroelectro-physiological research exploring the interface between changes in neural states and those of cognition. An example can be found in the work of Freeman (1994a) who suggests that specific state transitions (i.e., phase shifts) in oscillating neural circuits (detected by EEG) signal specific state transitions in cognition (as in a shift from the registration of a sensory impression to appreciation of its perceptual meaning, or as Allman, [1993] notes, as when brain wave patterns suddenly shift into a chaotic state during periods of intense concentration). The application of familiar and developing technologies and methodologies to new questions about the mind/brain interface is exciting but requires cautious interpretation of findings (see Rapp, 1994, for a caution in this regard).

The capacity of nonlinear dynamic systems to swiftly and creatively select multitask processing options creates the astonishing flexibility necessary to support a complex cognition. Whereas linear systems are periodic, predictable, and inflexible, nonlinear chaotic systems are the converse. If a system is required to produce a constant pure tone, for example, and cycle at only one frequency, then it will be rigidly linear in function. However, if a system is required to behave dynamically across time, then nonlinearity is desirable. Normally, a nonlinear system can produce near-identical repetitions of behavior (if desired) without becoming locked into a particular processing mode or "phase state." As it oscillates in a given mode, a normal dynamic system will often become attracted to another, though perhaps very similar, mode of operation and can then be observed to shift phase. Attendant changes in behavior usually accompany phase shifts in chaotic dynamic systems.

An example from communication neuroscience might help illustrate this concept. When ever-changing environmental conditions unpredictably necessitate activation of particular (local) neuronal pathways at specific moments in time, such as when auditory stimuli impinge on receptors, auditory pathways (versus others) can be flexibly and variably excited without the entire nervous system locking into perseverative behavior or losing its identity as a processor of electro-chemical information. If such a "listening" system should be drawn toward making an overt response, other neural pathways can be simultaneously activated to trigger behavioral states (speech or gesture, for example) that are very different from those of listening, but that are nevertheless globally consistent with the known capacities of the responding organism. If this is the way that chaotic systems work, then the possibilities for controlling them will lie in the determination of those factors that provoke system changes that elicit phase shifts and that result in transitions into new behavioral states. In the jargon of dynamic systems theory, those "factors" are known as strange attractors.

Strange Attractors

Logic dictates that nonlinearity would enrich a system's creative capacities at the cost of its behavioral predictability. Yet, this is not totally the case. Chaotic systems seek stability amidst constantly opposing forces of entropy but in fact undergo repeated state transitions (Freeman, 1994a). In the behavior of chaotic systems can be found essentially three degrees of freedom or three phase states of behavior: maintenence of an aperiodic but relative steady state (as opposed to a fixed point or periodic state), attraction toward a different steady state (creating a period of instability and turbulence), and assumption of new steady state (Gleick, 1987). Since this pattern of behavior will appear regular at a global level of observation, one can generally predict the fact of change in chaotic systems and the general conformation of change (i.e., those states to which a system tends to repeatedly return). This regularity provides, in addition to fractal architecture, for the essence of chaotic "order within disorder."

Although not a definition theoretical physicists would love, an attractor might be defined simply as a stable behavioral state (Gleick, 1987). In nature, preferred behavioral states change as organisms face problems of growth and interaction with the environment. Complex systems often face several attractor states (attractive behavioral solutions) during periods of instability and flexible, healthy organisms can move easily among choices. The environment presents targets achieved creatively by richly diverse behavioral trajectories through different fractal states. Equivalently, one could say that less adaptive systems may be also drawn toward several attractors during periods of instability, but be unable to recognize them as such, or fail to identify desirable alternatives. Occasionally, systems may become inert, locked in to a current behavioral pattern and unable to motivate movement in any direction at all. Neurologically damaged systems, for example, are often unable to make appropriate behavioral shifts in order to determine, initiate, or complete appropriate and/or simultaneous responses to stimuli.

The question of how nonlinear systems settle into one of the various possible steady states to which they are drawn during periods of turbulence is an interesting one. Herein lies the unpredictability of chaotic systems; it is found at local levels of observation, as individual system processing circuits transition unpredictably into one of several possible steady states. Herein also is found the echo to a question posed above in the discussion of fractals: Since transitioning systems (in whole, or part) are not drawn ultimately to all possible steady states but rather to some and then one, what determines the subset of possible states from which new stability is drawn and what is the mechanism that underlies that capacity for "choice"?

According to Pritchard and Duke (1995), the behavioral states that emerge from a system's normal activities are themselves attractors—and thus are self-reinforcing. The self-construction of those attractor states represents learning and problem solving, ideally conducted in such a way as to facilitate survival of the organism; environmental "affordances" drive opportunistic goal-directed behavior. Since many problems have multiple possible solutions, what is it that systems tend to want to learn? If we think of a child's developing neurolinguistic system, for example, as chaotic, we might rephrase this question as, What is it that children are drawn to learn about language and when are they drawn to learn it during development? If thinking instead about an adult whose previously normal language processing capacities have become reduced through focal stroke and aphasia, we might ask, What are the consequences of a loss of chaotic function and to what states are aphasic systems drawn during recovery? A key issue in answering these questions is identification of the natural constraints on language processing systems, for these determine in large part how a system will respond to stimuli as well as to which stimuli it will be attracted in both development and recovery.

II. CHAOS THEORY IN THE COMMUNICATION SCIENCES

Originally a construct from theoretical mathematics and physics, dynamic systems theory has found application in such diverse biological domains as heart function (Janse, 1995; Peng, Buldyrev, Hausdorff, Havlin, Mietus, Simons, Stanley, & Goldberger, 1994; Kanters, Holstein-Rathlou, & Agner, 1994) and evolution of the species (Fogel & Stayton, 1994; Viret, 1994; Woo, 1994). In fact, many human functions have been described as dynamic and nonlinear, including neurological (Duke & Pritchard, 1991; also Babloyantz & Lourenco, 1994 on the topic of attention), psychological (Barton, 1994; Butz, 1993; Langs & Badalmenti, 1994; Nandrino et al., 1994; Priel & Schreiber, 1994), perceptual (Richards, Wilson, & Sommer, 1994), vocal (Herzel, Berry, Titze, & Saleh, 1994; Nwokah, Hsu, Davies, & Fogel, 1999), and motoric (Thelen & Smith, 1996), among others.

Of particular interest to the present discussion is the rise of applications to the domains of normal cognition (Freeman, 1994b; Howe & Rabinowitz, 1994; van Gelder, 1998), normal speech development (Thelen, 1991), speech fluency (Smith, 1997), voice (Herzel et al., 1994), normal language development (Kent, 1981, 1984, 1992; Schwartz, 1992; Seidenberg, 1994; Vihman, 1993), and disordered language development (Mitchell, 1995). Although there is little research addressing chaos theory and language dissolution, hopefully, this will change. One of the most challenging explorations of chaos in the communication sciences will be in the realm of language: whether addressing normal or disordered states, or whether discussing processes of development or dissolution, it is challenging to map constructs founded in the hard sciences onto behavior whose biological substrates are, at best, inferred. Issues of philosophy aside [e.g., (a) the mind arises from the brain (cf. Edelman, 1989; Searle, 1984, 1992), (b) the mind influences the brain (cf. Eccles, 1994), and (c) the mind and brain are parasitically interdependent (cf. Locke, 1994)], language appears to be an emergent property of neural function and, in consequence, may also be understood as chaotic.

Chaos in Normal Language Processing

If normal language is a dynamic system, then aspects of its structure and/or function should resemble other kinds of dynamic systems. Specifically, it should be almost infinitely flexible and creative, sensitive to context and thus unpredictably emergent in content, yet globally coherent and internally (structurally) consistent. It should arise from mechanisms that can simultaneously, quickly, and accurately process many kinds of information while exploiting bidirectional feedback across self-similar levels of structure to minimize error formation, filtering it from production. If language arises from a dynamic cognitive system, it should be sensitive to organizational constraints and should produce behavior that, when repeated, is never quite exactly the same in every respect. It might also appear appropriately oriented around some behavioral parameter (such as a topical attractor) for a time, shifting toward new parameters as "attention" changes.

It can be argued that human language meets these requirements. It is probably the most creative of all cognitive functions, structurally capable of infinite recursion, and not requiring recapitulation of precise previous experiences for its generation in the present (i.e., new words and sentences can be created though never before heard). Adherance to fundamental global constraints allows the system to quickly create and comprehend new instantiations of itself, which in turn become attractive self-reinforcers. The language system need not have represented every single possible semantic, syntactic, or phonological construction in order to generate and appreciate novel forms. The system is self-organizing and emergent in the sense that using certain aspects of itself (particular words, for example) strengthens the likelihood of their use in the future, as if the act of processing itself influences its own outcomes. As discussed above, the nervous system can be characterized in many of these same terms and, too, is understood to be a nonlinear, deterministic, dynamic system.

Chaos in Language Development

Although self-organizing theories of language development are not in themselves new (cf. Edelman, 1987; Kent, 1981, 1984; Lindblom, Mac-Neilage, & Studdert-Kennedy, 1984; Thelen, 1989), recent characterizations of language development and disorders in children are increasingly couched in the specialized terminology of chaos (Kent, 1992; Lindblom, 1992; Mitchell, 1995; Schwartz, 1992; Thelen, 1991; Vihman, 1993). Whereas earlier studies sought to establish the self-organizing model as a legitimate biological approach to development (separate from competing structuralist and cognitive approaches), current studies appear more directed toward investigation of the mechanisms that underlie the self-organizing process. Examples follow.

Language development in children has been described as a process of auto-organization (Kent, 1984) wherein numerous small physical and cognitive advances combine at critical points in time to generate performance leaps much greater than could have been engendered by the influence of any single factor alone. Thelen (1991) described prespeech development in this way, characterizing it also as "softly assembled" behavior that emerges through a series of transitions to different stable attractor states (more commonly known as developmental "stages"). Acknowledging the interplay between neurological and behavioral factors in development, Thelen (1991) describes the maturational process as one that is nevertheless independent of biological critical periods. Locke (1994, 1997) has suggested, however, that there are sensitive periods ("stages") within early development when brain maturation and language input are especially primed to collide: prenatally, at 5–7 months, at 18–24 months, at 30–37 months, and at 3+ years. Although Locke (1983) asserts that language development is an essentially continuous process, he also argues that periods of reorganization are essential for the acquisition of new skills. His contention is that the failure of brain and language to meet adequately during these species-specific maturational windows will lead to interdependent deficits: acquisition of a less than optimal language system and establishment of a less than optimal neural infrastructure for language.

An example of Locke's (1994, 1997) thesis is found in his emphasis on the importance of an early receptive vocabulary for stimulating language-specific brain mechanisms at around 24 months of age. It is as if this early knowledge base provides the developmental pressure that will suddenly trigger activity of analytical language mechanisms at the same time that it provides the database on which those mechanisms can practice. Many researchers have commented on the "naming explosion" that usually follows acquisition of an initial 50-word expressive vocabulary, a process completed on average at about 22 months of age (see Weismer, Murray-Branch,

& Miller, 1994 for discussion). One might propose that between 8 and 24 months children exhibit a general pattern of steady vocabulary growth that segues into a period of instability (as when frozen forms decompose) and then terminates in new behavior: adoption of an analytical approach to language, and the rapid acquisition of new words. Analagous developmental patterns can be found in the domains of phonology, syntax, and morphology, as well.

If the behavioral elements of this developmental snapshot were framed within the conventions of nonlinear dynamics, the overall picture could be described as follows. Prior to the second birthday, a child's developing neurolinguistic system is attracted to a state of word learning and he acquires a fast-mapped, underanalyzed early nominal vocabulary over a period of months (Weismer et al., 1994). Words are understood phonologically as gestalt sound patterns and semantically as elements of encapsulated experience. During this prelinguistic period, the learning system is oscillating aperiodically in anticipation of change but it is considered stable since its behavior and the scope of its capacities are fairly consistent across time. The language-learning system processes information quickly and easily, expending time and energy economically and making good use of input and feedback mechanisms to hypothesize and self-correct when errors are produced.

Throughout the course of learning, this system repeatedly reorganizes in response to internal and external environmental pressures. Overcoming constraints at local and global levels of processing, forces of entropic disorganization will ultimately create wobble in the enlarging system and it will begin to transition to another phase state: It will seek that set of all possible phase states known as a strange or chaotic attractor and from it gravitate toward one that will vault it into new behavior. Attainment of a 50-word vocabulary seems to push the language acquisition system to a point of crucial instability; energy is added to the learning process and a developmental threshold is crossed that will permit more adaptive functioning (analysis). This change primes the learning system for its major challenge in the second and third years of life: acquisition of the units comprising formal conventional language and the rule subsystems that constrain their use. The general principle at work here seems to be, "Grow, then divide," for, just as in the creation of fractals, it seems as if the process of self-segmentation is at work at this stage of the language-learning process (Lindblom, 1992).

Within any period of turbulent instability, such as the transition to language, there lies the mystery of biological creativity: To what next state will a changing system most likely be drawn? Development from a self-organization perspective is a bottom-up (or rather, "upward blooming") process that proceeds in a way like that described earlier for evolution. It is not driven by efforts to achieve specific (cognitive) goals but rather unfolds in a fashion entirely dependent on the elements of its composition (i.e., its constraints) and the opportunistic affordances of its environment. Within the context of the present example, it seems that the majority of developing children shift into a neurocognitive state that permits the apperception of pattern, the appreciation of rule, and the analysis of the language code into its component parts (cf. Pinker, 1999). Is this condition a natural attractor state for humans at approximately 2 years of age?

The selection of a particular state from among several rough equivalents might mean that several slightly different learning paths can lead a system to the same destination (cf. Bates & MacWhinney, 1987). Recent evidence from research on vocabulary acquisition in children who are late talkers is a case in point yet also highlights the exceptions to the rule. It seems that some late-talking children reach the 50-word threshold at a later chronological age than most of their normal peers and yet catch up on language performance measures toward the end of their preschool years (cf. Weismer et al., 1994). Other children do not make these equalizing gains (Rescorla, Roberts, & Dahlsgaard, 1997). Why aren't the language-learning systems of latter group as strongly attracted toward analysis as robustly as their peers? How might a transition to that state be made more attractive for these children earlier in development and what manipulations might facilitate this shift for better language learning?

Despite the influence of individual differences in development, there are some cross-linguistic commonalities that might well be considered either universal constraints (predisposing language-learning systems to behave in predictable ways) or universal attractors (states to which most language-learning systems are drawn). Mohanan (1993) has argued for universal sound distribution and alternation patterns (i.e., place and voice assimilations) as attractors and Goldsmith (1993) has given the nod to phonological representations themselves. To this list might be added the "strong syllable + (optional) weak syllable" trochaic template for word learning so favored in early stages of development (McGregor & Johnson, 1997), the prelinguistic accumulation of a first 50-word vocabulary, Locke's (1994, 1997) developmental sensitive periods, CV syllable structure (Fudge, 1987), the most underspecified English consonant and vowel (/t/ and schwa, respectively) (Bernhardt, 1992a), and the Sonority Sequencing Principle—especially the Obstruent-Vowel (OV) form (Buckingham, 1989, 1990b; Christman, 1992a, 1992b, 1994; Clements, 1990; Kent, 1993). These phenomena often constrain normal systems or represent states to which they are drawn. Some also happen to be those to which damaged systems revert in aphasia, as will be discussed section following. These predilection behaviors are but some that determine how a language-learning system will behave and the directions in which it will change.

As in phylogeny, ontogenetic development is attracted toward complexity. The process of motor speech learning, for example, has been described as a series of states beginning with uncoordinated and undifferentiated vocal tract action, transitioning through patterned rhythmic movement, and reorganizing into a more complex state of coordinated coarticulation of differentiated vocal gestures (Davis & MacNeilage, 1990; Thelen, 1981). Mitchell (1995) discusses the importance of optimal timing in this process of motor speech learning and emphasizes the importance of readiness when planning intervention with speech-delayed children. From a dynamic systems perspective, readiness might be understood as that condition of "beginning wobble," when a small amount of energy applied to a system in a stable state will cause it to transition to another more complex state with relative ease. With respect to the above-mentioned list of postulated universals, readiness for increased complexity is seen when more "marked" language behaviors Consonant-Vowel-Consonant [CVC], Obstruent-Nasal-Vowel [ONV], and iambic forms, for example) begin to appear. It sounds easy and it sounds typical. Is this kind of flexibility always available to chaotic systems?

Chaos-Reduction in Language Dissolution

Deterministic dynamic systems dedicated at a global level of function to processing a particular kind of information are not externally directed goal-driven executors of behavioral prescriptions but rather are spontaneous creators of their structural configurations and operational functions (Thelen, 1991). They are always somewhat "disorderly" (Gleick, 1987) since their behavior is never quite precisely repeated. In them is also found a certain degree of background "noise," the level of which may contribute to phase state shifts and/or the creation of errors (Gleick, 1987; see also Hernandez, Valdes, Biscay, Jimenez, and Valdes, 1995 for application to EEG forecasting). The nonperiodic (nonlinear) and apparently random behavior of nonrepetitious systems is not total, for a certain predictability in pattern and/or structure exists across scale, but the hallmark of impairment is slippage into either excessive functional regularity or excessive unpredictability. What is critical to normal function is the maintenance of what has been called, "the edge of chaos," a state of dynamism that balances the opposing forces of regularity and entropy so that a system remains ready to flexibly transition into different appropriate phase states as environmental conditions warrant (Waldrop, 1992). Whereas a certain amount of disorderly chaos in biological systems is healthy, within naturally dynamic systems the appearance of behavior that is overly periodic (controlled) or aperiodic (random) may signal pathology (Gleick, 1987).

Many neuropathies that indirectly impair language, including epilepsy and stroke, can be viewed as bringing a normally chaotic nervous system under excessive control (Glanz, 1994; Regalado, 1995; Schiff, Jerger, Duong, Chang, Spano, & Ditto, 1994). Whereas language processing is normally a speedy, appropriately self-organizing, and relatively error-free affair accomplished by a flexible and synchronized nervous system (Paulesu, Frith, Snowling, Gallagher, Morton, Frackowiak, R. S. J., & Frith, 1996), aphasic language processing is much more slow and error prone, characterized contradictorily by both excessive regularity and variability in performance, and is the consequence of an inflexible and asynchronous neurology (Brown, 1980; see also Paulesu et al., 1996 with respect to asynchrony in dyslexia). Paraphasic word blends (cf. Buckingham & Christman, 1996) and abstruse neologisms are two rather bizarre aphasic symptoms that would seem to arise naturally from an unruly (i.e., randomly behaving, classically "chaotic") system running amok. It may be the case, however, that the converse is also simultaneously true: What may contribute to the creation of nonsense words is processing that is chaos-reduced or overly chaos-controlled.

It could be argued that the essence of dynamism is appropriate flexibility and that it is precisely this quality that has been lost in aphasia. Focal acquired lesions to the language cortex typically yield unitary, multimodality language-processing syndromes known as the "aphasias" (Schuell, Jenkins, & Jimnez-Pabn, 1964). Aphasia is an impairment of the ability to process (comprehend, synthesize, and formulate) propositional language due to adventitious focal cortical or subcortical brain damage. It is characterized by deficits in the accuracy, responsiveness, completeness, promptness, and efficiency with which preserved language knowledge is manipulated by neurolinguistic computational mechanisms (Davis, 1993; Duffy, 1994; Porch, 1994; Rosenbek, LaPointe, & Wertz, 1989; Schuell et al., 1964).

Although typologies abound and individual patient profiles may differ within "types," at least two grossly discrete aphasic syndromes are generally recognized: one characterized by nonfluent, dysprosodic speech supporting agrammatic language, and the other characterized by fluent, prosodic speech supporting paragrammatic language (Benson & Ardila, 1996). Morpho-syntactic deficits are typically associated with agrammatism and lexical-semantic deficits with paragrammatism although most aphasic speakers will evidence impairments across linguistic domains (e.g., semantics, syntax, phonology, morphology, pragmatics) and across language tasks (confrontation naming, verbal repetition, auditory comprehension, reading, writing, gesture/pantomime, spontaneous speech).

It is generally held that language competence (stored knowledge) is substantially better preserved than is language performance (access and manipulation of stored information) in aphasia (Davis, 1993; Tseng, McNeil, & Milenkovic, 1993). This may arise in part because the functionally redundant organization of the nervous system ensures that, if circuitry is lost (as from stoke), sequelae will typically present as partial (rather than total) cognitive-behavioral deficits. Mesulam (1990) underscores the fact that even the core neural areas for language processing (i.e., Broca's and Wernicke's zones) are not completely dedicated to spoken language, "but also participate in intersecting networks that coordinate praxis, writing, reading, and verbal memory" (p. 604). In fact, Kertesz (1991), Mesulam (1990), Small (1994), and others (cf. Hebb, 1949) have suggested that mentation is too distributed to ever be fully localizable. For Small (1994), language is not contained in PDP processing units just as for Mesulam (1990) and Kertesz (1991) it is not contained in Wernicke's and Broca's areas. Thus in the event of focal stroke to a core area, it is unlikely that language will be eliminated but it is therefore also likely that multimodality language deficits will ensue (cf. Schuell et al., 1964).

Although aphasia may be exacerbated by the presence of associated neurogenic sensory, motor, or cognitive concommitants, these (visual field cuts, apraxias, neglect syndromes, and so on) are nevertheless recognized as nonaphasic disorders. More ambiguous are the contributions of subtle and pervasive neurological sequelae (highly variable performance, slow response time, insensitivity to response cues, inability to allocate and mobilize attention, and perseveration) to aphasic language reduction (cf. Tseng et al., 1993). These behaviors reflect performance factors that contribute to aphasic symptomatology and they can be handled by an IA/PDP model of language processing when they are interpreted in terms of slow activation and slow decay (Dell, 1988; Harrman & Kolk, 1991; Miller & Ellis, 1987; Stemberger, 1985; Tseng et al., 1993, p. 292). Chaos theory, however, can enrich our understanding of aphasic performance deficits by putting these derailed mechanisms within the larger context of unsteady oscillatory systems. Examples will follow for three significant performance deficits usually seen across aphasia types: (1) reduction in speed of processing (Martin, Roach, Brecher, & Lowery, 1998), (2) reduction in accuracy of lexical access (including phonological assembly) (cf. Buckingham, 1981), and (3) reduction in the ability to switch and/or maintain phase states (i.e., perseveration [Buckingham, Whitaker, & Whitaker, 1979]; attention allocation deficit [Tseng et al., 1993]).

Table 2.1 proposes contrasts in the performance of chaotic (normal) language-processing systems and those that have become chaos-reduced (aphasic). First, whereas normal language is speedily processed, Martin et al. (1998, p. 322) note that the slow or weak word activation typical of aphasia is likely to yield, "increased probabilities of semantic errors,

TABLE 2.1
Characteristics of Normal (Chaotic) and Aphasic (Chaos-Reduced)
Language-Processing Systems Interpreted within
a Dynamic Systems Framework

Chaotic System	Chaos-Reduced System
Appropriate unpredictability within a globally ordered system:	Excessive unpredictability within an overly constrained system:
Speedy processing	Slow processing
Easy and accurate access and manipulation of language units	Difficult and inaccurate access and manipulation of language units
Flexible phase shifting that maintains "edge of chaos" oscillatory state	Inflexible phase shifting (perseveration) and unstable phase state maintenance
Appropriate self-organization; apparent global coherence	Inappropriate self-organization; apparent global disintegration
Coordinated neural phase states	Uncoordinated neural phase states
Exquisite sensitivity to initial conditions and feedback	Reduced or excessive sensitivity to initial conditions and feedback
Constraints facilitate performance	Constraints impair performance
Error detection and prevention	Error production

omission errors, circumlocutions, target-related neologisms and perseverations." Chaotic systems that have lost their characteristic dynamism tend to process increasingly slowly as they approach a state of static balance, just as a swinging pendulum (the quintessential periodic oscillator) will have the least velocity at its cyclic extremes and at rest. In fact, it has been said that for biological systems, static equilibrium is death (the flip side of the novel "chaos as health" notion) (Gleick, 1987).

In the normal scheme of things, a chaotically dynamic system will seek a state of stable instability: It will be attracted to a behavioral trajectory that is never exactly repeated but that is nevertheless limited in the degree to which it may vary from itself. To all outward appearances, the behavior of such systems seems random until the zoom lens of science reveals its fundamental hidden pattern. Attractor states are steady but the transitions from one to another are turbulent. Healthy systems neither become locked in to specific attractor states nor become lost in turbulence; to do so will reduce their function to either unusual periodicity (perseverated behavior) or aperiodicity (bizarrely random behavior). Each of these conditions represents a kind of unfortunate equilibrium (static and dynamic, respectively) that can have catastrophic consequences for dynamism. It might be said that, in aphasia, the language-processing system has lost its chaotic edge and must operate all too frequently at either extreme of its dynamic continuum, unpredictably combining (and/or repeating) phonemes, morphemes, and so on from restricted linguistic stores.

A second contrast in chaotic versus chaos-reduced systems may be found in the realm of deterministic self-organization. According to Hagoort (1993), part of the reason that information can normally be so rapidly accessed in the lexicon is because of its extremely efficient organization. This has been conceptualized by Harley (1998, pp. 308–309) as follows:

> it is better to think of the meaning of a word as an attractor in a semantic space defined by the semantic microfeatures. . . . The attractor is the lowest point in a larger basin of attracton; if an input points to anywhere in the basin of attraction, then because in a connectionist network similar inputs cause similar outputs, normally the correct meaning will be associated with that input. (p. 308)
>
> It might be profitable to take this analogy further, and think of a semantic input or lemma projecting to a basin of attraction in phonological space in lexicalization. (p. 309)

Perhaps what children establish when fast-mapping (Kent, 1993) new words or concepts are associations of terms with appropriate basins of attraction, establishing the sense of words and leaving fully specified reference to be accomplished at a later date. Something obverse might be happening in aphasia when lexical-semantic disturbances manifest as deficits in accessing the meaning of specific words or in activating their associates (Hagoort, 1993).

In any case, inaccurate word choices can arise from a disturbance of lexical representation (competence deficit) or from an inability to access an intact representation (performance deficit). The frequent tendency of aphasic speakers to exhibit particular difficulty naming specific words during confrontation tasks (Davis, 1993) while producing them easily in less pressured circumstances lends credence to performance factors as contributors to anomia (inability to name). Word substitution errors may yield either related or unrelated semantic paraphasias, and anomia itself may be masked by circumlocution and/or the presence of neology (Buckingham, 1981). Unrelated semantic paraphasia (e.g., "doorknob" for the target word "cat") and neologism production ("bangahachapee" for "cat") naturally imply a greater degree of postlesion disorganization than does related semantic paraphasia (e.g., "dog" for "cat"). Together, these errors suggest that a system's capacity for appropriate lexical-semantic self-determinism can be compromised along a continuum of malfunction.

In the normal case, the language-processing system would normally orient toward an appropriate basin of semantic attraction during a naming task, correctly selecting from within it a specific lemma (word meaning with syntactic markers) and its associated morpho-phonological form (see Levelt, 1989 for discussion of lemmas and lexical entries). Schuell and Jenkins (1961), who examined vocabulary in aphasic speakers, found that their more severely aphasic subjects produced more omissions and irrelevant responses on naming tasks than their less severe subjects (who produce more semantic associates). From a dynamic systems perspective, it might be said that word-search mechanisms within severely chaos-reduced (aphasic) systems selected lemmas from inappropriate basins of attraction (causing unrelated semantic errors) and/or perhaps also became unable to fully access their associated phonological forms (causing either no response or randomly generated one- or two-stage neologisms) (Buckingham, 1981, 1990a). Less severely compromised mechanisms, on the other hand, might have been attracted to erroneous words within proper basins of attraction and produced related semantic errors instead of targets. In any event, an inability to correctly identify basins of semantic attraction, select specific attractors, and/or assemble their phonological forms suggests a disruption in self- organization at semantic and/or phonological levels of representation.

Two fascinating examples of phonological derailment in aphasia are phonemic paraphasia and neologistic jargon, phenomena that may (Brown, 1977; Ellis, 1985; Kertesz & Benson, 1970; Lecours, 1982; Luria, 1970) or may not (Buckingham, 1977, 1979, 1981, 1982; Buckingham & Kertesz, 1974; Butterworth, 1979; Lecours & Lhermitte, 1972; Pick, 1931) arise from a common underlying linguistic pathology (phonemic distortion of correctly accessed lexical forms). Argument on this topic has addressed the importance of language-specific word and segment frequencies, the significance of hesitation in abstruse (bizarre) neology, the explanatory power of underlying anomia for jargon versus simple paraphasia, and the extent to which variations in recovery patterns illuminate underlying dysfunctions (see Christman & Buckingham, 1989 for review). With respect to mechanisms of phonemic paraphasia in particular, it has been important to account for the direction and possible intrasyllabic locations of sound errors, the featural differences of errors versus targets, the sizes of the linguistic units over which errors can occur, and the constraints on possible phonemic error mechanisms (see Buckingham, 1989, 1990a, 1990b, 1991).

As fashions in phonological theory have changed, explanations for the aforementioned (and for corresponding problems in developmental research) have been most recently couched in terms of nonlinear (Bernhardt, 1992a, 1992b; Bernhardt & Gilbert, 1992) and underspecified (Beland, Caplan, & Nespoulous, 1990) phonology (with current investigation of licensure (Wheeler & Touretzky, 1997) and optimality constructs (Bernhardt & Stemberger, in press; Stemberger, 1995). While both serial and parallel models of language processing have anchored discussions of disordered phonology, the popularity of PDP has most recently been greater.

Perhaps that is because of its "life-like" feel, the intuitive sense that real biological systems could, and perhaps do, operate like the model. Interestingly enough, recent advances in medical research are revealing human biological systems to be chaotic as well (Allman, 1993; Regalado, 1995).

How can paraphasia and neology with all of their apparent irregularity represent the reduction of chaos in a normally dynamic system? After all, many conditions for the maintenance of chaos seem to be met in disordered phonology. Neologisms may appear outwardly strange and disorganized, but they are actually constrained in their formation to a considerable extent; there is preservation of fundamental order (phonotactic and sonority sequencing) even within apparent disorder (Christman, 1994). Impaired phonological processing still seems emergent and sensitive to present conditions in aphasia: the activation of given phonemes, rimes, and even syllables in neology not only increases their likelihood of future use but also delimits activation of subsequent segments in a series. Verbal processing in fluent, logorrheic patients seems fast (almost pathologically so) though inaccurate (accurate processing is painfully slow and may actually trigger logorrhea in compensation for delay). Because some fundamentally dynamic characteristics appear intact in paraphasia and neology, it might be hard to appreciate how they represent the reduction of dynamism in aphasia.

A reduction in dynamism yields language that is unpredictable from an utterance-specific perspective, but that is actually highly constrained at a broad structural level of analysis (i.e., revealing reduced access to the full complement of word forms, sentence types, phonemes, syllable structures, morphemes, and so forth).

Perhaps a look at the overly constrained—and remarkably similar— phonological error profiles of two radically different aphasic populations would be illustrative. In a study investigating neologistic jargonaphasia in three fluent subjects with left hemisphere posterior lesions, Christman (1992b) examined the degree to which the demisyllable structure of neologisms (versus legitimate English words) conformed to markedness predictions of sonority theory (Clements, 1990). Among these, initial demisyllables of CV shape and Obstruent-Vowel sequence would be the least marked, whereas Nasal-Vowel, Liquid-Vowel, Glide-Vowel, and Vowel-only sequences, respectively, would be increasingly marked. Demisyllables having cluster onsets (OLV, ONV, OGV, OOV) would be more marked than those with singleton onsets. English initial demisyllables are constrained by sonority yet come in a variety of these (more and less) marked configurations. It was unknown whether the bizarre nonwords produced by fluent aphasic speakers would respect similar constraints.

Christman's (1992b) findings revealed a tendency toward over-constraint in the formation of these unpredictable words: Abstruse neologisms were overwhelmingly composed of CV initial demisyllables (78% avg.)

with Obstruent-Vowel sonority sequences (69% avg.). Target-related neologisms (phonemic paraphasia) showed similar patterns wherein CV initial demisyllables (77.5% avg.) had predominantly OV sonority sequences (69% avg.). Code and Ball (1994) replicated Christman's (1992b) sonority analysis with nonlexical recurring utterances in English and German (non-fluent) aphasia databases and found strikingly similar results: English CV initial demisyllables (75.5% avg.) typically had Obstruent-Vowel sonority sequences (57% avg.) as did German CV initial demisyllables (84% avg.), which also tended toward Obstruent-Vowel sonority sequences (75.5% avg.). In both fluent and non-fluent English and German aphasic populations mentioned earlier, nonwords were a primary feature of disordered language and they were built from a restricted corpus of demisyllable frames. In contrast, the normal English words produced by Christman's (1992b) subjects were configured with a greater variety of initial demisyllable shapes and sonority profiles as reflected in the less frequently occurring CV initial demisyllables (63%) that had Obstruent-Vowel sonority sequences (32%).

In their conclusion, Code and Ball (1994) agreed with Christman (1992b) that sonority may be a well-distributed constraint on syllable construction, represented at all levels of phonological processing, including motoric. This idea suggests a fractal structure to phonology, in that sense of a self-similar constraint repeating across scale at all levels of function. Alternatively, the unmarked nature of CV syllable structure and Obstruent-Vowel sonority sequences might merit their consideration as strong attractors in deterministic phonological processing.

A third contrast in normal versus chaos-reduced systems is found in the domain of state-shifting. As mentioned earlier, dynamic systems are responsive to internal and external environmental conditions. Responsiveness means that a system will repeatedly transition to those attractor states that will allow it to meet the continually changing current demands of its environment. This constant readiness to shift from one deterministic mode to another is the antithesis of perseveration, the state of being "locked in" to a mode (or a restricted set of modes) of operation no longer adaptive for current conditions (cf. Buckingham et al., 1979; Sandson & Albert, 1984; 1987; Santo-Pietro & Rigrodsky, 1986). Perseveration arises when episodes of pathological periodicity create dynamic "loss regions" in a formerly flexible system, a situation not totally unlike that which has been described for seizure activity in epilepsy (Regalado, 1995).

Continuous perseveration (Sandson and Albert, 1987) provides the clearest example of locked-in behavior in aphasia because it is characterized by uninterrupted strings of precisely repeated (periodic) behavior. An aphasic patient who says, for example, "smoke, smoke, smoke, smoke" (see Table 2.2 discussed later) in response to a particular stimulus has

TABLE 2.2
Perseverate Streaks in Fluent Jargonaphasia

Tell me what you do with:

1. Soap.	corterd... spordits....... corterd...... .cornerd, corner....... .jack..... ..corner... corner.... pretty...crook...corpse...cortered.
2. Pencil.	porter...cord...cord...cord...ice...pretty ice... pretty, pretty...Jidduhl... griddle..chittuhld...Urkyoolerz....crook....crook....corter.... cribbel.....corn...
3. Money.	corter... creea... crausd... people.... pressed...pressure.
4. Key.	pressduhyuh...cows...depressed...pressure...cowna...sit...sibbel.
5. Book.	callerd...countered...corner...flesh the stay cob... commond...countered.
6. Shoe.	measure the calm...catterd...connection...towerdoe...suhmoehuh...smoke, smoke smoke, smoke...shuttered...smoke...shuttered...canned...cutter, cutter, can.
7. Towel.	Ess...the..the..the..the..settered..check...chetter...can...cuttered...can...
8. Chair.	word..p..plea..top..can..corner..can..can..tor..coven..woo..keven.. word...word...nose.. ordered..opened..sittuht can..tomorrow can..that word..the word..the word..
9. Razor.	tomorrow..do..do..droove..teach..telled..word..word..cannuhd...ka...can.. word...cornered..corned..menstand...started
10. Brush.	started...started...beginners...famous...remembers...
11. Clock.	ourselves we...keepen we..words..cannuhd..cannuhd...cabled..cord.. cord..cord..keepenedna..opened..corner..kookuhmuh..natural...cuban... mickeled..cornered....remembering...
12. Umbrella.	wrinkle...world..mobile..open..cormon..try..try..cabin..tried..closa.. close..trouble..
13. Knife.	word...remember...open..open..cord..cabin..tried..could..cabined.. could..kribben...cabin..could..craj..can..
14. Glasses.	settled..cabined..cant tell..cant tell..could..could..
15. Table.	could..open..open..could..beautuh..could..

Subject M.S. (Christman, 1992b).

become, at least for some period of time, completely unable to switch to another attractor state (a different lexical item, in this case). What triggers the abrupt onset and offset of continuous perseveration? As Gleick (1987) notes, such bifurcations (abrupt changes in behavior) are typical of the way nonlinear systems operate. Many times, however, perseveration is more subtle than this and the "locking-up" phenomenon more easily disguised.

In fluent aphasia, segmental and syllabic perseveration are "rarely disso-ciated" from neology (Buckingham, 1989, p. 91). Of course, it is impossible to know exactly what will become perseverated in a neologistic string; what seems at first glance to be a collection of wildly different words, composed with a little too much flexibility and creativity, can actually be understood as strings of reduced forms composed from a restricted set of phonemes, syllable types, and, sometimes, even syllable tokens (cf. Christman, 1992b, 1994). When words or neologisms (in whole or part)

are perseverated into runs of recombined forms (creating neologistic port-
manteaus or word blends), this too can be understood as a kind of locked-in
behavior even though the repetitious behaviors may be intermittent rather
than continuous.

Examples of perseverate streaks can be found in Table 2.2, a collection of utterances culled from a larger sample produced by jargon subject
M.S. (Christman, 1992b), who interwove "families" of neologistic word
blends into verbiage describing the functions of various common objects.
The apparent alternation among a restricted set of alliterative and asso-
nantial blends, with a return to a base error form across time, is striking.
Throughout the sample, M.S. returned to the syllable /k r/ as a kind of
default pattern; when combined with other perseverated units and with
minimal feature changes in typically trochaic utterances, a theme of un-
cannily related forms runs across responses to the entire set of stimuli:
For example, "corterd, cornered, corner, corpse, corterd, porter, cord, corn,
corter, callerd, word, coven, ordered, cannuhd, corned, cannuhd, cabled,
cord, opened, corner, cuban, mickled, corner, corman, cabin, kribbened,
cabined," and so on. This kind of perseveration is described by Helm-
Estabrooks and Albert (1991) as partially recurrent and is identified by the
persistent (inappropriate) production of a previous behavior across intervening stimuli within a given response set. In terms of chaos theory, it might
be said that /k ɔ r/ (or perhaps a more abstract variant of it like /velar-low
vowel-alveolar/ sequence) has become a pathological phonological attractor that competes with others intermittently (like the /alveolar-mid high
front vowel-stop/ syllable in the words "jidduhl, griddle, chittuhled, sib-
ble" or like the form /prEs/ in the words "pressed, pressure, pressduhyuh,
depressed").

It is not surprising that this type of perseveration should appear in an
individual having fluent phonological jargonaphasia (like subject M.S.)
since it has been associated with left hemisphere temporo-parietal lesions
disturbing cholinergic neurotransmitter systems (Sandson & Albert, 1987).
It is also not surprising that a form like /k ɔ r/, or others like it, having
CV initial demisyllable shapes built of sharply contrastive OV sonority sequences, would become strong default phonological attractors given arguments presented in earlier sections of this chapter. It seems puzzling at first
that such disturbed language can be produced despite the preservation of
such basic abilities as assigning word stress, constructing syllable frames,
and selecting and sequencing phonemes. However, this is not unlike the
paradox of the fibrillating heart (Gleick, 1987, p. 284) in which though its
parts, "seem to be working, yet the whole goes fatally awry." Such is the
nature of disorder in complex systems. Since linear models cannot inform
effective treatments for disturbed dynamism, medical therapeutics may
depend critically upon the promise of chaos anticontrol for answers.

Chaos Anticontrol

If the loss of dynamism in a normally chaotic system creates error, then by extension, chaos anticontrol may bring release from pathological regularity and return to an errorfree state (Horgan, 1994; Regalado, 1995; Schiff et al, 1994). A standard where chaotic irregularity is considered good seems counterintuitive from a conventional perspective but is rather convincingly demonstrated in the realm of modern medicine. Cardiology and neurology are two disciplines in particular that have capitalized on chaos anticontrol in the creation of new medical therapeutics. With respect to heart function, normal heartbeat appears superficially to be a fairly regular phenomenon such that beats per minute can be determined easily in whole numbers. In actuality, there exist important miniscule time variations between beats that reveal normal pulse rates to be chaotically rather than periodically patterned. Research showing that older and/or physically diseased hearts have less chaotic beat rates than normal organs suggests that overly periodic or overly controlled beat rates are symptoms of pathology. This hypothesis is being tested in a new line of anticontrol research showing that muscular shock therapy can yield improvement in cardiac behavior through re-establishment of chaotic beat patterns (Allman, 1993).

Exciting new medical weapons of chaos anticontrol in the nervous system (such as an epilepsy "pacemaker") are currently under development, their potential suggested by their capacity to release an overly periodic, seizuring system to its former dynamism (Regalado, 1995). The term "pacemaker" for such a tool seems a misnomer, for anticontrol techniques rely on the retuning of a system's "loss regions" (errors created by periodicity) to their previously aperiodic state with precisely timed perturbations that maintain chaos (Regalado, 1995). It could be argued that at least some aspects of acquired language disorders arise from pathological restrictions on a normally chaotic neurology. If so, how might chaos anticontrol relate to less concrete human functions like disordered language processing?

The answer may perhaps be found in the simple prerequisite for identifying the "loss regions" in a dynamic system: a brief period of observation (Regalado, 1995). It is not necessary to completely understand the system, its exact initial conditions, for example, but rather to be able to identify behaviors that arise from excessive periodicity (though they may seem chaotic) and counteract them with appropriate stimulation. Just as epileptic seizures represent dynamism "loss regions" in the nervous system (Regalado, 1995), slow processing, anomia, neology, paraphasia, and perseveration may represent dynamism loss regions in the aphasic language system. As Schwartz (1992) has noted, what makes chaos theory so promising from a clinical perspective is the significance it accords to input (i.e., the system's sensitivity to initial conditions), a factor that is clinically manipulable, and its emphasis on the nonlinear nature of learning. Strengthening "phonological attractors" within a child's delayed language-learning system, for example, or interrupting the perseverative behavior of an aphasic speaker might ultimately translate to something quite commonplace like increasing the saliency of desired targets or providing critically timed cues in therapy but the theory will help us better understand why it is often the case that a little bit of stimulation can lead to sudden leaps in learning.

III. FUTURE CHAOS

How can language phenomena best be understood? Any theory of cognition that can predict the facts of its development and dissolution (allowing for individual variation) while modeling the normal neurolinguistic interface with a high degree of psychological and physiological reality will be a strong contender. Therein has lain much of the value of connectionistic models in their application to the study of these issues in both children and adults (see Berg, 1989, 1992; Christman, 1992a, 1992b, 1994; Dell, 1988; Miller & Ellis, 1987). It has been argued that certain principles of interactive activation and parallel distributed processing characterize neural structure and function and, together with principles from chaos theory, provide an integrated framework for understanding cognitive function that surpasses more linear and classically (vs. chaotically) deterministic approaches to modeling the mind/brain problem. Indeed, according to Parks et al. (1991, p. 208), "The relationship between . . . deterministic chaos findings and parallel distributed processing networks in brains and computers is one of the important questions on the cutting edge of cognitive neuroscience."

It has been argued that the nervous system is chaotic: self-organizing, locally unpredictable but globally stable, and orderly despite appearances, and it has been suggested that cognitive-linguistic behaviors arising from neural activity possess similar characteristics. Von Baeyer (1998) has noted that while modern dynamics investigates important relationships between radically diverse phenomena (of which language and brain certainly are two), its most fundamental goal is to investigate the very nature of all change. Perhaps chaos theory will help us better understand the central questions asked of all dynamic systems: Why do they change? and What drives them to change ?

In the future, it will be important to better understand the attractors that draw learning systems from one developmental state to another and to understand those that motivate the progressive reorganizations of aphasia recovery. It remains to be seen whether language processing is a phenomenon that can be characterized by the mathematics of chaos or whether reversing "chaos-reduction" is a supportable metaphor for what aphasia therapy does to facilitate recovery. It also remains to be seen whether chaos theory adds any practical twist to our daily interactions with individuals having communication disorders; but to the extent that it has broadened our understanding of human behavior, it has already been of great help. This is indeed a promising area of investigation in the communication neurosciences.

Since neural and linguistic processing systems are inherently dynamic and emergent from an IA/PDP perspective, then what can a dynamic systems (i.e., chaos) theory perspective add to our understanding of these normal and disordered complex human functions? Arising out of fractal structure, the beauty of emergent systems is found in their capacity for creativity, for making more out of less, and for creating terribly complex (as well as simple) structures/behaviors out of essentially simple elements. The seemingly incongruous notions of order within disorder and, alternatively, local disorder within global order, capture the chaotic essences of behavioral complexity (whether addressing "small-scale" neurochemisty or "large-scale" species evolution) in a way that connectionistic principles alone cannot. Recent application of dynamic systems theory to biology foretells what is likely to be a powerful and transforming approach to future study of human behavior, including the study of normal and disordered communication. As Basar (1990, p. 26) has noted, "I think, despite a number of difficulties, the new area treating chaos in brain function is one of the necessary quiet revolutions in neuroscience."

Connectionism has been criticized for characterizing behavior at a level of analysis that cannot capture the regularity and structure of human cognition nor account for its ability to generate unique patterns of activity (Parks et al., 1992). The issue is a broad one confronting the cognitive neurosciences: "To what degree must systems make reference to symbolic representations when processing information?", a question that can probably only be answered properly with respect to a specific level of function (e.g., sensory perception vs. linguistic production). Connectionism has also been criticized for being too unconstrained and failing to make unique predictions, such when PDP models have generated rules and behaviors never observed in natural languages (Parks et al., 1992). Finally, PDP models have suffered at the hands of those who claim that they do not handle well the processing of serial information and who claim that they are not stable (Parks et al., 1992). Perhaps what these complaints point to is the need for a larger chaotic context in which to place connectionistic mechanisms and thus understand complex behavior.

REFERENCES

Abraham, D. F. (1995). Dynamics, bifurcation, self-organization, chaos, mind, conflict, insensitivity to initial conditions, time, unification, diversity, free will, and social responsibility. In R. Robertson & A. Combs (Eds.), *Chaos theory in psychology and the life sciences* (pp. 155–173). Mahwah, NJ: Lawrence Erlbaum Associates.

Allman, W. F. (1993, June). The mathematics of human life. *U.S. News and World Report*, 84–85.

Babloyantz, A., & Lourenco, C. (1994). Computation with chaos: A paradigm for cortical activity. *Proceedings of the National Academy of Sciences of the United States of America, 91, 19,* 9027–9031.

Babloyantz, A., Salazar, J. M., & Nicolis, C. (1985). Evidence of chaotic dynamics of brain activity during the sleep cycle. *Physics Letters A, 111*, 152–156.

Barton, S. (1994). Chaos, self-organization, and psychology. *American Psychologist, 49*(1), 5–14.

Basar, E. (1990). Chaotic dynamics and resonance phenomena in brain function: Progress, perspectives and thoughts. In E. Basar (Ed.), *Chaos in brain function* (pp. 1–30). New York: Springer-Verlag.

Bates, E., & MacWhinney, B. (1987). Language, variation, and language learning. In B. MacWhinney (Ed.), *Mechanisms of language acquisition*. (pp. 157–193). Hillsdale, NJ: Lawrence Erlbaum Associates.

Beland, R., Caplan, D., & Nespoulous, J. L. (1990). The role of abstract phonological representations in word production: Evidence from phonemic paraphasias. *Journal of Neurolinguistics, 5*(2/3), 125–164.

Benson, D. F., & Ardila, A. (1996). *Aphasia: A clinical perspective*. New York: Oxford University Press.

Berg, T. (1989). Intersegmental cohesiveness. *Folia Linguistica, 23*(3/4), 245–280.

Berg, T. (1992). Phonological harmony as a processing problem. *Journal of Child Language, 19*, 225–257.

Bernhardt, B. (1992a). Developmental implications of nonlinear phonological theory. *Clinical Linguistics & Phonetics, 6*(4), 259–282.

Bernhardt, B. (1992b). The application of nonlinear phonological theory to intervention with one phonologically disordered child. *Clinical Linguistics & Phonetics, 6*(4), 283–316.

Bernhardt, B., & Gilbert, J. (1992). Applying linguistic theory to speech-language pathology: The case for non-linear phonology. *Clinical Linguistics & Phonetics, 6*(1&2), 123–146.

Bernhardt, B., & Stemberger, J. P. (in press). Multi-linear phonology and child phonological development. Manuscript, University of British Columbia & University of Minnesota.

Brown, J. W. (1977). *Mind, brain, and consciousness: The neuropsychology of cognition*. New York: Academic Press.

Brown, J. W. (1980). Brain structure and language production: A dynamic view. In D. Caplan (Ed.), *Biological studies of mental processes*. Cambridge, MA: MIT Press.

Buckingham, H. W. (1977). The conduction theory and neologistic jargon. *Language and Speech, 20*, 174–184.

Buckingham, H. W. (1979). Linguistic aspects of lexical retrieval disturbances in the posterior fluent aphasias. In H. Whitaker & H. A. Whitaker (Eds.), *Studies in Neurolinguistics. Vol. 4.* New York: Academic Press.

Buckingham, H. W. (1981). Where do neologisms come from? In J. W. Brown (Ed.), *Jargonaphasia*. New York: Academic Press.

Buckingham, H. W. (1982). Critical issues in the linguistic study of aphasia. In N. Lass (Ed.), *Speech and language: Advances in basic research and practice. Vol. 8.* New York: Academic Press.

Buckingham, H. W. (1989). Phonological paraphasia. In C. Code (Ed.), *The characteristics of aphasia*. London: Taylor & Francis.

Buckingham, H. W. (1990a). Abstruse neologisms, retrieval deficits, and the random generator. *Studies in Neurolinguistics, 5*, 215–235. (Special issue on "Phonological and Phonetic Aspects of Aphasia". R. Beland, J. Ryalls, & A. R. Lecours, Eds.).

Buckingham, H. W. (1990b). Principle of sonority, doublet creation, and the checkoff monitor. In J. L. Nespoulous & P. Villard (Eds.), *Phonology, morphology, and aphasia*. New York: Springer-Verlag.

Buckingham, H. W. (1991). The mechanisms of phonemic paraphasia. *Clinical Linguistics & Phonetics, (3/4)*, 41–63.

Buckingham, H. W., & Christman, S. S. (1996). Perseverative blends and splicing: Evidence for theories of syllable constituency. (Short Paper). *Brain and Cognition, 32*(2), 323–325.

Buckingham, H. W., & Kertesz, A. (1974). A linguistic analysis of fluent aphasia. *Brain and Language, 1*, 43–62.

Buckingham, H. W., Whitaker, H., & Whitaker, H. A. (1979). On linguistic perseveration. In H. Whitaker & H. A. Whitaker (Eds.), *Studies in neurolinguistics, Vol. 4*, New York: Academic Press.

Butterworth, B. (1979). Hesitation and the production of verbal paraphasias and neologisms in jargon aphasia. *Brain and Language, 18*, 133–161.

Butz, M. (1993). Practical applications from chaos theory to the psychotherapeutic process, a basic consideration of dynamics. Psychological Reports, 73(2), 543–554.

Calvin, W. H. (1996). *How brains think: Evolving intelligence then and now*. New York: Basic Books.

Cavanaugh, J., & McGuire, L. C. (1994). Chaos theory as a framework for understanding adult lifespan learning. In D. Sinnott (Ed.), *Interdisciplinary handbook of adult lifespan learning* (pp. 3–21). Westport, CT: Greenwood Press.

Chase, C. H., & Tallal, P. (1990). A developmental, interactive activation model of the word superiority effect. *Journal of Experimental Child Psychology, 49*, 448–487.

Christman, S. S. (1992a). Abstruse neologism formation: Parallel processing revisited. *Clinical Linguistics & Phonetics, 6*(1&2), 65–76.

Christman, S. S. (1992b). Uncovering phonological regularity in neologisms: Contributions of sonority theory. *Clinical Linguistics & Phonetics, 6*(3), 219–248.

Christman, S. S. (1994). Target-related neologism formation in jargonaphasia. *Brain and Language, 46*(1), 109–128.

Christman, S. S., & Buckingham, H. B. (1989). Jargonaphasia. In C. Code (Ed.), *The characteristics of aphasia*. London: Taylor & Francis.

Clements, G. N. (1990). The role of the sonority cycle in core syllabification. In J. Kingston & M. Beckman (Eds.), *Papers in Laboratory Phonology I: Between the Grammar and the Physics of Speech* . New York: Cambridge University Press.

Code, C., & Ball, M. J. (1994). Syllabification in aphasic recurring utterances: Contributions of sonority theory. *Journal of Neurolinguistics, 8*(4), 257–265.

Cohen, J. D., Servan-Schreiber, D., & McClelland, J. L. (1992). A parallel distributed processing approach to automaticity. *American Journal of Psychology, 105*(2), 239–269.

Damasio, A. R. (1989). Time-locked multi-regional retroactivation: A systems-level proposal for the neural substrates of recall and recognition. *Cognition, 33*, 25–62.

Davis, G. A. (1993). *A survey of adult aphasia and related language disorders* (2nd ed.). Englewood Cliffs, NJ: Prentice-Hall.

Davis, R. D., & MacNeilage, P. F. (1990). Acquisition of correct vowel production: A quantitative case study. *Journal of Speech and Hearing Research, 33*, 16–17.

Dell, G. S. (1988). The retrieval of phonological forms in production: Tests of predictions from a connectionistic model. *Journal of Memory and Language, 27*, 124–142.

Duffy, J. R. (1994). Schuell's stimulation approach to rehabilitation. In R. Chapey (Ed.), *Language intervention strategies in adult aphasia* (3d ed., pp. 146–174). Baltimore, MD: Williams & Wilkins.

Duke, D. W., & Pritchard, W. S. (Eds.) (1991). *Proceedings of the conference on measuring chaos in the human brain.* Singapore: World Scientific.

Eccles, J. C. (1994). *How the self controls its brain.* Berlin: Springer-Verlag.

Edelman, G. M. (1987). *Neural darwinism: The theory of neuronal group selection.* New York: Basic Books.

Edelman, G. M. (1989). *The remembered present. A biological theory of consciousness.* New York: Basic Books.

Edelman, G. M. (1993). Neural darwinism: Selection and reentrant signaling in higher brain function. *Neuron, 10,* 115–125.

Ellis, A. W. (1985). The production of spoken words: A cognitive neuropsychological perspective. In A. W. Ellis (Ed.), *Progress in the psychology of language, Vol. 2.* London: Lawrence Erlbaum.

Fogel, D. B., & Stayton, L. C. (1994). On the effectiveness of crossover in simulated evolutionary optimization. *Biosystems, 32*(3), 171–182.

Francis, S. E. (1995). Chaotic phenomena in psychophysiological self-regulation. In R. Robertson & A. Combs (Eds.), *Chaos theory in psychology and the life sciences* (pp. 253–265). Mahwah, NJ: Lawrence Earlbaum Associates.

Frank, G. W., Lookman, T., Nerengerg, M. A. H., Essex, C., Lemieux, J., & Blume, W. (1990). Chaotic time series analyses of epileptic seizures. *Physica D, 46,* 427–438.

Freeman, W. J. (1994a). Characterization of state transitions in spatially distributed, chaotic, nonlinear, dynamical systems in the cerebral cortex. *Integrative Physiological and Behavioral Science, 29*(3), 294–306.

Freeman, W. J. (1994b). Role of chaotic dynamics in neural plasticity. (Review). *Progress in Brain Research, 102,* 319–333.

Friston, K. J., Tononi, G., Reeke, G. N. Jr., Sporns, O., & Edelman, G. M. (1994). Value-dependent selection in the brain: Simulation in a synthetic neural model. *Neuroscience, 59*(2), 229–243.

Fudge, E. (1987). Branching structure within the syllable. *Journal of Linguistics, 32,* 359–377.

Glanz, J. (1994, August). Do chaos-control techniques offer hope for epilepsy? *Science, 265*(5167), 1174.

Gleick, J. (1987). *Chaos: Making a new science.* New York: Penguin.

Goldman-Rakic, P. S. (1988a). Changing concepts of cortical connectivity: Parallel distributed cortical networks. In P. Rakic & W. Singer (Eds.), *Neurobiology of eocortex* (177–202). Chichester: John Wiley.

Goldman-Rakic, P. S. (1988b). Topography of cognition: Parallel distributed networks in primate association cortex. *Annual Review of Neuroscience, 11,* 137–156.

Goldsmith, J. (1993). Harmonic phonology. In J. Goldsmith (Ed.), *The last phonological rule: Reflections on constraints and derivations* (pp. 21–60). University of Chicago Press: Chicago.

Gould, S. J. (1996). *Full house.* New York: Three Rivers Press.

Habib, M., & Demonet, J-F. (1996). Cognitive neuroanatomy of language: The contribution of functional neuroimaging. *Aphasiology, 10*(3), 217–234.

Hagoort, P. (1993). Impairments of lexical-semantic processing in aphasia: Evidence from the processing of lexical ambiguities. *Brain and Language, 45*(2), 189–232.

Hao, J., Vandewalle, J., & Tan, S. (1994). Predictive control of nonlinear systems based on identification by backpropagation networks. *International Journal of Neural Sustems, 5*(4), 335–344.

Harley, T. A. (1998). The semantic deficit in dementia: connectionistic approaches to what goes wrong in picture naming. *Aphasiology, 12*(4/5), 299–318.

Harrman, H.J., & Kolk, J. H. J. (1991). A computer model of the temporal course of agrammatic understanding: The effects of variation in severity and sentence complexity. *Cognitive Science, 15,* 49–87.

Hebb, D. O. (1949). *The organization of behavior.* New York: Wiley.

Helm-Estabrooks, N., & Albert, M. L. (1991). *Manual of aphasia therapy*. Austin, TX: Pro-Ed.

Hernandez, J. L., Valdes, J. L., Biscay, R., Jimenez, J. C., & Valdes, P. (1995). EEG predictability: Adequacy of non-linear forecasting. *International Journal of Bio-Medical Computing, 38*(3), 197–206.

Herzel, H., Berry, D., Titze, I. R., & Saleh, M. (1994). Analysis of vocal disorders with methods from nonlinear dynamics. *Journal of Speech and Hearing Research, 37*(5), 1008–1019.

Horgan, J. (1994, November). Brain storm: Controlling chaos could help treat epilepsy. *Scientific American, 271*(5), 24.

Howe, M. L., & Rabinowitz, F. M. (1994). Dynamic modeling, chaos, and cognitive development. *Journal of Experimental Child Psychology, 58*(2), 184–199.

Jacobs, A. M., & Grainger, J. (1992). Testing a semistochastic variant of the interactive activation model in different word recognition experiments. *Journal of Experimental Psychology: Human Perception and Performance, 18*(4), 1174–1188.

Janse, M. J. (1995). Chaos in the prediction of sudden death. *European Heart Journal, 16*(3), 299–301.

Kandel, E. R., Schwartz, J. H., & Jessell, T. M. (1991). *Principles of neural science* (3rd ed.). Norwalk, CT: Appleton & Lange.

Kanters, J. K., Holstein-Rathlou, N. H., & Agner, E. (1994). Lack of evidence for low-dimensional chaos in heart rate variability. *Journal of Cardiovascular Electrophysiology, 5*(7), 591–601.

Kelso, J. A. S. (1995). *Dynamic patterns: The self-organization of brain and behavior*. Cambridge, MA: MIT Press.

Kent, R. D. (1981). Articulatory-acoustic perspectives on speech development. In R. E. Stark (Ed.), *Language behavior in infancy and early childhood* (pp. 105–126). New York: Elsevier/North-Holland.

Kent, R. D. (1984). Psychobiology of speech development: Coemergence of language and a movement system. *American Journal of Physiology, 246*, 888–894.

Kent, R. D. (1992). The biology of phonological development. In C. A. Ferguson, L. Menn, & C. Stoel-Gammon (Eds.), *Phonological development: Models, research, implications*. Timonium, MD: York Press.

Kent, R. D. (1993). Sonority theory and syllable pattern as keys to sensory-motor-cognitive interactions in infant vocal development. In B. de Boysson-Bardies, S. de Schonen, P. Jusczyk, P. MacNeilage, & J. Morton (Eds.), *Developmental neurocognition: Speech and face processing in the first year of life* (pp. 329–340). Dordrecht: Kluwer Academic.

Kertesz, A. (1991). Tutorial review: Language cortex. *Aphasiology, 5*(3), 207–234.

Kertesz, A., & Benson, D. F. (1970). Neologistic jargon: A clinicopathological study. *Cortex, 6*, 362–386.

Langs, R., & Badalmenti, A. (1994). Psychotherapy: the search for chaos and the discovery of determinism. *Australian & New Zealand Journal of Psychiatry, 28*(1), 68–81.

Laplanc, D. (1994). Localization revisited in light of parallel distributed processing. (Letter). *Journal of Neurology, 242*, 47–48.

Lecours, A. R. (1982). On neologisms. In J. Mehler, E. C. T. Walker, & M. F. Garrett (Eds.), *Perspectives on mental representation*. Hillsdale, NJ: Lawrence Erlbaum.

Lecours, A. R., & Lhermitte, F. (1972). Recherches sur le langage des aphasiques: 4. Analyse d'un corpus de néologismes: notion de paraphasic monémique. *L'Encephale, 61*, 295–315.

Levelt, W. J. M. (1989). *Speaking: From intention to articulation*. Cambridge, MA: MIT Press.

Levinson, E. A. (1994). The uses of disorder: Chaos theory and psychoanalysis. *Contemporary Psychoanalysis, 30*(1), 5–24.

Lieberman, P. (1984). *The biology and evolution of language*. Cambridge, MA: Harvard University Press.

Lindblom, B. (1992). Phonological units as adaptive emergents of lexical development. In C. A. Ferguson, L. Menn, & C. Stoel-Gammon (Eds.), *Phonological development: Models, research, implications* (pp. 131–163). Timonium, MD: York Press.

Lindblom, B., MacNeilage, P. F., & Studdert-Kennedy, M. (1984). Self-organizing processes and the explanation of phonological universals. In B. Butterworth, B. Comrie, & Ö. Dahl (Eds.), *Explanations for language universals* (pp. 181–204). Berlin: Mouton.

Locke, J. L. (1983). *Phonological acquisition and change.* New York: Academic Press.

Locke, J. L. (1994). Gradual emergence of developmental language disorders. *Journal of Speech and Hearing Research, 37*, 608–616.

Locke, J. L. (1997). A theory of neurolinguistic development. *Brain and Language, 58*, 265–326.

Luria, A. R. (1970). *Traumatic aphasia.* The Hague: Mouton.

Mandell, A. J. (1985). From molecular biological simplification to more realistic central nervous system dynamics: An opinion. In J. O. Cavenar (Ed.), *Psychiatry: Psychobiological foundations of Clinical Psychiatry, 3:2.* New York: Lippincott.

Martin, N., Roach, A., Brecher, A., & Lowery, J. (1998). Lexical retrieval mechanisms underlying whole-word perseveration errors in anomic aphasia. *Aphasiology, 12*(4/5), 319–333.

McClelland, J. L., & Rumelhart, D. E. (1981). An interactive activation model of context effects in letter perception: Part 1. An account of basic findings. *Psychological Research, 88*, 375–405.

McClelland, J. L., & Rumelhart, D. E. (1986). *Parallel distributed processing: Explorations in the microstructure of cognition: Volume 2: Psychological and biological models.* Cambridge, MA: MIT Press.

McClelland, J. L., Rumelhart, D. E., & Hinton, G. E. (1986). The appeal of parallel distributed processing. In D. E. Rumelhart & J. L. McClelland (Eds.), *Parallel distributed processing, Vol. 1,* Cambridge, MA: MIT Press.

McGregor, K. K., & Johnson, A. C. (1997). Trochaic template use in early words and phrases. *Journal of Speech, Language and Hearing Research, 40*, 1220–1231.

McKenna, T. M., McMullen, T. A., & Shlesinger, M. F. (1994). The brain as a dynamic physical system. *Neuroscience, 60*(3), 587–605.

Mesulam, M-M. (1990). Large-scale neurocognitive networks and distributed processing for attention, language, and memory. *Annals of Neurology, 28*(5), 597–613.

Miller, D., & Ellis, A. W. (1987). Speech and writing errors in neologistic jargonaphasia: A lexical activation hypothesis. In M. Coltheart, G. Sartori, & R. Job (Eds.), *The cognitive neuropsychology of language* (pp. 253–271). London: Lawrence Erlbaum Associates.

Mitchell, P. R. (1995). A dynamic interactive developmental view of early speech and language production: Application to clinical practice in motor speech disorders. *Seminars in Speech and Language, 16*(2), 100–109.

Mohanan, K. P. (1993). Fields of attraction in phonology. In J. Goldsmith (Ed.), *The last phonological rule* (pp. 61–116). Chicago: University of Chicago Press.

Moran, M. (1991). Chaos theory and psychoanalysis: The fluidic nature of the mind. *International Review of Psychoanalysis, 18*(2), 211–221.

Mosca, F. (1995). Freedom in chaos theory: A case for choice in a universe without a bottom line. In F. D. Abraham & A. R. Gilgen (Eds.), *Chaos theory in Psychology: Contributions in psychology No. 27*(pp. 181–191). Westport, CT: Praeger Publishers/Greenwood Publishing Group.

Nandrino, J. L., Pezard, L., Martinerie, J., el Massioui, F., Renault, B., Jouvent, R., Allilaire, J. F., & Widlocher, D. (1994). Decrease of complexity in EEG as a symptom of depression. *Neuroreport, 5*(4), 528–530.

Nelson, K. E. (1991). Varied domains of development: A tale of LAD, MAD, SAD, DAD, and RARE and surprising events in our RELMS. In F. S. Kessel, M. H. Bornstein, & A. J. Sameroff (Eds.), *Contemporary constructions of the child: Essays in honor of William Kessen* (pp. 123–142). Hillsdale, NJ: Lawrence Erlbaum Associates.

Nwokah, E. E., Hsu, H-C., Davies, P., & Fogel, A. (1999). The integration of laughter and speech in vocal communication: A dynamic systems perspective. *Journal of Speech, Language, and Hearing Research, 42,* 880–894.

Parks, R. W., Long, D. L., Levine, D. S., Crockett, D. J., McGeer, E. G., McGeer, P. L., Dalton, I. E., Zec, R. F., Becker, R. E., Coburn, K. L., Siler, G., Nelson, M. E., & Bower, J. M. (1991). Parallel distributed processing and neural networks: Origins, methodology, and cognitive functions. *International Journal of Neuroscience, 60,* 195–214.

Parks, R. W., Levine, D. S., Long, D. L., Crockett, D. J., Dalton, I. E., Weingartner, H., Fedio, P., Coburn, K. L., Siler, G., Matthews, J. R., & Becker, R. E. (1992). Parallel distributed processing and neuropsychology: A neural network model of Wisconsin Card Sorting and Verbal Fluency. *Neuropsychology Review, 3*(2), 213–233.

Paulesu, E., Frith, U., Snowling, M., Gallagher, A., Morton, J., Frackowiak, R. S. J., & Frith, C. D. (1996). Is developmental dyslexia a disconnection syndrome? Evidence from PET scanning. *Brain, 119,* 143–157.

Peng, C. K., Buldyrev, S. V., Hausdorff, J. M., Havlin, S., Mietus, J. E., Simons, M., Stanley, H. E., & Goldberger, A. L. (1994). Non-equilibrium dynamics as an indispensable characteristic of a healthy biological system. *Integrative Physiological & Behavioral Science, 29*(3), 283–293.

Pick, A. (1931). Aphasia. Trans. J. W. Brown. Springfield: Thomas.

Pinker, S. (1999). Words and rules: The ingredients of language. New York: Basic Books.

Porch, B. E. (1994). Treatment of aphasia subsequent to the Porch Index of Communicative Ability (PICA). In R. Chapey (Ed.), *Language intervention strategies in adult aphasia* (3d ed., pp. 175–183). Baltimore, MD: Williams & Wilkins.

Priel, B., & Schreiber, G. (1994). On psychoanalysis and non-linear dynamics: The paradigm of bifurcation. *British Journal of Medical Psychology, 67*(3), 209–218.

Pritchard, W. S., & Duke, D. W. (1995). Measuring "chaos" in the brain: A tutorial review of EEG dimension estimation. *Brain and Cognition, 27*(3), 353–397.

Rambidi, N. G. (1993). Non-discrete biomolecular computing: An approach to computational complexity. *Biosystems, 31*(1), 3–13.

Rapp, P. E. (1994). A guide to dynamical analysis. *Integrative Physiological and Behavioral Science, 29*(3), 311–327.

Regalado, A. (1995, June). A gental scheme for unleashing chaos. *Science, 268,* 1848.

Rescorla, L., Roberts, J., & Dahlsgaard, K. (1997). Late talkers at 2: Outcome at age 3. *Journal of Speech, Language, and Hearing Research, 40,* 556–566.

Resnick, M. (1995). Beyond the centralized mindset. *Journal of the Learning Sciences, 5*(1), 1–22.

Richards, W., Wilson, H. R., & Sommer, M. A. (1994). Chaos in percepts? *Biological Cybernetics, 70*(4), 345–349.

Robertson, S. S., Cohen, A. H., & Mayer-Kress, G. (1993). Behavioral chaos: Beyond the metaphor. In L. Smith & E. Thelen (Eds.), *A dynamic systems approach to development: Applications* (pp. 119–150). Cambridge, MA: MIT Press.

Rosenbek, J. C., LaPointe, L. L., & Wertz, R. T. (1989). *Aphasia: A clinical approach.* Austin, TX: Pro-ed.

Rossler, O. E., & Rossler, R. (1994). Chaos in physiology. *Integrative Physiological and Behavioral Science, 29*(3), 328–333.

Rumelhart, D. E., & McClelland, J. L. (1986). Parallel distributed processing: *Explorations in the microstructure of cognition: Volume 1: Foundations.* Cambridge, MA: MIT Press.

Sandson, J., & Albert, M. L. (1984). Varieties of perseveration. *Neuropsychologia, 22,* 715–732.

Sandson, J., & Albert, M. L. (1987). Perseveration in behavioral neurology. *Neurology, 37,* 1736–1741.

Santo-Pietro, M. J., & Rigrodsky, S. (1986). Patterns of oral-verbal perseveration in adult aphasics. *Brain and Language, 29,* 1–17.

Sarraille, J. J., & Myers, L. S. (1994). FD3: A program for measuring fractal dimension. *Educational & Psychological Measurement, 54*(1), 94–97.

Schiff, S. J., Jerger, K., Duong, D. H., Chang, T., Spano, M. L., & Ditto, W. L. (1994, August). Controlling chaos in the brain. *Nature, 370*(6491), 615–620.

Schuell, H., & Jenkins, J. J. (1961). Reduction of vocabulary in aphasia. *Brain, 84*, 243–261.

Schuell, H., Jenkins, J. J., & Jimnez-Pabn, E. (1964). *Aphasia in adults.* New York: Harper and Row.

Schwartz, R. G. (1992). Clinical applications of recent advances in phonological theory. *Language, Speech, and Hearing Services in Schools, 23*, 269–276.

Searle, J. R. (1984). *Minds, brains, and science.* London: British Broadcasting Company.

Searle, J. R. (1992). *The rediscovery of the mind.* Cambridge, MA: MIT Press.

Seidenberg, M. S. (1994). Language and connectionism: The developing interface. *Cognition, 50*, 385–401.

Siegel, R. A. (1992). Commentary on "neural networks in pharmacodynamic modeling: Is current modeling practice of complex kinetic systems at a dead end." *Journal of Pharmacokinetics and Biopharmaceutics, 20*(4), 413–418.

Skarda, C. A., & Freeman, W. J. (1987). How brains make chaos in order to make sense of the world. *Behavioral and Brain Sciences 10*, 161–195.

Small, S. L. (1994). Connectionistic networks and language disorders. *Journal of Communication Disorders, 27*, 305–323.

Smith, A. (1997). Dynamic interactions of factors that impact speech motor stability in children and adults. In W. Hulstijn, H. F. M. Peters, & P. H. H. M. Van Lieshout (Eds.), *Speech production: Motor control, brain research, and fluency disorders.* Exerpta Medica International Congress Series 1146 (pp. 143–149). Amsterdam: Elsevier.

Smolensky, P. (1986). Neural and conceptual interpretation of PDP models. In J. L. McClelland & D. E. Rumelhart (Eds.), *Parallel distributed processing: Explorations in the microstructure of cognition. Vol. 2: Psychological and biological models* (pp. 390–431). Cambridge, MA: MIT Press.

Sternberger, J. P. (1985). An interactive model of language production. In A. W. Ellis (Ed.), *Progress in the psychology of language. Vol. 1* (pp. 143–184). London: Lawrence Erlbaum.

Sternberger, J. P. (1995, May). *Where does consonant harmony come from?* Paper presented at the 1995 child phonology meeting, Memphis, Tennessee.

Sternberger, J. P., Elman, J. L., & Haden, P. (1985). Interference between phonemes during phoneme monitoring: Evidence for an interactive activation model of speech perception. *Journal of Experimental Psychology: Human Perception and Performance, 11*(4), 475–489.

Sutherland, S. (1986, October). Parallel distributed processing. *Nature, 323*, 486.

Thelen, E. (1981). Rhythmical behavior in infancy: an ethnological perspective. *Developmental Psychology, 17*, 237–257.

Thelen, E. (1989). Self-organization in developmental processes: Can systems approaches work? In M. R. Gunnar & E. Thelen (Eds.), *Systems and development.* The Minnesota Symposia on Child Psychology, 2 (pp. 77–117). Hillsdale, NJ: Lawrence Erlbaum.

Thelen, E. (1991). Motor aspects of emergent speech: A dynamic approach. In N. Krasnegor, D. Rumbaugh, & M. Studdert-Kennedy (Eds.), *Biological and behavioral determinants of language development* (pp. 339–365). Hillsdale, NJ: Lawrence Erlbaum.

Thelen, E., & Smith, L. B. (1996). *A dynamic systems approach to the development of cognition and action.* Cambridge, MA: MIT Press.

Tseng, C-H., McNeil, M. R., & Milenkovic, P. (1993). An investigation of attention allocation deficits in aphasia. *Brain and Language, 45*(2), 276–296.

Van Eenwyk, J. R. (1991). Archetypes: The strange attractors of the psyche. *Journal of Analytical Psychology, 36*(1), 1–25.

van Geert, P. (1994). *Dynamic systems of development: Change between complexity and chaos.* London: Harvester Wheatsheaf.

van Gelder, T. (1998). The dynamical hypothesis in cognitive science. *Behavioral and Brain Sciences, 21*(5), 615–628.

Vihman, M. M. (1993). The construction of a phonological system. In B. de Boysson-Bardies, S. de Schonen, P. Jusczyk, P. MacNeilage, & J. Morton (Eds.), *Developmental neurocognition: Speech and face processing in the first year of life* (pp. 411–419). Dordrecht: Kluwer Academic.

Viret, J. (1994). Reaction of the organism to stress: The survival attractor concept. *Acta Biotheoretica, 42*(2–3), 99–109.

von Baeyer, H. C. (1998). All shook up. *The Sciences, Jan./Feb.*, 12–14.

Waldrop, M. M. (1992). Complexity: *The emerging science at the edge of order and chaos.* New York: Touchstone.

Weismer, S. E., Murray-Branch, J., & Miller, J. F. (1994). A prospective longitudinal study of language development in late talkers. *Journal of Speech and Hearing Research, 37*, 852–867.

Wheeler, D. W., & Touretzky, D. S. (1997). A parallel licensing model of normal slips and phonemic paraphasias. *Brain and Language, 59*, 147–201.

Woo, C. H. (1994). Rapid exploration of alternatives via chaos. *Biosystems, 32*(2), 93–96.

3

Diagnosis, Prognosis, and Remediation of Acquired Naming Disorders from a Connectionist Perspective

Deborah A. Gagnon
Cornell University

Nadine Martin
Temple University & Moss Rehabilitation Research Institute

Recent years have witnessed a revolution in both clinical and theoretical views of normal and impaired language production. In the clinic, functional tools of assessment (e.g., Kay, Lesser, & Coltheart, 1992) have provided a new way of analyzing language behavior; in theory, connectionism has redefined our understanding of how function is achieved. In this chapter, we describe connectionism and argue for the eventual clinical relevance of thinking in connectionist terms. We contrast methods of assessment and treatment that may be derived from connectionist models to methods that are already part of the language therapist's repertoire, both those that have been available traditionally (syndrome classification) and those that have emerged only recently (psycholinguistic analysis). We hope to convince students and practitioners in the speech and language rehabilitation field of the reasons why connectionist models offer an important advance over these previous approaches.

The first part of the chapter builds our general argument for connectionism as a framework for assessing and treating language disorders. The goals of language theory and therapy are made explicit in order to establish the relevance of theory to practical, clinical concerns, and vice versa. Next, structuralist, functionalist, and connectionist perspectives on language and disorder are discussed in relation to the stated goals of therapists and theorists. To anticipate our conclusion, we propose that a connectionist perspective currently provides the best framework for explaining language disorder and may ultimately provide the most suitable guide to treatment as well.

The second part of the chapter supports the argument for connectionism with examples of the practical application of its methodology (computer simulation) to assessment and treatment of naming disorders. We begin by describing a connectionist model of single-word production, which has been shown to be capable of accurately simulating a wide variety of fluent aphasics' error patterns in confrontation naming and predicts recovery patterns as well (Dell, Schwartz, Martin, Saffran, & Gagnon, 1997; Martin, Dell, Saffran, & Schwartz, 1994; Schwartz, Dell, Martin, & Saffran, 1994). This model illustrates the applicability of connectionism to goals that go beyond simply diagnosing a naming deficit, namely, explaining the underlying mechanism that leads to the deficit and predicting the evolution of language behaviors that accompany recovery. Next, recent experimental work that attempts to apply principles of connectionist theory to treatment is reviewed. In particular, research is introduced that demonstrates how thinking in connectionist terms may be useful in directing treatment for word-finding disorders (Laine & Martin, 1996; Martin & Laine, 2000; Martin, Laine, & Lowery, 1996). In short, the aim of this chapter is to demonstrate the appropriateness of connectionist models as potential diagnostic, prognostic, and remediatory tools in the treatment of language disorder.

STRUCTURE, FUNCTION, AND PROCESS

Treatment methods derive from theoretical bases, so before focusing on practical applications of language theory to language therapy, we review the three primary theoretical perspectives that have been applied to language disorder. The interconnection between language theory and therapy arises because both enterprises share common goals: to describe, predict, explain, and control (i.e., treat) language behavior. These goals provide a cohesive thread throughout the chapter as we continuously revisit them in assessing how well each of the three theoretical perspectives measure up. Note that describing, predicting, explaining, and controlling are also the goals of science in general. Thus, therapists as well as theorists may think of themselves as scientists who are interested in forming and testing hypotheses about the probable cause of a disorder. Specifically, the aims of the language theorist and therapist are:

1. *To describe patterns of language performance.* Description is the first aim of any science. To be scientific, description of language impairment must be objective, valid, and reliable. The diagnostic tools currently available to therapists more or less meet these conditions. They vary, however, in their focus of assessment, analysis of language

impairment, and degree of specificity. Given that description is the foundation on which the other three aims are met, it is important to determine which assessment method provides the optimal level of description for serving the further aims of prediction, explanation, and control.

2. *To make predictions about language performance.* The term "prediction" can apply in at least three different ways to language performance. First, one may wish to predict which behavioral symptoms tend to co-occur. For example, is the presence of semantic paraphasias in a patient's speech predictive of the presence of formal paraphasias as well? One may wish, instead, to predict a patient's change in language behavior over time, as behavior evolves from an acute state to a chronic state of impairment or to a recovered state. Finally, one may wish to predict from a patient's performance in one language task how that patient will perform on another language task. If the patient makes semantic paraphasias in naming objects, will he or she necessarily make this type of error in repeating the spoken names of those objects?

3. *To interpret different patterns of language performance in terms of "what" (structures, functions, processes) has been compromised.* A scientist wants to do more than simply describe and predict, he or she also wants to explain the phenomena of interest. What causes a particular behavior? What level of explanation is most suited to addressing questions of treatment? Because various levels of description exist, a single phenomenon may be explained in more than one way. For instance, a particular language impairment can be explained in terms of its neuroanatomical characteristics, behavioral characteristics, linguistic characteristics, psychosocial characteristics, and so on.

4. *To understand what external influences mediate change in language behavior.* This addresses the final goal of theory and therapy: control. A helpful treatment tool should allow one to study and evaluate the effect of specific treatment interventions on language behavior. Which of the three methodologies best provides this capability?

Following, the most prominent theoretical paradigms that have been applied to the study and treatment of language disorder are considered in light of these aims. The term "paradigm" refers to an overall perspective, or view, of the phenomena associated with a field of scientific inquiry. A paradigm directs theory building and evaluation, as well as development of more practical products, for example, assessment and intervention techniques in language therapy. The study and treatment of language disorder have historically been conducted under two main paradigms: one that views disorder in terms of neuroanatomical organization (structuralism) and the other in terms of psycholinguistic organization (functionalism). Connectionism may be considered as yet a third paradigm that has evolved from the functionalist perspective.[1]

Paradigms differ in terms of their degree of specificity and level of analysis, thus providing alternative views of the same phenomena. With regard to specificity, it seems apparent that treatment based on a more precise description of a patient's abilities and inabilities will be more effective (Howard & Patterson, 1989). Thus, specificity is one dimension on which each of the paradigms may be evaluated. There are also different levels of analysis at which language behavior may be described, and presumably, some levels are more suitable than others for directing treatment. We have already mentioned that the historical focus of analysis in language disorder has been on either neuroanatomical or psycholinguistic organization; connectionism offers yet another level of analysis. In what follows, the three main paradigms are described in terms of their underlying assumptions, goals, and methods and are evaluated in terms of which offers the greatest specificity and the most suitable level of analysis to meet the four aims of the therapist/theorist outlined previously.

Structuralism

Perhaps the most obvious description of language disorder is in terms of language abilities that are spared versus those that are impaired. For example, a patient might be able to repeat words, but not name objects. Or, a patient might be able to produce content words, but not function words. By testing on a number of tasks that assess a wide variety of language functions, a profile that describes the patient's deficit in terms of the relative sparing and impairment of linguistic abilities may be obtained. The *Boston Diagnostic Assessment Exam* (BDAE; Goodglass & Kaplan, 1983) is an example of an assessment tool that produces such a profile. Now suppose that certain profiles tends to show up again and again, across different patients. A group of symptoms that tends to co-occur and that characterizes a particular abnormality constitutes a syndrome. Thus, patients may be categorized according to the syndrome that best corresponds to the cluster of symptoms they demonstrate in assessment testing (Caplan, 1993; Ellis & Young, 1988; Shallice, 1988).

How might one explain the occurrence of a particular syndrome? Early aphasiologists noted that certain syndromes tend to arise from damage at certain neural loci (e.g., Lichteim, 1885; Wernicke, 1874). Thus, explanation of language and other cognitive disorders was traditionally made in relation to the site of neuroanatomic—or structural—injury (Albert, Goodglass, Helm, Rubens, & Alexander, 1981). For instance, the syndrome we know as

Wernicke's aphasia might be said to be "caused" by damage to Wernicke's area, the syndrome known as Broca's aphasia might be said to be "caused" by damage to Broca's area, and so on. Structuralism is the approach that describes language disorder in terms of disrupted behavioral functions and their associated neuroanatomical structures.

One criticism of syndrome classification is that it simply amounts to a checklist of symptoms, any of which may be absent in a patient who is assessed with a particular syndrome and present in a patient who is not assessed with this particular syndrome (Caplan, 1993). In other words, there are no necessary or sufficient behavioral features on which to base classification. This may sometimes lead to equivalent diagnoses of two patients who have no symptoms in common, thus failing to capture their very large and meaningful behavioral differences (Caramazza & Badecker, 1989; Schwartz, 1984). The converse problem also appears: A patient may not be uniquely classifiable because the particular cluster of symptoms he or she exhibits may fit into more than one syndrome category. In fact, Prins, Snow, and Wagenaar (1978) claim that "no more than twenty or thirty percent of dysphasic patients will fit neatly into one of the specific dysphasia syndromes."

The ability of the structuralist approach to predict outcomes of treatment or recovery is, therefore, limited. The limitation arises because change can only be measured in terms of moving from one syndrome classification to another. Any prediction about recovery is based on correlational data (i.e., on the co-occurring behaviors across patients at different points in recovery) and on noting general patterns of recovery (e.g., global aphasia often resolves into Broca's and Wernicke's into conduction or anomic). Specific predictions about the recovery pattern of a particular patient are not possible. Finally, the variability among patients within a particular syndrome class makes the approach impractical for predicting generalization of treatment. Thus, the syndrome classification approach to describing and predicting behavior does not satisfy many of the needs of the language therapist because it is focused more on specifying behavioral-neuroanatomical correlates and less on a description of language function within individual patients. Clinicians primarily work, after all, with clients on a patient-by-patient (not group) basis.

The structural level of explanation also provides little help in guiding treatment; indeed, structural models were never really intended to serve this function. After all, how can the language therapist, whose goal is to positively modify language function, be helped by knowing the cause of aberrant behavior in terms of neural structure? One possible way might be to correlate treatments with syndrome class. Melodic intonation therapy (MIT) represents one such effort to apply a neuroanatomic rationale to treatment (cf. Helm-Estabrook & Albert, 1991; Sparks, Helm, & Albert,

1974). Because language deficits typically arise from left hemisphere neural injury, the rationale behind this therapy is that stimulating language production with rhythmic and melodic cues should be useful in treating language disorder because these tasks engage intact neuroanatomic structures on (typically) the right side of the brain. In other words, language-related functions from the intact right side of the brain might be solicited in retraining left-brain functions. An approach such as this, however, is silent on the answers to some very practical types of treatment questions: How much stimulation should be provided? How soon should external support, or cues, be faded? Is the use of multimodal treatments beneficial? And so on. More generally, criticism of such approaches lies, again, in knowing that individuals classified with the same syndrome often vary a great deal in terms of their behavioral deficits. Thus, the same treatment will not be equally effective across all members of a category and the approach offers no mechanism for predicting who will and will not benefit from a particular treatment.

In short, a structural perspective is clearly not optimal for satisfying the aims put forth previously. Syndrome classification fails to capture the similarities and differences across individuals' behaviors at a meaningful (i.e., behavioral) level of analysis, and without this, it is difficult to predict, explain, or control language behavior. What is needed is a level of analysis in which differences and similarities among patients are informative with respect to the underlying behavioral deficit. It is the field of cognitive neuropsychology, to which we now turn, that we believe provides a more appropriate and useful level of analysis for meeting the aims of description, prediction, explanation, and control of language behavior.

Functionalism

The introduction of model-based analyses of functional disorder less than 25 years ago (Marshall & Newcombe, 1973) provided a very important turning point in the study of speech and language pathology. The term "functional" refers to the behavioral components involved in producing language. Functional descriptions of disorder are abstract in that they are neutral with respect to structural (neuroanatomic) medium. Thus, the functional models of cognitive neuropsychology shifted focus from a physical level of analysis to a behavioral—in this case, psycholinguistic—level.

If the aim of the neuroanatomist is to explain disordered behavior in terms of damaged "hardware," then the aim of the cognitive neuropsychologist is to describe disordered behavior in terms of corrupted "software." Software specifies the flow of information in a system. A first step in understanding word production, according to cognitive neuropsychology, is to develop an information flow model of the steps, or procedures, involved. Figure 3.1 depicts the possible flow of information in producing words: The

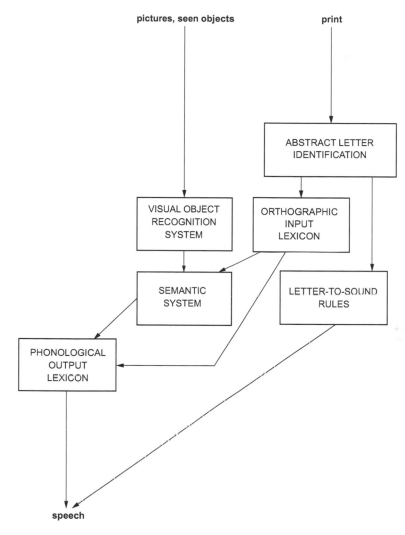

FIG. 3.1. Functional information flow model of single word production (from Kay, Lesser, & Coltheart, 1992). (Permissions Info: Figure 6 (p. 10) in Kay, J., Lesser, R., & Coltheart, M. (1992). *PALPA: Psycholinguistic assessments of language processing in aphasia.* Hove: Erlbaum.)

boxes represent hypotheses about components of the system (representations and/or procedures), and the arrows represent communication from one component to another. Specific patterns of impairment purportedly arise as a result of damage to a particular component or from a faulty connection between one component and another (see Caplan, 1992; Ellis & Young, 1988; Hillis, 1993a; Marshall & Newcombe, 1973; or Shallice, 1988, for more elaborate descriptions of the approach). Thus, the traditional functional, or psycholinguistic, approach takes a different tack on describing language dysfunction: The approach does more than just describe symptoms, it describes the organization of a behavioral system enabling identification of particular representations and processes that are compromised in neural injury.

The functional approach encourages the therapist to be a scientist and systematically test hypotheses about the functional locus of an individual's impairment. *The Psycholinguistic Assessments of Language Processing and Aphasia* (PALPA; Kay, Lesser, & Coltheart, 1992)—an assessment tool developed on the notion of a function-based analysis—makes use of such a systematic, converging approach to assessment. The goal in using this type of assessment tool is to identify, on a patient-by-patient basis, the component within an information flow model of language that has been compromised, not to group patients into discrete syndrome classes. Whereas syndrome classification fails to predict important behavioral similarities and differences among patients, functional classification seems to provide the appropriate level of detail for making clinically relevant classifications (Caplan, 1993).

The functional approach is not without its detractors. One criticism of the box-and-arrow models that result from functional analysis is that such models are limited to identifying the structures and processes that comprise the language system and the routes by which information is processed but not how these processes are realized (see Seidenberg, 1988, for a well-articulated version of this argument). In this sense, functional information-processing models are like road maps: They tell us which structures or routes are impaired and which are spared in the same way that a road map depicts buildings and roads and indicates which routes are available and which are unavailable for travel. This level of description could guide the therapist to a limited extent in that it can identify what functional components need to be targeted for treatment or, possibly, what alternative routes could be used to process information when one route is blocked. What a road map does not do, however, is specify the mechanics and dynamics of how to get there—it does not explain how to operate the car that will get you from one place to another. Similarly, a functional model does not tell the therapist how to treat a particular impairment since it provides no description of the dynamics of processing. Treatment is a dynamic process and requires a model that specifies the dynamic aspects of language processing.

An example of functional model-guided treatment is provided by Nettleson and Lesser (1991). Using functional assessment, Nettleson and Lesser identified the level of breakdown for six anomic subjects. Two of these subjects were thought to have problems related to the semantic system, two purportedly had problems accessing the phonological lexicon, and the last two had problems with phoneme assembly. The former two pairs of subjects were given model-appropriate treatment (semantic stimulation and phonological stimulation, respectively), while the latter pair was given model-inappropriate treatment. Three of the four model-appropriate subjects showed significant improvement in their naming performance, while neither of the model-inappropriate subjects showed significant improvement. This study was significant in that it underscored the inappropriateness of considering anomic patients as a homogenous group. Instead, the results of this study argue for assessing the level at which naming impairment arises for each patient individually and targeting that particular level for treatment in therapy.

The Nettleson and Lesser study also underscores, however, that functional models can tell us what processes are impaired and need to be targeted, but they cannot tell us how to target those impaired processes (see also Hillis, 1993b; Hillis & Caramazza, 1994). For example, when a patient fails a test that requires access to semantic information, this suggests that the patient may be having trouble accessing or using semantic information, or perhaps has corrupted semantic representations. How should we treat such a disorder? Do we stimulate semantic processes by providing an enriched semantic input? This might be appropriate if activation processes are weak or slowed. What if, however, activation of semantic information is adequate, but inhibition of related semantic information (representations) is not? In this latter case, enriching the semantic input would be detrimental. The approach to treatment in this case might be to reduce semantic confusion. But how do we minimize semantic confusion? What stimulation cues will prove to be effective? Functional models are silent on such questions because the answer lies in understanding the effects of external stimuli on access to and retrieval of language units and these models provide no help in predicting these effects.

In sum, traditional functional models lack the necessary specificity to answer specific treatment questions (Caramazza, 1989; Hillis, 1993a; Howard & Patterson, 1989) and their static nature makes them ineffective for predicting change. Although a functional level of analysis may provide a more satisfactory level of description, these two significant shortcomings prohibit such models from making testable and novel predictions or from directing control—all hallmarks of good science and useful clinical models. Connectionism, to which we now turn, pushes the functionalist movement in the direction of greater specificity and adds the important capacity to predict change.

Connectionism

In a sense, connectionism is simply a more fine-grained description of functional architecture. It is an approach to modeling cognitive processes in terms of networks of interconnected, simple, neuron-like units. The connectionist movement borrows heavily from neural structure and process as a metaphor, but it is important to point out that connectionist models are not meant as models of neural architecture. Connectionism is a form of functionalism and as such, is a medium- independent enterprise: The goal of functionalist methodology is to describe information flow at a level of description that is independent of whether that information is transmitted via neural tissue or, say, computer hardware. In fact, connectionist methodology uses computer simulation as a way of forcing an explicit, computational description of the processes and representations hypothesized to be involved in performing a particular cognitive function. This explicit instantiation is one of the characteristics that sets the connectionist approach apart from its predecessors in the functionalist movement.

There are certain key features that all connectionist models share. These include the notion of a network of units commonly arranged in levels that vary in terms of the type of information conveyed. Units at one level of the model are connected to units within and/or between levels. These connections can vary in strength, and information can flow in a backward and/or forward direction between levels. Central to all connectionistic thinking is the concept of activation, corresponding to the notion of information, or energy, being transmitted across units. Transmission implies a dynamic system, one that is always in flux. Thus, a central contribution of connectionist methodology is that it allows one to study changes in a system over time.

Connectionism is more than just a specification of what is inside the boxes of a functionalist information flow model, then. The dynamic, interactive nature of the connectionist system sometimes results in emergent behaviors that could not have been predicted on the basis of a static model. Also, connectionist theory includes constructs that can describe changes in behavior over time (e.g., activation that is weak can become stronger; activation that is decaying can become more enduring). Because computer simulations involve changes over time, predictions about future behavior can be made based on the status of the model at the present. This is an important addition over the previous two approaches since it provides a means of making predictions about future patterns of performance and ultimate state, or outcome (Code, Rowley, & Kertesz, 1994).

Information theory tells us that certain factors are influential in determining the manner in which information flows. These include both internal and external parameters of the information processing system, such as the contribution of internal noise, the rate at which information is transmitted and lost, and the nature of external inputs to the system. These factors are all explicitly specified in a computer simulation and thus, are all within the control of the modeler, allowing him or her to test alternative hypotheses about the effect of these factors on behavior. This explicitness is what gives the connectionist approach an advantage as a therapeutic tool: Its methodology provides a means of varying the very same factors that clinicians vary in practice and testing the effect of these various influences on language behavior (Plaut, 1996). So, another important advantage to connectionist models is that they allow one to configure different internal states of the system (via parameter settings) and to evaluate the effect of various external inputs. The former is analogous to configuring the system to reflect a particular individual's state and the latter is analogous to testing the effect of external intervention to the system, as happens in therapeutic intervention. Thus, connectionist models provide a means of testing the effect of individual differences and of treatment inputs on language performance.

The ultimate goal of connectionist methodology is to provide a sufficiency proof for a specific theory of cognitive function. One way to go about doing this is to develop a computer model that successfully simulates the behavior of a population of subjects on a particular task (e.g., normals' performance on a picture naming task). If one is then interested in understanding abnormal performance on that task due to brain damage, then the next step might be to "lesion" the normal model in some theoretically motivated way, corrupting the integrity of the model in such a way as to mimic the impairment. This may involve modifying or destroying "representations," the "connections" between them, or some parameter of the model. The effect of different manners and targets of corruption on processing efficacy is itself a theoretical and testable object of study. The simulation output can be compared and evaluated against that of the impaired individuals whose behavior one seeks to understand (e.g., anomic aphasics). The modeled theory gains support to the extent that the simulation performs similarly to these individuals' actual patterns of performance. This approach is illustrated in some detail below as we describe how we went about testing our own theory of word production (see also Bates, McDonald, MacWhinney, & Applebaum, 1991, for a similar approach).

Connectionism, then, provides an explicit description of functional process and representation that allows one to do "good science," for example, to make more precise predictions that can be objectively evaluated. The success of the undertaking is proportional to the degree to which performance by a computer model that incorporates the relevant properties of the theory matches human performance. The ultimate contribution of connectionism to clinical concerns may be that it is the only approach that actually ventures into the domain of prediction and control in a practical sense by including a provision for change and by providing an objective means of explicitly testing alternate treatment strategies.

Summary

At this point, it might be useful to summarize the types of questions that neuroanatomic, psycholinguistic, and connectionist models are capable of addressing. From a neuroanatomic perspective, one might ask: What are the behavioral symptoms of language disorder and how do they tend to co-occur across patients? What is the relationship between syndrome and neural anatomy? Functional information flow models ask which functional component is affected in producing disordered behavior and thus, answer the question of which behavior should be targeted in treatment, but offer no specific treatment suggestions. Structure- and function-based models address questions of "what" and "which." The answers to these questions are summarized in Table 3.1 for the major aphasic syndromes. Connectionism,

TABLE 3.1

The Classic Aphasia Syndromes, Clinical Profiles, Locus of Functional Deficit, and Locus of Structural Damage

Syndrome	Clinical Profile	Locus of Functional Deficit	Locus of Structural Damage
Broca's Aphasia	"Telegraphic speech"; missing function words & grammatical morphemes; often accompanied by articulatory difficulties	Speech stage (planning & production)	3rd frontal convolution; precentral gyrus
Wernicke's Aphasia	Fluent speech with phonemic, morphemic, & semantic paraphasias; impaired auditory comprehension	Phonological output lexicon	1st temporal gyrus
Anomic Aphasia	Word finding difficulty, primarily for nouns	Semantic and/or phonological systems	Inferior parietal lobe, or connections between parietal & temporal lobes
Global Aphasia	Disturbance of all language functions	All stages of language production	Perisylvian association cortex
Conduction Aphasia	Phonemic paraphasias in spontaneous speech & repetition	Disconnection between phonological & speech production stages	Arcuate fasciculus, and/or connections between frontal & temporal lobes

on the other hand, answers the "how" questions. How are representations accessed and connected with other representations? How do behaviors evolve? How shall we treat a disorder? Practical treatment questions that a traditional functional approach cannot address but that a connectionist model can address include: What is the best means of training to promote generalization? Is it better to stimulate with central exemplars of a category or more distant exemplars (cf. Plaut, 1996)? Is it better to provide a treatment context rich with close lexical competitors or a context sparse with respect to lexical competitors (Laine & Martin, 1996)? Connectionism offers a means of studying language retraining and relearning, which may be, ultimately, what language remediation is really all about.

Although we have been arguing for the superiority of connectionist models in meeting the needs of therapists, we do not wish to discredit the merits of the other approaches. As Dell et al. (1997, p. 832–833) state,

> Models in the cognitive neuropsychology of language can, at least in principle, range from purely functional information processing models to neural models. In our view, theory is advanced by the construction of models at many places along this range, and by considering their relationships.... Rather than consider models (at different levels) to be strict competitors... one should consider how their advantages might complement one another.

The same statement can be generalized to structural models as well, since these certainly generated a great deal of study and understanding that has led the field to its present position of trying to understand the relationship between structure and function. But this exceeds the scope of our present discussion. We move now to considering a particular connectionist model that aims to describe both normal and disordered word production. This model lies closer to the information-processing end in the range of cognitive neuropsychological models.

A CONNECTIONIST ACCOUNT OF ACQUIRED NAMING DISORDER

Description and Explanation

We are now ready to consider a specific example of how connectionist modeling can aid in understanding and treating a particular form of language deficit. In this example, the deficit of interest is acquired naming disorder. The model that is described is a model of lexical retrieval that offers an explanation for both normal and aphasic performance in single word production as observed in a confrontation–picture naming task.

Difficulty in retrieving words (anomia) is a pervasive symptom of aphasia. Most current functional theories assume that word retrieval is a two-step process (Kempen & Huijbers, 1983; Levelt, 1989). In the first step, a word's semantic specification is retrieved from memory; at the second stage, its phonology is retrieved. The detail of how information is retrieved at each step varies across theories, but this basic two-stage conception of word retrieval is almost universally accepted because the support for it is overwhelming. Evidence comes in the form of:

- *speech errors* that are strictly semantically related to targets or strictly phonologically related to targets (e.g., Garrett, 1980)
- *priming experiments* that reveal a time period during word retrieval when only semantic information about the word is available and another when only phonological information is available (e.g., Schriefers, Meyer, & Levelt, 1990)
- *tip-of-the-tongue phenomena* (e.g., Badecker, Miozzo, & Zanuttini, 1995; Meyer & Bock, 1992)
- *experimental studies* of multiword utterances (Ferreira, 1993; Kempen & Huijbers, 1983; Meyer, 1994; Schriefers, 1992).

When individuals with anomic tendencies attempt to name objects, the nature of their errors tends to vary. The errors of some individuals may be marked by a prevalence of semantic errors (giraffe —> elephant) or formal errors (squirrel —> school), others may tend to produce unrelated responses (frog —> bowl), some may make many neologistic errors (octopus —> /saktapul/), and still others may have a tendency to produce mixed errors (errors that share a semantic and phonological relationship to the target, e.g., skeleton —> skull). Most tend to make some combination of these five error types, but it is important to note that not all combinations are equally likely and that some are predicted not to occur at all by the model. We will return to this point later. The more immediate questions that arise are: Why do individuals vary in the nature of their responses? and What determines the types of response a particular individual will make?

A classic structuralist (localist) explanation of such individual differences is that there are distinct areas of the brain that contain either semantic information or phonological information about words, so that a lesion could affect one or the other or some combination of these areas to result in a particular pattern of response. Using this rationale, a strict structuralist explanation would be hard pressed to explain normals' speech errors because normals, by definition, are without lesion. Neuroanatomic models embrace a noncontinuity assumption, that is, neural damage should produce a fundamentally and qualitatively different system than that found in normals. The traditional functional perspective allows for continuity between disordered and ordered systems, but it lacks the specificity to describe how such continuity may be achieved.

The model that we and our colleagues developed (Dell et al., 1997; Schwartz et al., 1994) adopts a continuity stance and provides a connectionist account of the variety of patients' error patterns. The following steps were taken in developing and testing this model. First, a simulation model of normals' single word production performance was developed. Normals' speech errors were systematically collected from the *Philadelphia Naming Test*, a confrontation–picture naming test consisting of 175 picturable objects (Roach, Schwartz, Martin, Grewal, & Brecher, 1996). Sixty normal subjects (defined as having no speech or hearing impairment) were tested. By and large, their responses were correct, but these subjects did make a few of the five types of errors mentioned previously. The proportion of responses that correspond to the 6 response types (correct plus 5 error types) across our 60 normal subjects is provided in Table 3.2. This response pattern formed the basis for parameterizing the computer model. "Parameterizing" means specifying, in quantitative terms, the representations and processes of the cognitive architecture (structure) within a computer model.

The theoretical model contains three levels of representation (see Fig. 3.2): semantic, lexical, and phonological. Each level contains "units" representing semantic features, lexical items, and phonemes, respectively. The instantiated model consists of only 10 semantic units, 5 lexical units, and 9 phonological units. A reduced model was necessary for practical computational reasons that are not useful to go into here, but it is important to know that the units were very carefully chosen so that the random output of the model would reflect the real-world opportunities for the five error types to occur.[2] In Fig. 3.2, the target word is "cat," and the other four

TABLE 3.2
Naming Data from 60 Control Subjects and Simulated Probabilities
(Dell et al., 1997)

	Response Category					
	Correct	Semantic	Formal	Nonword	Mixed	Unrelated
Data from controls	0.969	0.012	0.001	0.000	0.009	0.003
Simulated probabilities	0.966	0.021	0.000	0.001	0.012	0.000

.6% of all responses were descriptions or no responses.

Permissions Info: Table 4 (p. 811) in Dell, G. S., Schwartz, M. F., Martin, N., Saffran, E. M., & Gagnon, D. A. (1997). Lexical access in aphasic and nonaphasic speakers. *Psychological Review, 104*, 801–838.

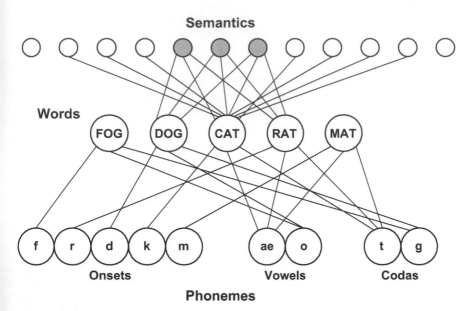

FIG. 3.2.   The Dell et al. (1997) model of lexical retrieval. (Permissions Info:
Figure 1 (p. 805) in Dell, G. S., Schwartz, M. F., Martin, N., Saffran, E. M.,
& Gagnon, D. A. (1997). Lexical access in aphasic and nonaphasic speakers.
Psychological Review, 104, 801–838.)

lexical items in the model represent items that are semantically related
("dog"), formally related ("mat"), mixed ("rat"), and unrelated ("fog"). A
neologism results from the substitution of a phoneme unit at the phonological level, for example /l/ replacing /k/ to produce "lat."

Naming in this model consists of activating the ten semantic units corresponding to "cat." "Activating," in computational terms, simply means
boosting the numerical value of the unit in question. The units at each level
in the model are connected via facilitatory links to those they correspond
to at the next level. "Facilitating," in computational terms, simply means
increasing the numerical value of the receiving unit. The activation from
the semantic units is said to spread to the lexical node for "cat"; as well,
the unit for "dog" becomes somewhat activated because it shares three out
of the ten semantic units with "cat." Spreading activation is implemented
in the computer simulation via a computational equation that takes into
account the size of the initial activation jolt, the number of time steps that
have elapsed, the amount of intrinsic "noise" (random perturbations) in
the system, the connection strength between the sending and receiving
units, and the decay rate (how quickly a unit reverts back to a resting level
of activation) of the units.

After a set number of time steps during which activation has been allowed to spread, the lexical unit with the highest activation level is chosen for production. Being "chosen" in the simulation means that activation of all units is set to zero and the selected unit receives a "jolt" of activation, just as the semantic units had previously. This activation is again allowed to spread for a given number of time steps down to the phonological units. Again, after the specified time period, the most highly activated phonemes are selected for production.

It was noted above that theorists by and large agree on a two-step conception of word retrieval but differ in the particulars. One way in which they differ is in how activation spreading between levels is conceived. So far, we have described a model in which activation is only allowed to spread in a forward direction. In fact, our model also allows for activation to spread backward, from lexical to semantic units and from phonological to lexical units. There are theoretical motivations for this feature of the model that again go beyond the present discussion. The effect of this feedback, however, is to promote formal and mixed errors. Feedback from phonemes to the lexical level increases the activation of lexical items to the extent they contain these phonemes and increases the likelihood that an item phonologically related to the target (formal or mixed error) will be chosen for production.

The simulation of normal performance consisted of repeating the procedure described above (applying activation to semantic units, selecting lexical units, selecting phoneme units) a total of 1,000 times. The resulting response pattern across these 1,000 trials is provided in Table 3.2 (the model cannot produce a "description" or "no response"). Although there are slight differences, by and large the model closely reproduced normals' actual response patterns. Thus, we were satisfied that the model captures the important and relevant aspects of normals' word retrieval. The primary determinant of normals' errors in the model is "noise" (random perturbations of activation across units); because noise is random, it is possible on any given trial that the wrong lexical unit will have a higher activation value than the target unit at the time of selection and an error will be committed. In normal speakers, as we have seen, naming errors are rare. In the model, this is because the balance between connection strength and decay rate is optimal.

Next, we sought to simulate aphasic performance on the same task, in which the proportion of incorrect responses is much higher. We tested 23 aphasic patients on the same naming test and determined the proportion of their responses corresponding to each of the six response types. The response patterns of 21 of these patients are provided in Table 3.3 (first row for each patient).[3] We wondered whether our model could successfully simulate each of the patients' patterns. Note that the considerable variation

TABLE 3.3

Naming Data and Predictions (Dell et al., 1997). The First Row for Each
Patient Shows the Proportions Obtained, the Second Row, the
Proportions Predicted

Patient	Naming Response						RMSD
	Correct	Semantic	Formal	Nonword	Mixed	Unrelated	
W. B.	0.94	0.02	0.01	0.01	0.01	0.00	
	0.93	0.04	0.01	0.02	0.01	0.00	0.010
T. T.	0.93	0.01	0.01	0.00	0.02	0.00	
	0.93	0.04	0.01	0.02	0.01	0.00	0.015
J. Fr.	0.92	0.01	0.01	0.02	0.02	0.00	
	0.93	0.04	0.01	0.02	0.01	0.00	0.014
V. C.	0.87	0.02	0.01	0.03	0.01	0.00	
	0.88	0.05	0.02	0.04	0.01	0.00	0.014
L. B.	0.82	0.04	0.02	0.09	0.01	0.01	
	0.82	0.04	0.03	0.08	0.01	0.02	0.007
J. B.	0.76	0.06	0.01	0.05	0.02	0.01	
	0.78	0.06	0.04	0.08	0.01	0.03	0.021
J. L.	0.76	0.03	0.01	0.06	0.03	0.01	
	0.83	0.06	0.03	0.06	0.01	0.01	0.033
G. S.	0.70	0.02	0.06	0.15	0.01	0.02	
	0.69	0.07	0.06	0.14	0.01	0.03	0.022
L. H.	0.69	0.03	0.07	0.15	0.01	0.02	
	0.69	0.07	0.06	0.14	0.01	0.03	0.018
J. G.	0.55	0.06	0.08	0.18	0.04	0.03	
	0.57	0.10	0.11	0.16	0.02	0.04	0.025
E. G.	0.93	0.03	0.00	0.01	0.02	0.00	
	0.95	0.03	0.00	0.00	0.02	0.00	0.009
B. Me.	0.84	0.03	0.01	0.00	0.05	0.01	
	0.85	0.09	0.01	0.02	0.03	0.00	0.028
B. Mi.	0.83	0.05	0.01	0.01	0.02	0.01	
	0.84	0.08	0.02	0.03	0.02	0.01	0.016
J. A.	0.78	0.04	0.00	0.02	0.03	0.01	
	0.89	0.07	0.01	0.02	0.02	0.00	0.047
A. F.	0.75	0.02	0.03	0.07	0.06	0.04	
	0.77	0.11	0.03	0.05	0.04	0.00	0.043
N. C.	0.75	0.03	0.07	0.08	0.01	0.00	
	0.77	0.11	0.03	0.05	0.04	0.00	0.041
I. G.	0.69	0.09	0.05	0.02	0.03	0.01	
	0.73	0.13	0.04	0.05	0.04	0.01	0.027
H. B.	0.61	0.06	0.13	0.18	0.02	0.01	
	0.59	0.11	0.11	0.14	0.02	0.03	0.030

(Continued)

164

TABLE 3.3
(Continued)

			Naming Response				
ent	*Correct*	*Semantic*	*Formal*	*Nonword*	*Mixed*	*Unrelated*	*RMSD*
	0.56	0.14	0.01	0.02	0.11	0.01	
	0.73	0.13	0.04	0.05	0.04	0.01	0.077
..	0.28	0.04	0.21	0.30	0.03	0.09	
	0.27	0.11	0.20	0.29	0.03	0.10	0.030
R.	0.08	0.06	0.15	0.28	0.05	0.33	
	0.18	0.09	0.20	0.37	0.03	0.13	0.102

across patients' response patterns indicates that this would be a stringent test of the model.

In order to simulate the effect of neural damage, we had to theoretically motivate what "lesioning" the model means. Parsimony motivates an account of all patterns of naming responses by manipulating the fewest number of these parameters. Toward this end, we chose to modify just two parameters: connection strength and decay rate. Connection strength can be thought of as how strongly connected units at different levels of the system are. Decay rate can be thought of as an indication of the representational integrity of units, or how long they remain activated. We hypothesized that pathological values of connection strength and decay rate would have different implications for the types of naming errors produced. In the case of a pathologically high decay rate, we would expect feedback activation to play a greater role in determining which lexical unit becomes selected. This is because feedback takes time; if lexical activation is decaying too rapidly, then the activation returning from the phoneme level should play a larger role in determining which lexical item gets selected, resulting in greater-than-expected rates of formal and mixed errors that tend to be promoted by such feedback. Pathological connection strength implies something different: Units are not as well connected to those units at other levels that are consistent with them. Thus, we should see more "nonsensical" errors in patients with this type of deficit (e.g., unrelated and nonword errors that bear little or no semantic or phonological relationship to the target word). Note that the "lesions" in this model cannot be mapped onto a neural lesion site: The question in this type of model is not where the lesion is located but rather, what type of dysfunction (processing damage) is incurred. Also, the lesions are global in that they affect all units, levels, and connections equally. In contrast, a local lesion would be one that affected, for example, the connection weight between lexical and phoneme units but not between semantic and lexical, or decay rate of lexical units to the exclusion of semantic and phonemic units.

For each patient, we tested various combinations of connection strength and decay rate values (keeping all other parameter values at normal levels) in the computer model to obtain the best fit to each patient's actual pattern of responses (cf. second row for each patient in Table 3.3). We did this in exactly the same way we had for the normal patterns, only for each patient individually. From this exercise, we discovered that the full range of variation among patients' response patterns could be captured from varying just these two parameters (compare first and second rows for each patient in Table 3.3). Importantly, those patients characterized with a connection strength "lesion" (patients W. B. through J. G. in Table 3.3) had proportionally more unrelated and neologistic responses; those patients characterized as having a decay rate "lesion" (patients E. G. through W. R. in Table 3.3) were seen to have proportionally more phonological and mixed errors. The root mean square deviation (RMSD) for each patient in the right-hand column of Table 3.3 gives an indication of the degree of "fit" (similarity) between the actual and the simulated response patterns. Using a chance estimation procedure (cf. Dell et al., 1997), it was determined that a RMSD value smaller than .22 was indicative of a good actual-simulated fit. All of our patients were fit substantially better than chance (Median: .026; Range: .007–.102); not even our most poorly fit patient (W. R.) came close to the .22 criteria. Thus, overall, the fits of the simulation patterns to the patient patterns were quite good.

Prediction

The model fits the patients' response patterns well, but can it predict things we did not already know about them? For example, can it predict how the pattern of responses will evolve as a patient recovers from his or her initial deficit? We made the theoretical claim that recovery should mean movement back toward the normal pattern of responses (see also Harley & MacAndrew, 1992; Martin et al., 1994) and that the type of lesion a patient has (connection weight or decay rate) should not change during the course of recovery. In other words, a decay rate patient should remain a decay rate patient so that, for example, the proportion of formal and mixed errors should decrease without seeing a corresponding increase in neologistic or unrelated responses (i.e., the emergence of a connection strength pattern). To test this claim, we administered the same naming test to ten of the original patients within nine months of the original test (Median: 3 months; Range: 1.5–9 months). Using the modeled parameter

TABLE 3.4
Recovered Naming and Predictions (Dell et al., 1997)

Patient	Correct	Semantic	Formal	Nonword	Mixed	Unrelated	RMSD
			Naming Response				
J. B.	0.87	0.01	0.01	0.03	0.03	0.00	
	0.89	0.04	0.01	0.04	0.01	0.00	0.018
A. F.	0.94	0.01	0.01	0.02	0.02	0.01	
	0.94	0.03	0.01	0.02	0.00	0.00	0.012
G. S.	0.91	0.00	0.02	0.05	0.01	0.00	
	0.91	0.04	0.01	0.03	0.01	0.00	0.019
L. H.	0.76	0.01	0.09	0.10	0.02	0.01	
	0.78	0.06	0.04	0.08	0.01	0.03	0.032
J. G.	0.90	0.02	0.01	0.03	0.03	0.00	
	0.91	0.04	0.01	0.03	0.01	0.00	0.012
H. B.	0.75	0.05	0.06	0.09	0.02	0.01	
	0.75	0.09	0.05	0.07	0.02	0.02	0.019
J. F.	0.74	0.09	0.01	0.02	0.09	0.02	
	0.77	0.11	0.03	0.05	0.04	0.00	0.030
G. L.	0.36	0.02	0.19	0.32	0.03	0.03	
	0.35	0.10	0.17	0.28	0.02	0.08	0.043
W. R.	0.19	0.08	0.21	0.19	0.01	0.26	
	0.18	0.09	0.20	0.37	0.03	0.13	0.092
J. L.	0.96	0.02	0.01	0.01	0.01	0.00	
	0.97	0.02	0.00	0.00	0.01	0.00	0.007

values for each patient, the model was allowed to evolve to mimic recovery in naming. Comparing the resulting pattern to patients' actual recovery patterns (Table 3.4), RMSD values indicate that the model was again successful in simulating response patterns (Median: .019; Range: .007–.092). More important, the patterns support the assumption that disordered response patterns would migrate back toward the normal pattern and that patients would, by and large, maintain their connection strength or decay rate "diagnosis": Eight patients retained the same "diagnosis" and one (J. L.) recovered to a normal level of performance. Only one patient (A. F.) changed from a decay rate response pattern to a connection strength response pattern, though this patient recovered to a very high level of correctness (94%) where differences between the two patterns are minimal and reliable predictions would be very difficult to make.

Thus, our model is able to predict performance over time (see also Harley, 1996, for discussion on recovery of language function in terms of a connectionist model). What about performance across tasks? To test this, 11 of the original patients were asked to participate in a repetition task using the same target names from the naming test. Again, response patterns were determined for each patient. Using his or her original connection strength and decay rate parameter settings, we then simulated repetition performance by activating lexical-level units directly (assuming perfect input from the phonological level) and running the simulation as before. Simulation response patterns were compared to actual repetition patterns (Table 3.5) and, again, RMSD values indicate these were quite similar (with the exception of W. R.; Median: .024; Range: .000–.273).

TABLE 3.5
Single Word Repetition and Predictions (Dell et al., 1997)

Patient	Correct	Semantic	Formal	Nonword	Mixed	Unrelated	RMSD
			Repetition Response				
T. T.	0.98	0.00	0.02	0.00	0.00	0.00	
	0.97	0.00	0.01	0.02	0.00	0.00	0.010
V. C.	0.95	0.00	0.01	0.04	0.00	0.00	
	0.95	0.00	0.01	0.04	0.00	0.00	0.000
L. B.	0.91	0.00	0.03	0.06	0.00	0.00	
	0.90	0.00	0.02	0.08	0.00	0.00	0.010
J. L.	0.89	0.00	0.02	0.03	0.00	0.00	
	0.92	0.00	0.02	0.05	0.00	0.00	0.015
J. G.	0.91	0.00	0.02	0.05	0.01	0.01	
	0.75	0.00	0.07	0.17	0.01	0.00	0.084
E. G.	0.94	0.00	0.03	0.01	0.00	0.00	
	0.99	0.00	0.00	0.00	0.00	0.00	0.024
B. Mi.	1.00	0.00	0.00	0.00	0.00	0.00	
	0.95	0.00	0.02	0.03	0.01	0.00	0.025
J. A.	0.90	0.00	0.02	0.08	0.00	0.00	
	0.97	0.00	0.01	0.02	0.00	0.00	0.038
I. G.	0.95	0.00	0.02	0.02	0.00	0.01	
	0.89	0.00	0.03	0.05	0.02	0.00	0.029
J. F.	0.94	0.00	0.02	0.03	0.01	0.00	
	0.89	0.00	0.03	0.05	0.02	0.00	0.023
W. R.	0.90	0.00	0.03	0.06	0.01	0.00	
	0.36	0.00	0.19	0.42	0.03	0.00	0.273

Permissions Info: Table 10 (p. 827) in Dell, G. S., Schwartz, M. F., Martin, N., Saffran, E. M., & Gagnon, D. A. (1997). Lexical access in aphasic and nonaphasic speakers. *Psychological Review, 104*, 801–838.

Summary

In conclusion, the model apparently captures normal and aphasic subjects' naming behavior quite well and is capable of predicting changes in performance both over time and tasks. Within the model, an anomic aphasic may have a deficit in activation transmission (determined by connection strength) and/or representational integrity (determined by decay rate). Note that this is a very different explanation of pathology than the one provided by a structural or even a traditional functional view. The deficit is described neither in terms of neural locus nor general functional loss. Instead, the deficit is described in terms of a very specific functional loss. In fact, both representation and process are so explicit as to be instantiatable in a computer simulation.

At this point, we believe that parameter lesions offer a better account of the underlying impairment common to members of a subgroup than traditional classifications have because they better serve a predictive function. A question we have not yet delved into is how well the parameter subgroups correlate with the classic syndrome categories: How do the parameter diagnoses relate to traditional aphasia diagnoses, if at all? Another interesting exercise would be to reverse the direction of prediction and use the model to predict a cluster of response patterns that are not represented in our current group of patients. Such patients should, in theory, exist. The model also predicts that certain response patterns should never be observed (e.g., a coupling of high neologism rate with high semantic rate), leading to a potential means of falsifying the theory. Finally, with regard to recovery, a few questions still remain, including: What is the rate of approach to the normal pattern? And what determines the point at which recovery towards the normal pattern stops? These are questions that neither a structuralist nor a traditional functionalist approach could ever hope to answer.

The success of the modeling exercise supports certain key features and assumptions of our theory: (1) interactivity, (2) continuity, and (3) globality. Interactivity refers to the way in which units are connected between levels. In our model, these connections are bidirectional: Activation flows both forward and backward between levels. Continuity was discussed briefly earlier and is perhaps the most relevant to clinical interests. Continuity pertains to whether normal and aphasic language performance falls along a continuum. This is not just a theoretical issue; the answer bears on the question of whether remediation of language function is even worthwhile. For if aphasia involves a qualitatively different way of processing language, then it may be futile to attempt retraining to a normal level of function; it may make more sense to develop alternative, or augmentative, means of communication. The Dell et al. (1997) work supports the notion that normal and aphasic language behavior is continuous and thus, that retraining is useful. Aphasic behavior was simulated from only quantitative parameter changes to the normal model; no qualitative architectural modifications were made. Also, resulting behaviors were not qualitatively different, only quantitatively different; both types of subjects made similar errors and the pattern of their errors were predictable if one assumed continuity. Globality refers to the extensiveness of the parameter variations: Are changes made to only certain units and/or certain levels? Or are they applied equally to all units and/or all connections? We were able to successfully simulate aphasic naming patterns by making global parameter changes to just two parameters: connection strength and decay rate. Although this seems to support the notion that brain injury exerts a global influence, we expect more extensive tests of the model to discredit this view (see Dell et al., 1997, for discussion). At the moment, we consider this feature of the modeling exercise to be a simplifying assumption, but also one that just so happens to work, so far.

Methodologically, the Dell et al. (1997) model makes a unique contribution in that it represents an attempt to simulate the performance of individuals instead of groups of patients or syndromes (see also Bates et al., 1991). The model's fits of the patients were used to test predictions about their behavior on other tasks and at future times. They were also used to group subjects, forming the basis for classification and analysis of group data. Finally, the very success of the effort confirms its value. It is now possible to see why connectionism provides a more useful understanding of disorder. Next, we turn to applications of connectionism in fulfilling the final goal of therapy and theory: control.

CONNECTIONIST THEORY-INTO-THERAPY

Control

A claim of the functionalist school is that its approach will be more useful to the treatment of language disorder than the structuralist school's approach has been. Applying functional theory to therapy has been a challenge, however, and so far, model-based deficit analyses have had little impact on the development of actual treatment techniques (Hillis, 1993a; Howard & Patterson, 1989). Connectionism, which offers a more specific and dynamic form of functionalism, seems poised to fulfill this practical function. In this section, we describe how empirical tests of a connectionist model of picture naming have formed the basis for what appears to be a promising treatment procedure for anomia (Laine & Martin, 1996; Martin & Laine, 2000; Martin, Laine, & Lowery, 1996).

A study by Laine and Martin (1996) provides the background for our story. The motive for this study was to provide support for the interactive nature of lexical retrieval processes. As described previously, interactivity refers to the nature of information flow between levels in a processing system. Activation can either travel in a forward direction only (e.g., semantic to lexical to phonological) or it can flow both forward and backward (e.g., phonological to lexical to semantic). Moreover, activation can cascade from one level to another, that is, flow from one level to the next before processing is completed at the earlier stage; or it can flow in a discrete fashion, that is, transmit activation to the next level only after processing is finished at the current level. The nondiscrete versus discrete nature of cognitive systems is a topic of great interest to theorists. In particular, whether levels of representation are "encapsulated" resulting in modular, discrete processing components, or whether levels are nondiscrete such that different levels of representation are active at the same time, is of great theoretical import and bears strongly on how one views the cognitive architecture in general.

Laine and Martin used a modified version of a multitarget naming task developed by Martin, Weisberg, & Saffran (1989) for their study. In Martin et al. (1989), subjects were provided with a matrix of six pictured objects and asked to name the objects while verbally navigating the matrix (see Fig. 3.3). The subject's task would be to start at a designated location, name the object at that location, verbally indicate where the next object on the path was located, name it, and so on. The purpose of this procedure was to obtain naming samples within the context of spontaneously produced speech, while limiting the complexity of semantic and syntactic contexts (Levelt, 1983). A typical response follows (prompted by a matrix with the same objects as in Fig. 3.3, but in a different configuration):

> We're gonna start on the top row, right hand corner, we have a blue tie . . . a blue scarf. Two below the scarf, we have a picture of a yellow glove. Diagonally up two blocks to the left, we have a picture of a yellow boot. Two blocks below the boot, we have a picture of a orange scar . . . s . . . sweater. Diagonally up a block to the left hand side, we have a picture of a blue necktie. Below the necktie, we have a picture of a green sock. (Martin et al., 1989)

The critical manipulation in the Martin et al. (1989) study was the nature of the relationship between objects in the matrix. These relationships were of three types: Objects could share a semantic relationship to one another (e.g., house, church, barn, store, tent, castle), a phonological relationship (e.g., school, skull, square, scale, screw, squirrel), or no identifiable relationship (e.g., hand, car, watch, pencil, banana, zebra). Two additional "mixed" conditions combined objects that were semantically related with one half also sharing a phonological relationship (e.g., boot, glove, necktie, sock, scarf, sweater) and objects that were phonologically related with one half

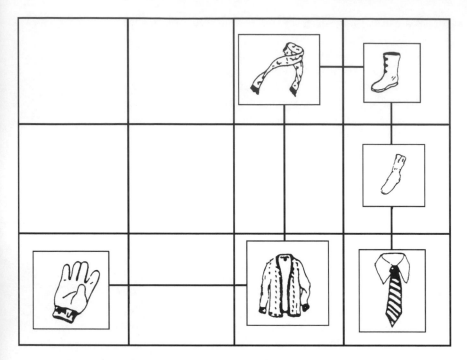

FIG. 3.3. Sample matrix from Martin, Weisberg, and Saffran (1989). (Permissions Info: Figure 3 (p. 473) in Martin, N., Weisberg, R. W., & Saffran, E. M. (1989). Variables influencing the occurrence of naming errors: Implications for models of lexical retrieval. *Journal of Memory and Language, 28,* 462–485.)

also sharing a semantic relationship (e.g., cannon, candle, camel, candy, cabbage, carrot). The measures of interest were the error rates across these conditions and the nature of subjects' errors when a nontarget name was given. Errors that were phonologically related to the target (e.g., the target is "school" and the subject says "square" or "squid"), semantically related (e.g., target is "boot" and subject says "glove" or "hat"), or had a mixed relationship to the target (e.g., target is "sock" and subject says "scarf" or "slipper") were of particular interest. Related substitutions such as these indicate an influence of lexical competitors at the level of processing at which the target and response are related.

Martin et al. (1989) predicted that if semantic, lexical, and phonological levels are independent of one another (i.e., processing between them is discrete), then the probability of making a mixed error (lexical item that is both semantically and phonologically related to the target) should be no greater than chance, that is, the probability of a semantic error being phonologically related to the target plus the probability of a phonological error being semantically related to the target. This is because in a discrete model, a mixed error has two opportunities to arise: once at the phonological level and once at the semantic level. If levels are nonindependent (i.e., nondiscrete), then the probability of making a mixed error should be greater than chance; that is, the probability of a mixed error should be compounded due to the interacting semantic and phonological influences. This prediction could be tested using this procedure by comparing the proportion of mixed errors in the "mixed" conditions to the summed probability of such errors in the semantic only condition and the phonological only condition. To make a long story short, Martin et al. (1989) found the evidence they were looking for—the incidence of mixed errors in the mixed condition was greater than the sum of the incidence in semantic only and phonological only conditions—thus supporting the nondiscrete type of information flow model.

Subjects in the Martin et al. (1989) study had been unimpaired speakers. Laine and Martin (1996) suggested that applying the multitarget naming procedure to an anomic subject might be informative on the discreteness issue as well. They combined the multitarget naming procedure with a repetition priming procedure for use with an anomic patient, I. L., who had been extensively evaluated in a prior study using the type of function-based deficit analysis that was described above (Laine, Kujala, Niemi, & Uusipaikka, 1992). In naming, I. L. provided semantic descriptions and circumlocutions and made few semantic errors, but was impaired in actually providing the verbal names for objects. This situation is very similar to the tip-of-the-tongue state we all are familiar with in which one has access to a word's meaning but not its sound structure (aside from perhaps initial sounds). Furthermore, I. L. could accurately repeat words that were spoken to her, including those she could not use in naming, and made few phonemic paraphasias. Thus, it appeared that both semantic and phonological information about words were intact, but that I. L. had an inability to retrieve the phonological specification of words from their semantics. In terms of Fig. 3.1, it was the link between the semantic system and the phonological output lexicon that was in question for I. L. Because the discrete versus nondiscrete views have very different predictions as to how I. L. would perform in naming, Laine and Martin (1996) studied her performance on this task in order to shed further light on the issue.

I. L. participated in a modified version of the multitarget naming task. The procedure varied from that used by Martin et al. (1989) in a couple of important ways. First, an additional "mixed" condition was included in which all six objects in the array were both semantically and phonologically related. In this study, Laine and Martin (1996) were not only interested in testing the rate of mixed errors relative to semantic errors and phonological errors, they were also interested in determining whether multidimensional overlap would have a facilitative or a detrimental effect on I. L.'s naming performance. Second, I. L. was provided with training. Instead of simply verbally navigating a matrix as normal subjects had done, testing began with I. L. naming each item that the experimenter pointed to, in order to establish her baseline naming performance. Then, the examiner would point to each object, name it, and ask I. L. to repeat the name. Training involved repeating this procedure four times. Following training, I. L. was again asked to name each object the experimenter pointed to, to obtain a posttraining measure of naming.

In short, Laine and Martin (1996) again found support from I. L.'s error patterns for the nondiscrete type of model they favor. However, it is the implication of the repetition training procedure used that is most pertinent to the present discussion. Though not intended to be a therapy study, Laine and Martin (1996) noted that their findings have implications for the design of treatments for anomia. First, the training procedure had a definite impact on the nature of I. L.'s naming responses. Before training, most of her responses were semantic circumlocutions. Following training, her responses evolved toward word errors of either the contextual (nontarget items in the matrix) or noncontextual (nontarget items not found in the matrix) variety. In other words, I. L.'s errors evolved toward responses that could be considered more "on target." Also, her nonword responses were phonological approximations to the target word, indicating successful lexical access. Second, there was an apparent effect of lexical context—the nature of the relationship among the array objects—on the nature of I. L.'s naming errors. Semantic relatedness among an array of objects, for instance, decreased the rate of noncontextual, phonologically related errors produced. The implication is that such implicit training techniques could be used in therapy in addition to the use of explicit retraining of semantic-phonological relationships.

Two implications of the Laine and Martin (1996) findings are of particular note with regard to a connectionist viewpoint. Laine and Martin note that nondiscrete processing, of which they obtained evidence, imparts a dynamic character to lexical retrieval. Connectionism, we have argued, makes the dynamics of lexical retrieval more explicit. There can be no doubt that a connectionist perspective, with its focus on specificity and dynamics, will be helpful in illuminating the effects of the training procedure. Second, an implemented connectionist model would open up to exploration the effect of lexical context on naming errors, as well as the interaction of this factor with degree of aphasic severity and functional locus of deficit. We can ask the question of what types of objects to use in a procedure such as Laine and Martin's to achieve a particular change and expect an answer from a connectionist implementation.

Treatment of naming disorders often involves some kind of cue or verbal stimulation that presumably will facilitate retrieval of words that the patient can no longer independently retrieve in a consistent manner. This stimulation provides a context in which naming can occur. Some cues are directly related to the phonological form of the intended word (e.g., shared initial phonemes). Other cues facilitate retrieval of phonological form indirectly by stimulating the target word's semantic representation (e.g., Howard, Patterson, Franklin, Orchard-Lisle, & Morton, 1985; Le Dorze, Boulay, Gaudreau, & Brassard, 1994). Treatment research is directed toward several questions concerning the cues that facilitate naming. First, it is useful to know what kind of cues facilitate retrieval, that is, what kind of cue or context is immediately effective in eliciting production of a word. Equally important is the identification of cues that are neutral or detrimental to naming. Important dimensions include the size of the unit serving as a cue (word, sound, phrase), the relationship the cue holds to the target (phonological, semantic, identical), and the modality in which the cue is presented (auditorally, orthographically).

Once a cue or context is identified as facilitating, there are several further issues concerning the effectiveness of that treatment. How long will the cue's effect last? Duration can be measured as a function of time or number of intervening utterances. Most of the research to date indicates that although phonological cues are often immediately very effective, the effects are not enduring (e.g., Patterson, Purell, & Morton, 1983). Semantically based cues have longer lasting effects than treatments that stimulate the phonological form of a word (Howard et al., 1985), but are even more effective if they are combined with some sort of phonological stimulation (e.g., Le Dorze et al., 1994). Another important issue regarding treatment efficacy is the generalization of a facilitating effect. Will the effects of the cue generalize to untrained items? If so, what untrained items will be affected? Connectionist models can make very specific predictions about this issue. Most models presume that facilitating cues raise activation levels of the target word. Some models—connectionist models included—make the further assumption that facilitation extends to other related words via spreading activation. Thus, generalization effects should be expected primarily for related items (e.g., Plaut, 1996). Finally, it is important to consider that even though a cue may be facilitating for some patients, it may not be so for all patients. Presumably, a cue's effect will vary depending on the functional locus of a patient's deficit (e.g., semantically vs. phonologically based anomias). This means that a cue or context that is effective for one patient will not be universally effective for all patients with naming problems. Conversely, when a cue is demonstrated to be ineffective for one patient, it does not mean that it will not be effective in facilitating naming in another patient.

Most of the issues noted previously address dynamic aspects of language production. The overriding goal of treatment is to effect temporary or permanent change in accessibility of a word's representation. "Change" is the key word that signals the need for connectionist models. Although structural and functional models can inform us of what problems to treat in therapy, as noted earlier, they do not suggest "how" to promote change. The connectionist viewpoint has opened up a world of opportunities to answer some questions of very real concern to therapists. Martin and colleagues decided to focus on the questions of what type of cues facilitate word retrieval, how the effect of cue type interacts with anomia type, and how long a cue's effect lasts. Motivated by the treatment possibilities that Laine and Martin (1996) seemed to open up, Martin and Laine (2000) and Martin, Laine, and Lowery (1996) decided to study the facilitation of word retrieval more specifically using the Laine and Martin training and testing procedure on other anomic subjects. A primary goal of these experiments was to learn if the contextual priming technique would be useful as a means of treating word retrieval disorders. Let's see how Martin and colleagues used a connectionist-driven model to develop tests of these issues.

Relearning in a connectionist framework can be viewed as a strengthening of connections that were previously weakened by brain damage (Harley & MacAndrew, 1992; Martin et al., 1994). The effect of repetition training, on this view, is to strengthen connections between semantics and phonology for named objects. As a second step in exploring the effects of the contextual priming procedure used with I. L., Martin and Laine (2000) replicated the I. L. findings with two other patients. Like I. L., these patients had severe naming difficulty, but their underlying source of impairment differed from I. L. and from each other. Background testing determined that one subject, L. M., demonstrated adequate semantic processing but had difficulty in phonologically encoding words. The other subject, J. L., demonstrated a severe semantic impairment and difficulty in phonological encoding. Unlike I. L., both subjects produced phonological errors in naming. The aim of the replication was to see if effects of the type of context (semantic vs. phonological vs. mixed) depended on the underlying source of lexical retrieval impairment.

Measurements of contextual priming effects included rates of correct responses and contextual and noncontextual errors. Baseline measures prior to training indicated that both J. L. and L. M. were unable to name correctly most of the pictures in all conditions. Following training, the proportion of correct responses increased, but again, this varied depending on the relatedness context in which the repetition training procedure took place. Also, the rates of contextual and noncontextual word errors varied across conditions. Specific findings in the replication study include the following: For L. M., whose deficit primarily affected phonological encoding, the effect of a semantically related context on correctness was neutral (relative to the unrelated context) and the phonologically related context was detrimental. For J. L., who had both semantic and phonological impairment, the phonological context was clearly beneficial compared to the other contexts. These patterns of responses were an indication that sensitivity to contextual priming might involve an interaction of the source of lexical impairment (semantic vs. phonological) and the kind of lexical features shared among the trained items. Follow-up studies (discussed later) provide further evidence of this interaction.

As in the case of I. L., Martin and Laine (2000) also examined the effects of context on rates of contextual and noncontextual word errors. One effect that was observed in the case of I. L. was that semantically related contextual priming consistently reduced the rate of phonologically related noncontextual errors compared to other conditions. That is, phonologically related word errors from outside the set of trained items, which were common in unrelated and phonologically related conditions, were significantly reduced when pictures being trained shared only semantic features. In the replication study described earlier, this effect was also observed for both J. L. and L. M.

What do these measures indicate? Laine and Martin (1996) hypothesized that the general effect of repetition priming is to raise the activation of and thus make more accessible a subset of lexical representations relative to other representations in the network. Relatedness among the target set presumably promotes spreading activation among target word representations. Evidence for such spreading activation should come in three forms: increased number of correct responses, increased number of related contextual and noncontextual responses, and reduced number of unrelated noncontextual responses. The increase in correct responses and the contextual errors reflect increased activation of these items due to direct priming (by virtue of the training procedure) and spreading activation from the target to these related items (by virtue of their relation to the target). Noncontextual errors do not result directly from priming, but rather are a more pure measure of spreading activation from the target word to neighboring representations. Whether all three of these effects are observed probably depends on the severity of the impairment, but also, in part, on the locus of the impairment.[4]

For example, when a subject's impairment involves accessing or encoding phonological representations, phonological errors should be common in both unrelated and phonological contexts. In semantic contexts, however, three effects that indicate spreading activation among the word representations should be observed. First is the effect that was observed in all three patients: a reduction in phonologically related noncontextual errors. This may occur simply because activation spreading between the target and semantically related words is so much greater than any activation spreading between the target and phonologically related word representations, even if phonologically related errors are typically the most common response in other conditions. Second, we might also see an increase in semantically related noncontextual errors. This effect would be the clearest indication that the procedure has the effect of promoting spreading activation within the lexical network. Finally, we might see an increase in the rate of correct responses relative to the unrelated condition. This effect would be due to increased activation of the target because of the repetition priming plus feedback from primed semantically related word representations.

In a third study, Martin, Laine, and Lowery (1996) administered a modified version of the Laine and Martin (1996) procedure to three new anomic subjects. The procedure was modified to include immediate and delayed posttests to assess endurance of the contextual priming effect. Additionally, in the semantic context condition, several categories were tested. Of the three patients tested, one patient, G. L., demonstrated good semantic processing with impaired phonological abilities (both input and output). The other two subjects, W. R. and J. W., demonstrated good phonological abilities, but impaired semantics. For these three subjects the results suggest that the procedure is facilitative when the relationship context plays to the strength of the subject's word retrieval abilities. That is, when a subject has adequate semantic abilities, but impaired access to phonological representations, the semantic context is either neutral or mildly facilitating and the phonological context is detrimental. When a subject has impaired semantic processing, but adequate phonological processing abilities, the semantic context is detrimental and the phonological context is facilitating.

With respect to longevity effects, G. L. demonstrated long-term effects of the procedure. In a three month posttest, G. L. maintained all gains in naming ability that were evident just following treatment. Of the two semantically impaired subjects, only J. W. sustained improvements in naming that followed treatment, but his performance over time showed an unusual pattern. J. W.'s naming benefited remarkably when pictures were presented in a phonological context (all trained and nontrained items had the same initial phoneme). On the pretraining test, J. W. was only able to name 3 out of 15 pictures (collapsed over 3 training sets). On the final posttest given on the same day of each training session, he named correctly 11 out of 15 pictures. At the 48-hour posttest, however, J. W. named only 4 out of 15 pictures correctly, suggesting that the phonological context had no more than an immediate effect. However, when tested on these same items approximately 3 months following the training sessions, J. W. was able to name 10 of the 15 target pictures. It remains to be determined why gains made following training are maintained for some subjects but not others.

The results of these preliminary applications of the contextual priming procedure to a training program for naming leave us with some promise of the feasibility of such an approach, but also leave us with a number of questions. It does seem evident that the contextual priming procedure facilitates or inhibits naming depending on the type of impairment (i.e., locus of functional impairment) and the context being exploited (a semantic vs. phonological relation between pictures in a training set). The studies suggest an interaction between these two variables such that subjects are differentially sensitive to the type of context depending on the source of their naming impairment. For patients with semantic impairment, it appears that semantically unrelated contexts promote better naming performance. In some cases, phonological relationships help also. For those patients with phonological impairment, it appears that phonologically unrelated contexts promote better performance and in some cases, semantic relationships among the (phonologically unrelated) pictures appear to improve performance.

The "apparent" interactions described earlier need to be substantiated in future studies. Additionally, there are several considerations that may complicate the neatness of these predictions. First, the two semantically impaired patients showed category-specific effects of training in the semantic context conditions. That is, although semantically related sets generally proved detrimental to naming, they each showed excellent performance on at least one of the categories. The facilitating categories were not the same for each subject, so the effect cannot be attributed to item-specific factors. Also, the categories that were beneficial were of low frequency, while those categories that were problematic for the subjects were high in frequency. Thus, the effect cannot be tied to frequency of the items in the target set. A second factor to consider is the effect may vary depending on the type of processing impairment as described by Dell et al. (1997). It may be the case that the effect is facilitating if the processing impairment is due to slowed activation but detrimental when the processing difficulty involves rapid decay of activation. Both of these factors—locus of impairment (semantic or phonological) and type of processing impairment (premature decay and slowed activation)—are being considered in future investigations using the contextual priming procedure.

Martin and colleagues are not alone in adopting a connectionist orientation toward treatment. For instance, Plaut and Shallice (1993), using a connectionist model of deep dyslexia (Hinton & Shallice, 1991), examined different rehabilitation strategies and discovered a dependency on lesion site in relearning and generalization. Plaut (1996) also demonstrated the efficacy of a counterintuitive stimulation technique in treating anomia with the aid of a connectionist model. Namely, using computer simulation, he predicted that stimulating with peripheral category members (e.g., for birds: penguin, rooster, ostrich, kiwi) would result in better relearning and generalization of naming than stimulating with more central category members (e.g., for birds: robin, canary, finch, wren).

Before closing this section, we discuss the results of two additional studies whose results may be interpreted within a connectionist framework as well. The first regards a cuing treatment procedure developed by Aurginac and Saffran (1996). Most work with explicit phonological cuing techniques (i.e., the patient is aware of being presented with a cue) indicates that initial phoneme cues work best in aiding aphasics' lexical retrieval. The strong preservation of initial phonemes in tip-of-the-tongue phenomena and speech errors indicates that initial phonemes must be represented particularly strongly in lexical representation and easily explains the initial phoneme cuing effect. Initial phoneme cues may work best, however, under conditions in which the cue is actively used in lexical search; in that case, initial phoneme cues correspond to a particularly salient part of the lexical address. But what happens when the subject is not aware of using a cue in lexical search? Aurignac and Saffran (1996) found that under such implicit cuing conditions, the final phonemes were actually more beneficial. In their study, aphasic subjects were presented with a photograph of an individual labeled with the possessive form of a name (e.g., Mr. Clown's) paired with a pictured object (e.g., mountain). Subjects were asked to produce the proper name followed by the name of the object (e.g., "Mr. Clown's mountain"). These proper names and object names shared either initial phonemes (e.g., Dean's Duck), initial consonant and vowel (e.g., Fawn's Fork), final consonant (e.g., Tim's Broom), rime (e.g., Gwen's Pen), or were phonologically unrelated (e.g., Tim's Cane). Aurignac and Saffran found that fewer errors were committed in subjects' naming when targets (objects) were preceded by a prime (proper name) from the rime condition than when preceded by a prime from any of the other conditions.

Aurignac and Saffran (1996) note that these results are interpretable within the framework of interactive activation models of word retrieval and that the effect reflects the sequential activation of phonemes in a word (e.g., activation of onset, then vowel, then coda). When the initial phoneme of the prime and target is the same, activation from the phonological level will feed back to the lexical level, increasing competition for the filling of subsequent phoneme slots. Conversely, when target and prime share rimes, phonological feedback will tend to promote the activation of both words because the phonemes activated via feedback are the same in both words and thus, competition is minimal.

In the second study, Jokel and Rochon (1996) describe a patient, P. D., with a naming impairment they believe to be localized to phonological output processes. On pretesting, P. D. was able to name only 10% of 134 pictures presented to her and perseverated on 49% of her responses. She was, however, at ceiling (100%) for word-picture matching, repetition, and oral reading of these same items. A tripartite treatment program consisting of repetition, reading, and sentence completion training was developed in an attempt to improve P. D.'s phonological access in oral naming. In all three training conditions, P. D. was presented with pictures of objects. In repetition training, each picture was presented with a spoken label and P. D. was asked to repeat the spoken word. In reading training, each picture was presented with its written label and P. D. was asked to read the name. In sentence completion training, each picture was presented with an incomplete sentence and P. D. was asked to complete the spoken sentence.

Using confrontation-naming performance in pre- and posttraining and percent of perseverative responses in pre- and posttraining as measures, Jokel and Rochon (1996) discovered that the only condition in which P. D. showed improvement was in the reading condition. In fact, naming performance worsened (not significant statistically) following sentence completion training and perseverative responses increased following repetition training. Why should reading improve naming performance? Jokel and Rochon hypothesize that since the same output forms and processes are shared in oral reading and oral naming, perhaps pairing orthographic information with a picture lowers activation thresholds (Hillis & Caramazza, 1994) for phonological forms. But they also offer another interpretation, more in line with connectionist thinking. They suggest that the improvement may arise via "simultaneous activation of lexical-semantic and phonological forms" (Martin et al., 1994). Such a process would serve to strengthen the connections between semantics and phonology, leading to improved naming. More work such as Jokel and Rochon's that compares various treatment conditions is obviously needed to decide between these alternatives, but the connectionist account provides a testable prediction: Any training procedure that serves to strengthen semantic-phonological connections should help patients such as P. D.

Summary

The work described in this section is a good example of the reciprocal relationship that is possible between psycholinguistic theories and treatment strategies: Psycholinguistic models can be used to develop treatment strategies and, in turn, outcome of treatment interventions can help to refine psycholinguistic theories. Thus, connectionist modeling holds great promise in providing answers to the practical questions of speech and language rehabilitators. In turn, therapists may provide outcome information that is critical to the development of these very same models.

LIMITATIONS AND THE FUTURE

Now that the utility of connectionist models in addressing the four goals of description, prediction, explanation, and control of language behavior has been argued and demonstrated, it is time to finally admit to their limitations. First, we do not wish to imply that this approach is immediately available to the therapist. Indeed, connectionist models are unapproachable at this point for practical use in the clinic. There is the problem of real-life application of functional approaches in general, namely, the time constraints of the therapist in delivering rehabilitatory care. Conducting a functional analysis is time-intensive and in this day and age of time-limited care, the amount of time allotted to assessment is becoming increasingly limited. Also, the therapist cannot look at functional analyses in isolation; functional communication (an entirely different issue) must be taken into account as well. Functional assessment approaches are, however, the current direction of the field and this chapter is an attempt to introduce that direction to present and future clinicians. Just as the theorist must be in touch with the real world of therapy to best make a contribution, the therapist must be in touch with the theoretical world of the theorist to best effect change in patients' language behavior.

A second criticism of the connectionist approach in particular lies in the fairly arbitrary choices the connectionist modeler must make in model design. These choices, while arbitrary, usually have great impact on the model's behavior. For instance, the networks used are usually very small. Entirely different behaviors might emerge from larger networks. But as networks become larger, it becomes increasingly difficult to understand their behavior as they approach the complexity of neural behavior itself. In other words, there is a tradeoff between practicality and reality. Finally, as a result of this need for reductionism in model design, the problems themselves that may be studied are greatly reduced versions of real-world problems. The Dell et al. (1997) model discussed earlier, for instance, only handles production of single words and only in response to a pictured input. Longer utterances would require a theory of processing over time, opening up a whole other dimension of modeling that itself is currently the object of intense speculation. Therefore, the present state of connectionist modeling is entirely too simplistic to be of real value in the clinic. Until the models begin to address real-life behavior issues, connectionism is in the same danger as traditional functionalism if all it does is merely redescribe the data. Good models, as depicted previously, enable us to make testable and novel predictions, not merely describe.

In the future, we can expect connectionism to enter the debate concerning the status of "syndromes." We expect to see an evolution from modeling phenomena (syndromes) to modeling individual case studies (e.g., as in Martin et al., 1994). In the future, local lesion site will become important. In the global lesion type of model such as Dell et al.'s (1997), only type of lesion is important. As approaches such as this one evolve, however, more detailed and realistic architectures will emerge, making the relationship between patients and disorders concrete and the location of lesion site increasingly relevant. Ultimately, disorder will again be related to structure, in this case, to neural pathway.

SUMMARY AND CONCLUSIONS

In the past couple of decades, language theorists have focused on describing language performance in terms of functional models that specify the architecture of the cognitive system in terms of stages of information processing and how these stages are connected, or arranged, relative to one another. The potential clinical benefit of the functional approach over a structural approach is that it forces a systematic, functional assessment of language impairment that was heretofore missing. This allows treatment to be directed specifically at the implicated component and to be tailored specifically to the individual. Meanwhile, a newer approach to understanding mental processes—connectionism—has appeared on the theoretical scene. Connectionism represents a natural evolution toward ever more precise theoretical accounts by providing a more explicit description of how information is transmitted and transformed from one representational format to another. It also adds a dynamic dimension to the characterization of cognitive process. The explicit and dynamic nature of connectionist characterization provides this approach with a number of advantages over previous classes of models in meeting the four goals of therapy and theory: to describe, predict, explain, and ultimately control (treat) language behavior.

Connectionism has already had an impact upon our understanding of normal language performance (e.g., Dell, 1986; Dell & O'Seaghdha, 1991). In this chapter, we have seen how it may also be an important addition to the study of the neuropsychology of language and to the treatment of language disorder. Although connectionist models promise to provide an even greater understanding of aphasic as well as normal language behavior for both theorist and therapist, it will be some time before the implements of this approach are seen in a clinical setting. When this happens, however, we can expect a tremendous advantage to the current practice of syndrome classification in providing therapeutic direction. It is our belief that a psycholinguistic analysis of disorder, with its focus on functional description, is more helpful to the clinician than traditional syndrome classifications have been, and that a connectionist approach, with its greater specificity and emphasis on the dynamics of language processing, will eventually do even better.

NOTES

1. It is a matter of debate as to whether connectionism represents a true paradigm shift, in the Kuhnian sense of the word (Kuhn, 1970). We use the term "paradigm" here loosely and informally; we are not intending to make any substantive philosophical or theoretical claim that connectionism represents a "true" paradigm shift.

2. In order for random output to correspond to opportunity in the real world, a second lexical "neighborhood" was also sampled. This second neighborhood differed from the first only in that it included one more mixed neighbor (to make six lexical units) and one more phonological unit (corresponding to the new phoneme introduced by the new lexical neighbor). Across 1,000 simulation runs, the first neighborhood was sampled in 90% of the trials and the second neighborhood in 10% of the trials. The interested reader may refer to Dell et al. (1997) for a more detailed description of, and rationale for, this procedure.

3. Two of the tested patients could not be modeled because they had too many non-naming responses. Non-naming responses are beyond the realm of a model that is, after all, a model of naming behavior.

4. Additionally, although not addressed in Laine and Martin (1996), the effects of this procedure might vary because of the type of "processing" impairment that lies at the root of the lexical retrieval failure. The characterization of aphasic impairment by Dell et al., (1997) as perturbations of connection strength and decay rate introduces another perspective from which to view the effects of manipulations such as priming.

AUTHORS' NOTES

Correspondence may be directed to D. A. Gagnon, D-LIT, 107 Olin, Cornell University, Ithaca, NY 14853 (*deb.gagnon@cornell.edu*) or to N. Martin, Center for Cognitive Neuroscience, Temple University, Philadelphia, PA 19140 (*nmartin@astro.ocis.temple.edu*). This work was supported by NIDCD grants DC00191 and DC01924.

REFERENCES

Albert, M. A., Goodglass, H., Helm, N. A., Rubens, A. B., & Alexander, M. P. (1981). Introduction. In G. E. Arnold, F. Winckel, & B. D. Wyke (Eds.), *Disorders of human communication 2.* New York: Springer-Verlag.

Aurignac, M., & Saffran, E. M. (1996). Implicit cuing and lexical retrieval. *Brain and Language,* 55, 159–162.

Badecker, W., Miozzo, M., & Zanuttini, R. (1995). The two-stage model of lexical retrieval: Evidence from a case of anomia with selective preservation of grammatical gender. *Cognition,* 57, 193–216.

Bates, E., McDonald, J., MacWhinney, B., & Applebaum, M. (1991). A maximum likelihood procedure for the analysis of group and individual data in aphasia research. *Brain and Language, 40,* 231–265.

Caplan, D. (1992). *Language: Structure, processing, and disorders.* Cambridge, MA: MIT Press.

Caplan, D. (1993). Toward a psycholinguistic approach to acquired neurogenic language disorders. *American Journal of Speech and Language Pathology, 2,* 59–83.

Caramazza, A. (1989). Cognitive neuropsychology and rehabilitation: An unfulfilled promise? In X. Seron & G. Deloche (Eds.), *Cognitive approaches in neuropsychological rehabilitation.* Hillsdale, NJ: Erlbaum.

Caramazza, A., & Badecker, W. (1989). Patient classification in neuropsychological research. *Brain and Cognition, 10,* 256–295.

Code, C., Rowley, D., & Kertesz, A. (1994). Predicting recovery from aphasia with connectionist networks: Preliminary comparisons with multiple regression. *Cortex, 30,* 527–532.

Dell, G. S. (1986). A spreading activation theory of retrieval in sentence production. *Psychological Review, 93,* 283–321.

Dell, G. S., & O'Seaghdha, P. G. (1991). Mediated and convergent lexical priming in language production: A comment on Levelt et al. *Psychological Review, 98,* 604–614.

Dell, G. S., Schwartz, M. F., Martin, N., Saffran, E. M., & Gagnon, D. A. (1997). Lexical access in aphasic and nonaphasic speakers. *Psychological Review, 104,* 801–838.

Ellis, A. W., & Young, A. W. (1988). *Human cognitive neuropsychology.* Hillsdale, NJ: Erlbaum.

Ferreira, F. (1993). The creation of prosody during sentence production. *Psychological Review, 100,* 233–253.

Garrett, M. (1980). Levels of processing in sentence production. In B. Butterworth (Ed.), *Language production.* Vol. 1 New York: Academic Press, 177–220.

Goodglass, H., & Kaplan, E. (1983). *The assessment of aphasia and related disorders* (2d ed.). Philadelphia: Lea & Febiger.

Harley, T. A. (1993). Connectionist approaches to language disorders. *Aphasiology, 7,* 221–249.

Harley, T. A. (1996). Connectionist modeling of the recovery of language functions following brain damage. *Brain and Language, 52,* 7–24.

Harley, T. A., & MacAndrew, S. B. G. (1992). Modelling paraphasias in normal and aphasic speech p. 378–383. *Proceedings of the 14th annual conference of the Cognitive Science Society.* Hillsdale, NJ: Erlbaum.

Helm-Estabrook, N. A., & Albert, M. L. (1991). *Manual of aphasia therapy.* Austin, Texas: Pro-Ed.

Hillis, A. E. (1993a). Contributions from cognitive architecture. In R. Chapey (Ed.), *Language intervention strategies in adult aphasia.* Baltimore: Williams & Wilkins.

Hillis, A. E. (1993b). The role of models of language processing in rehabilitation of language impairment. *Aphasiology, 7,* 5–26.

Hillis, A. E., & Caramazza, A. (1994). Theories of lexical processing and rehabilitation of lexical deficits. In M. J. Riddoch & G. W. Humphreys (Eds.), *Cognitive neuropsychology and cognitive rehabilitation.* Hove: Erlbaum.

Hinton, G. E., & Shallice, T. (1991). Lesioning an attractor network: Investigations of acquired dyslexia. *Psychological Review, 98,* 74–95.

Howard, D., & Patterson, K. (1989). Models for therapy. In X. Seron & G. Deloche (Eds.), *Cognitive approaches in neuropsychological rehabilitation.* Hillsdale, NJ: Erlbaum.

Howard, D., Patterson, K., Franklin, S., Orchard-Lisle, V., & Morton, J. (1985). The facilitation of picture naming in aphasia. *Cognitive Neuropsychology, 2,* 49–80.

Jokel, R., & Rochon, E. (1996). Treatment of an aphasic naming impairment: When phonology met orthography. *Brain and Cognition, 32,* 299–301.

Kay, J., Lesser, R., & Coltheart, M. (1992). *PALPA: Psycholinguistic assessments of language processing in aphasia.* Hove: Erlbaum.

Kempen, G., & Huijbers, P. (1983). The lexicalization process in sentence production and naming: Indirect election of words. *Cognition, 14,* 185–209.

Kuhn, T. S. (1970), *The structure of scientific revolutions (2d ed.).* Chicago: University of Chicago Press.

Laine, M., Kujala, P., Niemi, J., & Uusipaikka, E. (1992). On the nature of naming difficulties in aphasia. *Cortex, 28,* 537–554.

Laine, M., & Martin, N. (1996). Lexical retrieval deficit in picture naming: Implications for word production models. *Brain and Language, 53,* 283–314.

Le Dorze, G., Boulay, N., Gaudreau, J., & Brassard, C. (1994). The contrasting effects of a semantic versus a formal-semantic technique for the facilitation of naming in a case of anomia. *Aphasiology, 8,* 127–141.

Levelt, W. J. M. (1983). Monitoring and self-repair in speech. *Cognition, 14,* 41–104.

Levelt, W. J. M. (1989). *Speaking: From intention to articulation.* Cambridge, MA: MIT Press.

Lichteim, L. (1885). On aphasia. *Brain, 7,* 433–484.

Marr, D. (1982). *Vision.* San Francisco: Freeman.

Marshall, J. C., & Newcombe, F. (1973). Patterns of paralexia: A psycholinguistic approach. *Journal of Psycholinguistic Research, 2,* 175–199.

Martin, N., Dell, G. S., Saffran, E. M., & Schwartz, M. F. (1994). Origins of paraphasia in deep dyslexia: Testing the consequences of a decay impairment to an interactive spreading activation model of lexical retrieval. *Brain and Language, 47,* 609–660.

Martin, N., & Laine, M. (2000). Effects of contextual priming on word retrieval in anomia. *Aphasiology, 14.*

Martin, N., Laine, M., & Lowery, J. (1996). *Differential effects of contextual priming on semantically- and phonologically-based word retrieval deficits.* Manuscript.

Martin, N., Weisberg, R. W., & Saffran, E. M. (1989). Variables influencing the occurrence of naming errors: Implications for models of lexical retrieval. *Journal of Memory and Language, 28,* 462–485.

Meyer, A. S. (1994). Timing in sentence production. *Journal of Memory and Language, 33,* 471–492.

Meyer, A. S., & Bock, K. (1992). The tip-of-the-tongue phenomenon: Blocking or partial activation? *Memory and Cognition, 20,* 715–726.

Nettleson, J., & Lesser, R. (1991). Therapy for naming difficulties in aphasia: Application of a cognitive neuropsychological model. *Journal of Neurolinguistics, 6,* 139–157.

Patterson, K., Purell, C., & Morton, J. (1983). Facilitation of word retrieval in aphasia. In C. Code & D. J. Muller (Eds.), *Aphasia therapy.* London: Arnold.

Patterson, K. E., Seidenberg, M. S., & McClelland, J. L. (1989). Connections and disconnections: Acquired dyslexia in a computational model of reading processes. In R. G. M. Morris (Ed.), *Parallel distributed processing: Implications for psychology and neurobiology.* London: Oxford University Press p. 131–181.

Plaut, D. C. (1996). Relearning after damage in connectionist networks: Toward a theory of rehabilitation. *Brain and Language: Special Issue on Cognitive Approaches to Rehabilitation and Recovery in Aphasia, 52,* 25–82.

Plaut, D. C., & Shallice, T. (1993). Deep dyslexia: A case study of connectionist neuropsychology. *Cognitive Neuropsychology, 10,* 377–500.

Prins, R. S., Snow, C. E., & Wagenaar, E. (1978). Recovery from aphasia: Spontaneous speech versus language comprehension. *Brain and Language, 6,* 192–211.

Roach, A., Schwartz, M. F., Martin, N., Grewal, R. S., & Brecher, A. (1996). The Philadelphia Naming Test: Scoring and rationale. *Clinical Aphasiology, 24,* 121–133.

Schriefers, H. (1992). Lexical access in production of noun phrases. *Cognition, 45,* 33–54.

Schriefers, H., Meyer, A. S., & Levelt, W. J. M. (1990). Exploring the time-course of lexical access in production: Picture-word interference studies. *Journal of Memory and Language, 29,* 86–102.

Schwartz, M. F. (1984). What the classical aphasia categories can't do for us, and why. *Brain and Language, 21*, 3–8.

Schwartz, M. F., Dell, G. S., Martin, N., & Saffran, E. M. (1994). Normal and aphasic naming in an interactive spreading activation model. *Brain and Language, 47*, 391–394.

Schwartz, M. F., Saffran, E. M., Bloch, D. E., & Dell, G. S. (1994). Disordered speech production in aphasic and normal speakers. *Brain and Language, 47*, 52–88.

Seidenberg, M. (1988). Cognitive neuropsychology and language: The state of the art. *Cognitive Neuropsychology, 5*, 403–426.

Sevald, C. A., & Dell, G. S. (1994). The sequential cuing effect in speech production. *Cognition, 53*, 91–127.

Shallice, T. (1988). *From neuropsychology to mental structure.* Cambridge, England: Cambridge University Press.

Sparks, R., Helm, N., & Albert, M. (1974). Aphasia rehabilitation resulting from melodic intonation therapy. *Cortex, 10*, 303–316.

Tyler, L. K. (1992). *Spoken language comprehension: An experimental approach to disordered and normal processing.* Cambridge, MA: MIT Press.

Wernicke, C. (1874). Der aphasische symptomencomplex. Breslau: Cohn and Weigart. (Translated in Eggert, G. H. (1977). *Wernicke's works on aphasia.* The Hague: Mouton.)

Modeling Disordered Perception

D. Michael Daly

As duck hunters know, even a bird brain can tell good models from the real thing. Acoustic precision in birds is hardwired, either specified genetically or acquired and fixed during development. In the order *passerines* there is evidence of "song bird circuitry" specialized for learning and producing species-specific, even subspecies-specific whistles, and for distinguishing a bird's own song (Vates, Vicario, & Nottebohm, 1997; Whaling, Solis, Doupe, Soha, & Marler, 1997). Zebra finches have anatomic connections between auditory and vocal systems with parallel projections from auditory thalamus to at least two distinct areas of forebrain (Vates, Broome, Mello, & Nottebohm, 1996; Schmidt & Perkel, 1998). Isolation, deafness, or focal lesioning can selectively disrupt song acquisition during a "sensitive period" (Bottjer, Miesner, & Arnold, 1984; Scharff & Nottebohm, 1991).

A simple polysynaptic nervous system can reliably distinguish among brief acoustic transients. Hardwiring confers "behavioral specificity." Organisms with more complex nervous systems sample their environment in detail and defer processing to more "plastic" central locations. In mammals, sounds induce motion along the basilar membrane of a cochlear apparatus. The locations in motion vary with frequency: Higher frequency sounds displace the basilar end; lower frequencies displace the apical end. Each ear projects to cortex bilaterally; however, for some movements, input from the contralateral ear is represented more richly. The "tonotopic" arrangement of movements for fine-grained analysis of changes in sounds is maintained through laminar thalamic nuclei to cortex and among cortical areas in the geniculo-cortical system (Crosby, Humphrey, & Lauer, 1962).

A different "diffuse" arrangement allowing disparities of movements, and used for locating and orienting to sounds in space, is maintained in the collicular-tegmental system. Such "encephalization" allows a bat to echolocate while growing, to fly over a river in the rain, and to hunt while other bats hunt.

Bats use acoustic transients with constant frequency (CF) and frequency modulated (FM) components and silence for echolocation. The insectivorous horseshoe bat alters the pitch of its chirps on the fly. With echo frequencies relatively constant, subtle changes in echoes from CF components distinguish rate of insect wing beat and wing size; changes in FM components characterize target velocity (e.g., an insect's velocity in flight, or the bat's velocity on landing). The "acoustic fovea" of bats includes a proportionately larger representation on basilar membrane tuned to the 20–80 kHz frequencies used in echolocation. This fovea is preserved in auditory pathways and auditory cortex; frequency processing in cortex is sharpened by active inhibition (Riquimareaux, Giaoni, & Suga, 1989, 1990). In flight, bats listen for insect wing beats; localization involves the collicular-tegmental system.

Humans use brief acoustic transients to communicate; these, too, consist of combinations of CF and FM components and silence. Several lines of evidence suggest that the types of sounds used in languages include a universal "core" with specifiable dependent classes of sounds (Greenberg, Osgood, & Jenkins, 1966; Stevens, 1972, 1989). Whether these types reflect anatomic constraints or physiological constraints, or are an artifact of explanation, it is clear that we can synthesize sounds that have some acoustic features like speech sounds (Daly, Daly, Wada, & Drane, 1980) and use these to test auditory processing independently of language spoken.

Simplistically, a sound like the vowel e can be assembled using three steady state formants (F_1-F_2-F_3). Adding FM transients with formant frequency rise produces a sound like be; allowing the same transient frequencies to rise over a longer time produces a sound like we. Adding FM transients with F_2 frequency fall instead of rise produces a sound like ge; allowing the same transient frequencies to change over a longer time produces a sound like ye. Varying direction and duration formant change and onset is sufficient to generate the matrix of sounds shown in Fig. 4.1.

With systematic variation of "transient duration," perception can change abruptly (Liberman, Delattre, Gerstman, & Cooper, 1956). The schematic acoustic spectra in the upper portion of Fig. 4.2 show sounds of a **GY** set. Transient duration is increased from 20 msec. at *stimulus value 1* to 130 msec. at *stimulus value 12* in 10-msec steps. Patients listen through headphones to sets of randomized sounds and indicate classification of each sound with a

Sound Spectra

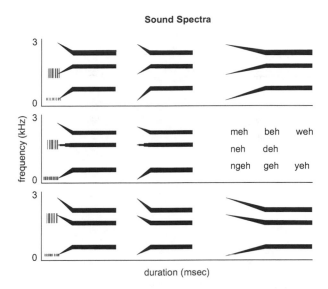

FIG. 4.1. Diagrammatic acoustic spectra of three-formant sounds (F_1, F_2, F_3).

Left column: *nasals* (narrow band noise precedes onset of resonant frequency changes). Center column: *stops* (brief, rapidly changing formant frequencies/amplitudes). Right column: *continuants* (slowly changing formant frequencies/amplitudes).

Top row: *labials* (rising F_2). Middle row: *dentals* (modestly rising or falling F_2). Bottom row: *velars* (falling F_2).

motor act (e.g., pointing). Responses can then be arranged in multidimensional contingency tables and analyzed.

The lower portion of Fig. 4.2 shows composite classifications for this set of sounds. For each stimulus value, the left ordinate shows the percentage of stimuli identified as *ge*. The dashed curve combines responses from right and left ears for eight normal subjects ($n > 300$/value). The solid gray and black curves combine responses from eight patients with complex partial seizures (CPS). Each was free of seizure-related complaint during testing; four had undergone excisional surgery when seizures proved medically intractable. Their left ear results appear in gray; the right ear results in black. Patients and controls consistently classified the sounds of *values 1* through *4* as *ge*, and those of *values 8* through *12* as *ye*. At the transition, they classified sounds at *values 5* and *6* less consistently.

One can also assemble a **BDG** set. With transient duration fixed, rapid F_2 frequency rise produces a sound like *be*, minimal F_2 rise or fall produces a sound like *de*, and rapid F_2 fall again produces *ge*. Stimulus values might reflect 100 Hz changes in F_2 starting frequency. Results would show transitions between *be* and *de*, and between *de* and *ge*.

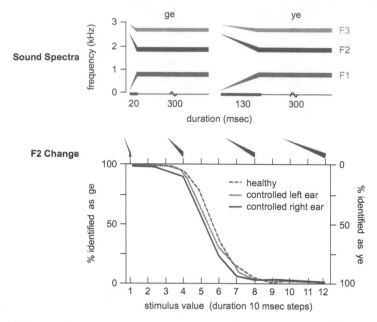

FIG. 4.2. Top: diagrammatic acoustic spectra of sparse acoustic stimuli (SAS).

Ordinate: frequencies in kHz of first three formants (F_1, F_2, and F_3). Abscissa: time in msec.

Bottom: cumulative responses to sets of **GY** stimuli illustrated in upper section Left ordinate: percent of stimuli identified as *ge*. Right ordinate: percent of SAS identified as *ye*.

Abscissa: stimulus value, representing duration of formant change from *value 1* (20 msec) to *value 12* (130 msec). Gray and black tracings: cumulative responses for right and left ear presentations (respectively) from eight women with medically controlled complex partial seizures; four had undergone excisional surgery. Each was free of ictal and medication induced complaint during testing. Black dashed tracing: cumulative responses from eight age-matched females free from neurologic complaint.

Diagonal lines at top of graph indicate duration of F_2 change for corresponding stimulus value. For stimulus values less than 5, subjects classified SAS as *ge*, and for values greater than 5, subjects classified SAS as *ye*. For *values 6* and 7, subjects classified less consistently.

With tonotopic organization, stimuli of **GY** cover similar extents of auditory cortex but at differing rates; likewise, stimuli of **BW** cover similar extents of auditory cortex (different from **GY**) but at differing rates. Stimuli of **BDG** cover differing extents of auditory cortex. With appropriate sets, **BW**s can provide unlateralized measures of cortical temporal processing, **GY**s reflect processing in cortex contralateral to the ear stimulated, and **BDG**s are sensitive to disruptions of cortical connectivity.

AUDITORY ANOMALIES AND LANGUAGE ACQUISITION

Speakers presume that listeners hear what was said. If the presumption holds for those in the central portion of a Gaussian distribution of listeners, those at the extremes hear more, or less, than was spoken. A small group of audiometrically normal subjects reports variations occur with **BW** or **GY**. At the shortest durations they detect no change and report hearing e; their stop-continuant boundaries are appropriate. We have tested two polyglot individuals who can consistently distinguish at least five classes of sounds (Daly, Daly, & Drane, 1985). One, a 33-year-old woman with normal hearing thresholds bilaterally, could consistently classify **GY** at the right ear as one of three sounds (g-colored, an intermediate sound, and y-colored). She classified these same sounds to left ear as one of six sounds (four g-colored, two y-colored). The other, a 33-year-old man with mild high-frequency loss bilaterally, could consistently classify **GY** as one of five sounds (e, two g-colored, and two y-colored) regardless of ear. He could classify **BW** as one of five sounds (e, two b-colored, a w-colored, and a ue-colored). As shown in the left panel of Fig. 4.3, he reported predominantly br-coloring with the left ear, but r-coloring with the right ear.

Both individuals could appropriately distinguish the **BW** and **GY** sounds using only two classes. Analogous abilities may appear in other sensory systems. Craig (1977) in evaluating vibrotactile readers for the blind encountered individuals with unusual abilities to distinguish rapidly changing stimuli on skin. For the auditory system, these results require that subtle, brief deformations of basilar membrane be preserved, or at least recoverable, centrally. Given such representation, modest differences in cochlea or cochlear functioning might account for differences between ears in either subject.

Hearing too little or otherwise processing aberrantly can impede language use in some modalities; it can also disrupt language acquisition (Daly, 1995). In some cases, these problems are familial. A 6-year-old boy was referred with a diagnosis of "functional dysarthria." One sibling, mother, and maternal grandmother reported similar problems. Their speech was difficult for unaffected individuals to understand; yet they understood each other with less difficulty. Affected individuals had difficulty drawing or tracing circles, turning a screwdriver or rolling hair curlers, and pedaling a bicycle; they were "athletically challenged." They could not "carry a tune," although all had age-appropriate audiometric thresholds. None had qualified to play a musical instrument in the middle school or high school band. The maternal grandmother and mother had received school-based speech therapy; all three generations reported that speech improved spontaneously at 10–11 years. All performed at or above grade

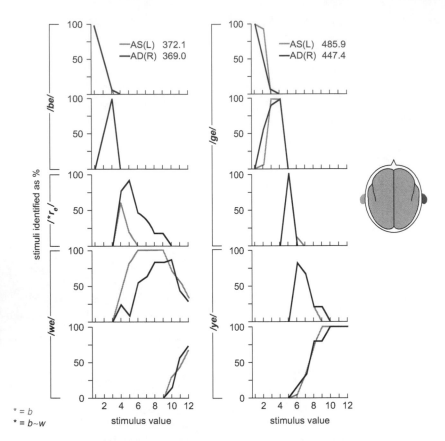

FIG. 4.3. Results from a 33-year-old man who could consistently resolve five classes of sounds in **BW** and **GY** sets (cf. Fig. 4.2).

Left column: **BW**. Right column: **GY**. AS: left ear presentation. AD: right ear presentation. L: left hand responses. R: right hand responses. Gray traces: left ear/left hand. Black traces: right ear/right hand.

Left ordinates: stimuli identified as indicated. Right ordinates: now represent stimuli identified as any other sound. G^2 value compares corresponding contingency table with chance performance. In each condition, $p(X^2 > G^2) < 0.00001$.

level on core subjects; the mother completed college-level Spanish using reading/writing classes to supplant conversational classes. Unaffected individuals were free of these problems. This kinship is shown in Fig. 4.4; gray centers identify tested members.

The father (II, center) understood his mother (I, right), sister (II, right), and the middle son (III, center); he reported that his wife (II, left) "speaks

Apraxia and Aberrant Perception

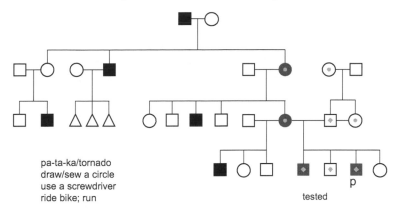

pa-ta-ka/tornado
draw/sew a circle
use a screwdriver
ride bike; run

tested

FIG. 4.4. Four-generation kinship with a history of apraxia and aberrant perception.

p: propositus. Gray center: tested individual. Filled symbols: affected members (by history only if not tested). Mother described women's difficulty with hair curlers as "they go every which way. None of us can make them turn the same direction or roll evenly." She described the difficulty with screwdrivers as inability to hold the screwdriver on the screw head and then turn the handle in the appropriate direction. See text for details.

funny." The middle son was the "outsider" of the children: He was active in sports; he spoke and wrote clearly. The problem occurred in children by two husbands; the distribution is consistent with an autosomal dominant mode of inheritance. Figure 4.5 shows the summed results for left ear, right ear, and binaural testing with **BW** (gray) and **GY** (black).

Unaffected members performed without difficulty; they understand unaffected family members and people outside this family without difficulty. The affected family members are another matter. The maternal grandmother and mother heard only *e* and *ye* in **GY**. They reported as vocalic *e* what controls report as *ge*. Both reported sounds in **BW** were clearer than **GY**. Both heard *veh* for *beh*, yet neither consistently distinguished sounds in **BW**. They understand each other, but both have some difficulty understanding eldest and youngest boys, and greatest difficulty understanding the middle boy. For any of the boys to understand his siblings requires effort. The eldest and middle boys disagreed sharply about classifications of sounds when tested concurrently. The youngest hears "yet me a yar of yape yelly" for "get me a jar of grape jelly." The source and nature of this family's complaints are complex; a parsimonious account entails central nervous system involvement.

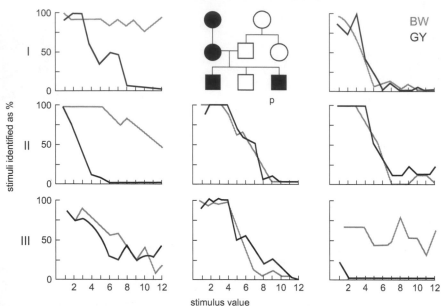

FIG. 4.5. Cumulative results for individuals from three generations of kinship in Fig. 4.4.

I, II, III: generational index of lineage in top center.

Left to right rank of graphs corresponds to position in lineage. Left ordinates percent of stimuli identified as *ge* for **GY** (black trace); *be* for **BW** (gray trace). **BW** is sum of left, right, and binaural **BW** presentations; **GY** is sum of left, right, and binaural **GY** presentations. Note that maternal grandmother (I, left) and mother (II, left) reported **GY** sound as *e* or *ye*. **p**: propositus (III right) reported all but some of the shortest **GY** stimuli as *ye*. (Reprinted with permission from Norris, JA, and Hoffman, PR (1999). The SDS developmental model of integrated functioning, Baton Rouge, LA: EleMentory.)

TRANSIENT ANOMALOUS PERCEPTION

Human primary auditory cortex fills a small six-layered volume in each temporal lobe. It is largely inaccessible from the surface; size and orientation make imaging difficult. Secondary and association areas extend anteriorly in the temporal lobes and posteriorly into the parietal lobes. The cortical auditory system exploits physiologic and anatomic processes common to other sensory systems (de Felipe & Jones, 1988). Excitatory thalamocortical afferents terminate predominantly in layer 4 on both excitatory and inhibitory neurons; excitatory callosal fibers from homologous areas terminate on these same inhibitory interneurons. Efferents from layers 5 and 6 project to dorsal thalamic nuclei and to the inferior colliculi. Corticocortical and local interlaminar fibers arise from layers 3 and 2.

The inhibitory elements (Cipollini & Keller, 1989), smooth or sparsely spined short axon cells, include axo-axonal chandelier cells (Fonseca, Soriana, Ferrer, Martinez, & Tunon, 1993), basket cells (a primary source of inhibition for iso-frequency organization (McMollen, 1990) and motion/direction selectivity (Kisvarday, Martin, Friedlander, & Somogyi, 1987), two local fast-response interneurons (the vertically oriented bitufted cells (McCormick, Connors, Lightall, & Prince, 1985) and horizontally oriented multipolar cells (Winer, 1984), as well as bipolar, neurogliaform, and giant cells of the deeper layers. These are demonstrably GABA-ergic; bipolar cells may also be peptide-ergic.

The inhibitory transmitter GABA acts in cortex through receptors distinguished pharmacologically as $GABA_A$ and $GABA_B$. $GABA_A$ activity is enhanced with muscimol, blocked with the convulsant bicuculline (BIC). The receptor complex, distributed over postsynaptic dendrite, soma and axon initial segment, increases membrane chloride conductance and is pregnane steroid sensitive. $GABA_B$ activity is enhanced with Baclofen blocked with faclophen (but not BIC). On presynaptic terminals, the $GABA_B$ receptor decreases monoamine and excitatory amino acid release; on postsynaptic membranes it increases potassium conductance. In slices of human temporal cortex, $GABA_A$ modulates early IPSP components; $GABA_B$ modulates late IPSP components (McCormick 1989).

GABA-ergic inhibition shapes receptive field properties of cortical neurons (Hicks & Dykes, 1983; McCasland & Hibbard, 1997; Schwark, Li, & Fuchs, 1994). In the visual system disinhibition with BIC decreases orientation and direction sensitivity so that cells respond readily to stimuli that had been ineffective (Daniels & Pettigrew, 1973; Rose & Blakemore, 1974; Sillito, 1974). With complete disinhibition, excitatory receptive fields become large and round; orientation and direction selectivity are virtually abolished (Tsumoto, Ecksrt, & Creutzfeldt, 1979). $GABA_A$ disinhibition can also transiently alter developmentally abnormal stereopsis. In monocularly deprived kittens, BIC temporarily restores binocular receptive fields with normal orientation and direction sensitivity for the deprived eye, but with concomitant loss of specificity for the other eye. Cells again respond monocularly when BIC effects dissipate (Burchfiel & Duffy, 1981). In monkeys, monocular deprivation markedly diminishes immuno-staining for $GABA_A$ receptor proteins in lattices of layer 4 cortex enervated by that eye. The effect appeared within 5 days of deprivation and persisted over 30 days of deprivation (Hendry et al., 1994).

Studies with GABA or GABA-agonists are more intricate. Iontophoretic GABA depresses spontaneous firing and elevates thresholds of cutaneous cells of cat somatosensory cortex. Receptive field thresholds increase more at the periphery than at the center, effectively reducing field size and narrowing field tuning (Kaneko & Hicks, 1988). $GABA_A$ agonists can also reversibly alter behavior of awake animals. Iontophoretic muscimol in monkey multimodal finger regions disrupts coordinated finger movements (Hikosaka, Tanaka, Sakamoto, & Iwamura, 1985). In bats, muscimol applied to the CF areas impairs ability to resolve frequency differences less than 100 Hz; applied to the FM areas it impairs ability to resolve time sensitive differences less than 20–30 msec. In each case larger frequency or time differences are unaffected (Riquimareaux, Gaioni, & Suga, 1992).

On the modular level of columns or slabs, diminished inhibition decreases stimulus specificity; enhanced inhibition increases specificity. At either extreme, otherwise appropriate stimuli are not differentiable.

In aggregates of slabs, inhibition modulates the extent of excitation (Horikawa, Hosokawa, Kubota, Nasu, & Taniguchi, 1996) and appears to synchronize synaptic level activity. Small decreases in inhibition—less than 20%—can double the extent of horizontally propagated field potentials. With even small decreases, direction of propagation becomes unpredictable in slices of rat sensory cortex (Chagnac-Amitai & Conners, 1989). Schwartzkroin and Haglund (1986), using thick slices of human temporal lobe, examined synaptic events that involve repetitive discharge of GABA-ergic inhibitory "interneurons." They found activity of fast inhibitory "interneurons" preceded postsynaptic "pyramidal" activity, and that both orthodromic and antidromic stimulation elicited IPSPs. They also reported "repetitive stimuli did not evoke after-discharge from human cortex or mesial temporal lobe" but "appeared to 'clamp' the cell at a relatively hyperpolarized potential." Interestingly, such synchronized activity can give rise to long-lasting inhibition in projected neurons even in the absence of excitatory amino acids (Michelson & Wong, 1990).

Active inhibition shapes receptive field properties of auditory neurons and the frequency-intensity sensitivities of the several cochlear representations in cortex (Suga, Zhang, & Yan, 1997). In secondary areas, persistence or decay of inhibition shapes direction of frequency change and inherently rate of change, because this involves "adjacent" extents of cochlear representations.

Sir Charles Symonds (1962) in describing the "epileptic disorder of function" observed that

> (Seizures) . . . may be regarded as occasional expressions of a fundamental and continuous disorder of neuronal function. The essence of this disorder is loss of the normal balance between excitation and inhibition at synaptic junctions. . . . (This) . . . disorder of function may be assumed to be present continuously. (p. 314)

Patients with focal seizures in auditory cortex have reported that sounds they had heard as stops (such as *deh*) become nasals (*neh*), then laterals or bleats (*leh* or *dleh*), and finally undifferentiated buzzes (Daly, Daly, Drane, & Wada, 1987). Misperceptions affect the transient portions of sounds and abate with control of seizures. Such changes are consistent with diminished inhibition (Daly, Wada, & Daly, 1980). We have noted other perceptual changes that are consistent with increased inhibition (Daly, Daly, Wada, & Drane, 1980; et al., 1981). One surgical and four nonsurgical patients illustrate these effects.

Disinhibition

At age 3-1/2 years this patient developed unilateral subacute hemispheric encephalitis. She suffered recurring partial motor seizures that began in either the left hand or foot. By age 4 years, she had suffered recurring bouts of partial *status epilepticus* and had developed left spastic hemiparesis. CT scans revealed extensive atrophy of the right cerebral hemisphere. She underwent two-stage removal of the right hemisphere sparing 2 cm at the occipital pole. Postoperatively she had left homonymous hemianopsia and a cortical sensory deficit; her spastic hemiparesis persisted.

In 15% of such patients seizures eventually develop in the remaining hemisphere. This patient reports two types occur now. In one, all objects lose color, and in a few moments, "everything becomes black." She feels she will fall but does not. Throughout, voices do not change character. A second type occurs without warning; her mother reports that the child's eyes open, neck extends, and left shoulder elevates. With right hand she may reach over to restrain left arm (and abort the seizure); failing this she fumbles with right hand, becomes unresponsive, then may be briefly confused. Spontaneous seizures of this type have occurred during testing.

We tested her at age 8 years. The right panel of Fig. 4.6 combines interictal performance over a year. Although she reports hearing clearly, performance with the right ear (contralateral to remaining hemisphere) is neither random nor equivalent to standard; the left ear (ipsilateral to remaining hemisphere) is at chance levels. The three left panels show performance immediately before and following a spontaneous seizure. In the top panel before seizure, performance with the left ear is random. Testing with the right ear had just begun when she had difficulty understanding, stared, fumbled, and was briefly unresponsive. As she began responding, she pointed slowly and with small hand movements.

Immediately following the seizure, performance with the right ear is random, as if auditory cortex in the remaining hemisphere had been ablated. This resolved rapidly. By panel 3 right ear performance is remarkably

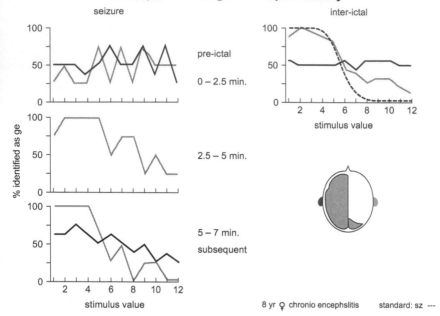

FIG. 4.6. Perception in case with right hemispherectomy and seizures in-
volving remaining hemisphere.

　　Right panel cumulative interictal performance on **GY**. Left ear (black trace)
presentations. Right ear (gray trace) presentations Normal controls (black
dashed trace). Left panel: right ear (gray traces) immediately following arrest and continuing approximately 7 minutes in 2.5 min epochs. Left ear
(black traces) before and following right ear testing. Head illustrates extent
of resection.

like the standard. In panel 2, the shift of curve toward larger stimulus values reflects a 30-sec period when longer duration sounds she had identified as *ye* she now reported as *ge*. A similar 2-minute episode, again with
right ear, followed an unaborted seizure on another occasion. During these
episodes, she included some but not all of the longest values, preclud-
ing appeal to perseveration. These shifts are consistent with augmented
inhibition.

Augmented Inhibition

Similar prolonged lateralized episodes have occurred in nonsurgical patients. The patients shown in the upper and middle portions of Fig. 4.7
experienced unilateral shifts lasting over 10 minutes. For each patient the

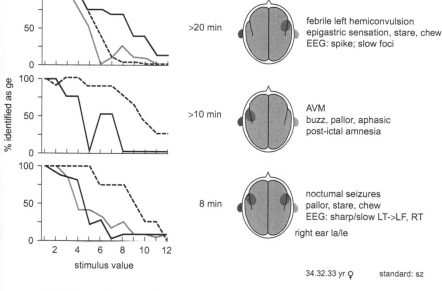

Episodic Aberrant Perception (3 Cases)

duration | lesion

>20 min — febrile left hemiconvulsion
epigastric sensation, stare, chew
EEG: spike; slow foci

>10 min — AVM
buzz, pallor, aphasic
post-ictal amnesia

8 min — nocturnal seizures
pallor, stare, chew
EEG: sharp/slow LT->LF, RT
right ear la/le

34.32.33 yr ♀   standard: sz

FIG. 4.7. Episodes of aberrant perception in three cases.
In each head the dark gray area illustrates location of electrographic abnormality. See text for details.

shift, shown with a dashed line, appeared at the ear contralateral to primary
focus. The patient shown in the bottom portion reported misperceptions
consistent with disinhibition for the ear contralateral to presumed primary
focus; she was unaware of the shift with the other ear.

The upper results are from a 34-year-old woman who had suffered repeated left hemiconvulsions associated with fever at 11 months. Her spells
began with a rising epigastric sensation, followed by stare, oral automatism, and fumbling. An EEG revealed foci of slow waves and of spikes in
the right anterior temporal area. During testing she had intervals marked
with pallor, lip smacking, and facial twitches, but reported no seizure. Her
shift appears with left ear/right hemisphere.

The middle results are from a 32-year-old woman with left temporal
arteriovenous malformation. Her spells begin with buzzing in the right
ear, followed by pallor and brief stare; she might then become aphasic.
Postictally she may be amnestic for the interval. Prolonged EEG monitoring
revealed sharp and slow transients recorded over left temporal region.
During testing, she had intervals marked by pallor, dilated pupils, and

small chewing motions; these might end with a brief smile or transient apraxia. She became aware that the proportions of sounds differed between ears during testing, but denied experiencing aura or seizure. Her shift appears with the right ear/left hemisphere.

The bottom results are from a 33-year-old woman who since childhood has had nocturnal seizures. These begin with forceful expiration and cry, then rigidity, and oral automatism. She has had brief daytime seizures with dizziness or cephalic sensation. In these, sounds become distant and her speech becomes garbled. Postictally she is amnestic for the interval. EEG showed sleep sensitive sharp waves over the left anterior temporal region and isolated sharp transients in right homologous area. During testing, the left ear boundary extended 50 msec. Following a brief arrest when she failed to respond, she made small chewing motions, her pupils alternately dilated and constricted over 10 sec., then a series of fast blinks followed. When asked to speak responses, boundaries with the left ear continued extended. With the right ear, she now reported as *la* or *le* sounds she previously had called *ge*. Twice during this, she was again briefly unresponsive. The episode ended abruptly; performance before and following this is shown with solid lines.

Active inhibition for a specifiable time confers asymmetry of "preference" in current accounts of motion-direction sensitivity (Daly & Lazar, 1990; Kautz & Wagner, 1998; Koch & Grothe, 1998). Accepting that movement of these stimuli across cortex elicits some rate-dependent level of inhibition, then maintaining that level with increased inhibition would require slower movement. With greatly increased levels, rapid movements might pass undetected.

The results shown in Fig. 4.8 are from a 32-year-old woman who since age 12 has had complex partial seizures. Her spells begin with a visual hallucination of a small tree at consistent location in the right visual field; followed by difficulty understanding speech and inability to speak, unresponsiveness, and an automatism. Postictally she may be amnestic for part of the interval. She has also experienced episodes with visual distortion too brief to characterize and often associated with rotational vertigo; she reports the visual environment seems to "freeze." Telemetered intensive monitoring confirmed episodes with visual distortion were without apparent ictal or electrographic concomitant. She has had episodes in which she has a recurring thought, which she is later unable to recall ("forced thinking"). Interictal deficits on language tests parallel frequency and severity of seizures. She has right inferior quadrantanopsia. EEG studies including telemetry reveal focus of slow wave activity in left posterior temporal region.

The panels include results during recurring episodes of "forced thinking." In the left panel (**GY**) where controls typically detect change longer

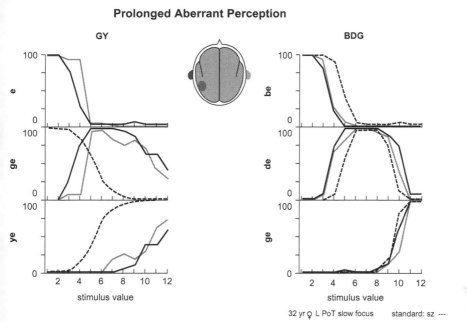

Prolonged Aberrant Perception

GY   BDG

32 yr ♀ L PoT slow focus   standard: sz ---

FIG. 4.8. Aberrant perception with episodes of "forced thinking."
Left panel: **BDG** Right panel: **GY**. Left ear (black trace) presentations.
Right ear (gray trace) presentations. Seizure-free controls (black dashed
trace). In the head, dark gray area illustrates location of electrographic abnormality.

than 20 msec, she rarely detected any less than 35 ms, reporting these as *e*.
Where controls report fewer *ge* sounds, she began to report *ge* sounds.
e-ge boundaries are consistently well-defined. *ge-ye* boundaries varied;
she was often unaware of these changes unless she found only one sound
in a set. In the right panel (**BDG**) with sounds of set duration, the *be-
de* and *de-ge* boundaries increased approximately 200 Hz beyond controls. She reported the sounds had been clear and identical in any group,
"like a stuck record"; she was unaware that boundaries were markedly
shifted.

The perceptual shifts in these patients are consistent with enhanced
inhibition. The laterality of episodes is consistent with "surround inhibition," the volume of enhanced GABA-mediated inhibition, which arises
around acute or chronic foci in penicillin, iron, cobalt, and alumina models
of experimental seizures. Auditory anomalies in brain remaining after
hemispherectomy reflect disease in the remaining hemisphere as well as
connectivity altered through loss of callosal fibers. Such alterations can
persist even with young, 'plastic' brains. In both surgical and nonsurgical

patients, the underlying disease gives rise to perceptual aberrations that fluctuate in intensity and that need not correlate with self-reported seizure frequency. The aberrations reflect change in the balance of excitation and inhibition. One class of aberrations reflects insufficient inhibition (Novotny, Hyder, Behar, Petroff, & Rothman, 1997), even disinhibition; another reflects enhanced, excessive inhibition. In the course of treatment, diminished hippocampal involvement may improve the accuracy of self-reported seizure counts. As the standards in Fig. 4.2 confirm, such aberrations ameliorate and even clear with effective treatment.

SYSTEMIC CHANGES WITH VIGILANCE

In mammals, "states" such as wake and sleep involve several distinct systems. "Vigilance"—capacity to remain alert while awake—involves "diffusely" projecting collections of neurons in areas such as the ascending reticular system, the diffuse thalamic systems, and basal forebrain regions; it may involve the tonic action of cells within areas such as the locus coeruleus (Aoki, Go, Venkatesan, & Kurose, 1994; Darracq et al., 1995). "Sleep" involves other populations of neurons (e.g., in midline-raphe nuclei, in caudal areas of raphe). Neither sleep nor wakefulness is a unitary state (Beatty & Wagoner, 1978): People who have studied all night for exams know that one can be awake without being alert. Whatever the account of states, it is clear that interactions of such systems (Hofle et al., 1997; Hutsler & Gazzaniga, 1996) affect the stability of processing in cortical sensory systems (Daly & Daly, 1994; Daly, Daly, Drane, Frost, & Kellaway, 1980; Daly, Hodson, & Gibson, 1991; Rouiller, Hornung, & De Ribaupierre, 1989).

Familial hypersomnia typically involves excessively and persistently impaired vigilance (Yoss, Moyer, & Hollenhorst, 1970; Yoss, Moyer, & Ogle, 1969) and possibly episodic cataplexy (muscle weakness provoked by emotion), sleep paralysis (brief bouts of inability to move in the transition between sleep and wakefulness), or hypnogogic hallucinations (vivid visual or auditory sensations that can accompany sleep paralysis) (Daly & Yoss, 1978). A 29-year-old woman was unable to remain alert while reading, driving, or attending church. Her husband confirmed her accounts, and denied experiencing such difficulty himself. Their 12-year-old son was unable to remain alert while reading or watching TV, or, by teachers' accounts, in the classroom. On questioning, the woman's father and mother reported similar difficulties: They had stopped for coffee four times on the 90-mile drive for testing. Figure 4.9 shows cumulative results from approximately 20 minutes of testing.

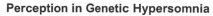

Perception in Genetic Hypersomnia

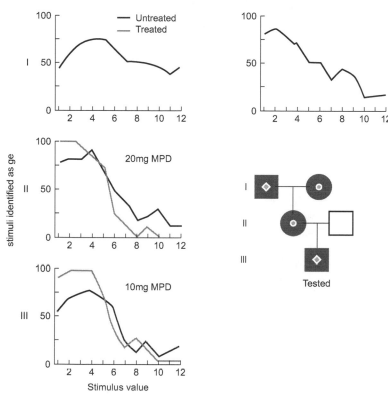

FIG. 4.9. Three-generation kinship with familial hypersomnia.
   p: propositus. Gray center: tested individual. Gray traces: untreated. Black traces: 20 min following sublingual dose of methylphenidate (MPD) indicated.

Each affected family member performed aberrantly when untreated. Untreated performances fluctuated markedly within the test interval; cumulative tracings mask the fluctuations. The trends in untreated performance for both women and the boy preclude appeal to "inattention" or "micro-sleep" (Valley & Broughton, 1983). The woman and her son had been independently diagnosed; both had been treated with methylphenidate. The treated portion of the tracings (GII and GIII) show results of testing approximately 20 minutes after sublingual medication (Mo 20 mg; So 10 mg; untreated vs. treated p $(X^2 > G^2) < 0.001$). Changes in performances were dose dependent up to levels that sustained vigilance and consistent with absorption and elimination kinetics for the compound.

Vigilance-sensitive perceptual changes are independent of static auditory anomalies and transient aberrations. Impaired vigilance can co-occur with either static or transient anomalies, confounding diagnosis. Again, as comparison with the control standard in Fig. 4.2 confirms, vigilance-sensitive perceptual changes abate and even clear with effective treatment.

MODELING TECHNIQUES

We have considered three classes of auditory anomalies:

1. Static anomalies in which a person distinguishes changes in sounds that speakers of his native language typically cannot distinguish, or fails to distinguish changes in sounds that speakers of his native language typically do distinguish. The conditions under which these anomalies become clinical problems depend in part on the conventions of a speaker's linguistic community.
2. Dynamic anomalies in which perception changes as the balance of excitation and inhibition in the auditory cortex changes. The sources of these anomalies are manifold. They arise with focal changes in auditory cortex, or with changes in other connected areas.
3. Anomalies in which stability of perception fluctuates. These can arise with "systemic" changes that alter cortical processing.

The aspects of auditory processing presented here constrain the types of models that can be applied to auditory processing and to the auditory system: Auditory processing occurs in time-sensitive, nonlinear dynamic systems.

Artificial neural networks are computational models described by types of nodes, types of connections between nodes, and learning/training and recall/generalization algorithms. Nodes have or compute values; they can be arranged as a sheet (where values put out are computed directly from values put in) or as layers of sheets (where values put out of one sheet are the values put into an adjacent sheet). Connections between nodes may flow in one direction only (feedforward) or may include values put out with new values put in (feedback). Learning/training algorithms converge on stable values put out for specific values put in. Recall algorithms describe how new values "similar" to those put in during training become "similar" to values put out with training.

A multilayer neural network with at least one intermediate layer (Multi-Layer Perceptron) can model any continuous function to a specifiable degree of accuracy (Hornik, 1991). Given a set of features that unambiguously represents all patterns of a set, MLP can acquire conditional probabilities that distinguish the patterns. MLP, like multivariate nonlinear regression models, can represent interactions among variables (Kasabov, 1996). MLP, however, are time-insensitive. To the extent that change over time can be determined from a sequence of values, sequences of "previous" values can be summed and put in, creating a time delay neural network. Alternately, values from a layer might be held then fed back to the preceding layer, leaving time-sensitive traces. If such recurrent neural networks are formally equivalent to finite automata, the input languages they accept must be equivalent to regular sets and to Type 3 grammars. Both time delay and recurrent neural nets (Norris, 1990) have been used in speech recognition engines.

Other lines of research offer time-sensitive alternatives. Oscillatory "objects" can be assembled from "excitatory" and "inhibitory" nodes. States of these objects are specified with triples of amplitude, frequency, and phase. The richer representation need not be mapped onto a traditional neural network; for example, it can be annealed to avoid the local minima problem (Inoue & Nagayoshi, 1992).

In some cases apparently random processes can be described and modeled as deterministic chaos. Simplistically, the path of a chaotic process is traced in a phase space of appropriate dimensions. The accumulated path is in fact a trajectory, since each visit to some area of the phase space comes from different preceding conditions. A chaotic process is inherently "temporal" but aperiodic. Aihara, Takake, and Toyoda (1990) have reported chaotic nodes with exponentially decaying refractoriness and graded outputs. Dingle, Andrea, and Jones (1993) have designed chaotic nodes where output values range from linear to periodic to chaotic depending on magnitudes put in. Neither chaotic nodes nor oscillatory objects offer time-sensitivity as a computational "free-ride."

REFERENCES

Aihara, K., Takake, T., & Toyoda, M. (1990). Chaotic neural networks. *Physics Letters A, 144,* 333–335.

Aoki, C., Go, C. G., Venkatesan, C., & Kurose, H. (1994). Perikaryal and synaptic localization of alpha 2A-adrenergic receptor-like immunoreactivity. *Brain Research, 650*(2), 181–183.

Beatty, J., & Wagoner, B. L. (1978). Pupillometric signs of brain activation vary with level of cognitive processing. *Science, 199,* 1216–1219.

Bottjer, S. W., Miesner, E. A., & Arnold, A. P. (1984). Forebrain lesions disrupt development but not maintenance of song in passerine birds. *Science, 224,* 901–904.

Burchfiel, J. L., & Duffy, F. H. (1981). Role of intracortical inhibition in deprivation ambylopia: Reversal with microiontophoretic bicucculline. *Brain Research, 206,* 479–492.

Chagnac-Amitai, Y., & Conners, B. W. (1989). Horizontal spread of synchronized activity in neocortex and its control by GABA mediated inhibition. *Journal of Neurophysiology, 61*(4), 747–757.

Cipollini, P. B., & Keller, A. (1989). Thalamocortical synapses with identified neurons in monkey primary auditory cortex: A combined Golgi/EM and GABA/peptide immunocytochemistry study. *Brain Research, 492*, 347–353.

Craig, J. C. (1977). Vibrotactile pattern perception: Extraordinary observers. *Science, 196*, 450–454.

Crosby, E., Humphrey, T., & Lauer, E. W. (1962). *Correlative Anatomy of the Nervous System.* New York: MacMillan. pp. 273–275.

*Daly, D. B., & Daly, D. M. (1994). Acoustic evaluation of pharmacodynamics. *Journal of the Acoustical Society of America, 96*(5), 3281–3282.

*Daly, D. D., Daly, D. M., Drane, J. W., Frost, J. D., & Kellaway, P. (1980). Effects of vigilance on cortical processing. *Society of Neuroscience Abstracts, 6*, 812–813.

*Daly, D. D., Daly, D. M., Drane, J. W., Pippenger, C., Porter, J. C., & Wada, J. A. (1981). GABAergic disinhibition and reversible secondary epileptogenesis in man. In J. A. Wada (Ed.), *Kindling II* (pp. 219–233). New York: Raven Press.

Daly, D. D., & Yoss, R. E. (1978). Narcolepsy. In P. J. Vinken & G. W. Bruyn (Eds.), *Handbook of Clinical Neurology* (v15, pp. 836–852). New York: Elsevier.

Daly, D. M. (1995). Anomalous central auditory processing in man. *Society of Neuroscience Abstracts, 21*, 2113.

Daly, D. M., Daly, D. D., & Drane, J. W. (1985). Central representation and categorical perception. *Journal of the Acoustical Society of America, 77*(1), S108.

Daly, D. M., Daly, D. D., Drane, J. W., & Wada, J. A. (1987). Inhibitory mechanisms and cortical processing, *Journal of the Acoustical Society of America, 82*(1), S58.

Daly, D. M., Daly, D. D., Wada, J. A., & Drane, J. W. (1980). Evidence concerning the neurobiologic basis of speech perception. *Journal of Neurophysiology, 44*(1), 200–221.

Daly, D. M., Hodson, A., & Gibson, K. M. (1991). Central auditory processing in a patient with SSADH deficiency. *Society of Neuroscience Abstracts, 17*, 892.

Daly, D. M., & Lazar, M. (1990). Ictal and interictal changes in auditory processing. *Thirteenth Annual Penfield Memorial Lecture,* Tokyo: Japanese Neurosurgical Society.

Daly, D. M., Wada, J. A., & Daly, D. D. (1980). Hemispheric processing and callosal mechanisms in patients with epilepsy. In J. A. Wada & J. K. Penry (Eds.), *Epilepsy: The tenth international symposium* (p. 534). New York: Raven Press.

Daniels, J., & Pettigrew, J. (1973). Gamma-aminobutyric acid antagonism in visual cortex: different effects on simple, complex, & hypercomplex neurons. *Science, 182*, 8–11.

Darracq, L., Gervasoni, D., Peyron, C., Chouvet, G., Jouvet, M., Fort, P., & Luppi, P. H. (1995). Effects of iontophoretic injections of strychnine and bicuculline on the activity of the noradrenergic neurons of the rat locus coeruleus during the sleep-waking cycle. *Society of Neuroscience Abstracts, 21*, 450.

de Felipe, J., & Jones, E. G. (1988). *Cajal on the cerebral cortex.* Oxford: New York. pp. 250–275.

Dingle, A., Andreae, J., & Jones, R. (1993). The chaotic self-organizing map. In N. K. Kasabov (Ed.), *Artificial Neural Networks and Expert Systems* (pp. 15–18). Los Alamitos: IEEE CS Press.

Fonseca, M., Soriano, E., Ferrer, I., Martinez, A., Tunon, T. (1993). Chandelier cell axons identified by parvalbumin-immunoreactivity in the normal human temporal cortex and in Alzheimer's disease. *NeuroScience, 55*(4), 1107–1115.

Greenberg, J. H., Osgood, C. E., & Jenkins, J. J. (1966). Memorandum concerning language universals. In J. H. Greenberg (Ed.), *Universals of Language* (pp. xv–xxvii). MIT Press: Cambridge.

Hendry, S. H., Huntsman, M. M., Vinuela, A., Mohler, H., de Blas, A. L., & Jones, E. G. (1994). $GABA_A$ receptor subunit immunoreactivity in primate visual cortex: distribution in macaques and humans and regulation by visual input in adulthood. *Journal of Neuroscience, 14*(4), 2383–2393.

Hicks, T. P., & Dykes, R. W. (1983). Receptive field size for certain neurons in primary somatosensory cortex is determined by GABA-mediated intracortical inhibition. *Brain Research, 274*, 160–170.

Hikosaka, O., Tanaka, M., Sakamoto, M., & Iwamura, Y. (1985). Deficits in manipulative behaviors induced by local injections of muscimol in the first somatosensory cortex of the conscious monkey. *Brain Research, 325*(1–2), 375–385.

Hofle, N., Paus, T., Reutens, D., Fiset, P., Gotman, J., Evans, A. C., & Jones, B. E. (1997). Regional Cerebral Blood Flow changes as a function of Delta and Spindle activity during Slow Wave Sleep in humans. *Journal of Neuroscience, 17*, 4800–4810.

Horikawa, J., Hosokawa, Y., Kubota, M., Nasu, M., & Taniguchi, I. (1996). Optical imaging of spatiotemporal patterns of glutamatergic excitation and GABA-ergic inhibition in the guinea-pig auditory cortex in vivo. *Journal of Physiology (London), 497*(3), 629–633.

Hornik, K. (1991). Approximation capabilities of multilayer feedforward networks. *Neural Networks, 4*, 251–264.

Hutsler, J. J., & Gazzaniga, M. S. (1996). Acetylcholinesterase staining in human auditory and language cortices: regional variation of structural features. *Cerebral Cortex, 6*(2), 260.

Inoue, M., & Nagayoshi, A. (1992). Boltzmann machine learning in an analog chaos neurocomputer. In *Proceedings of the Second International Conference on Fuzzy Logic and Neural Networks* (pp. 559–562). Iizuka: Japan.

Kaneko, T., & Hicks, T. P. (1988). Baclofen and gamma-aminobutyric acid differentially suppress the cutaneous responsiveness of primary somatosensory cortical neurons. *Brain Research, 443*, 360–390.

Kasabov, N. K. (1996). *Foundations of neural networks, fuzzy systems, and knowledge engineering* (p. 550). MIT Press: Cambridge.

Kautz, D., & Wagner, H. (1998). GABA-ergic inhibition influences auditory motion-direction sensitivity in barn owls. *Journal of Neurophysiology, 80*(1), 172–182.

Kisvarday, Z. F., Martin, K. A. C., Friedlander, M. J., & Somogyi, P. (1987). Evidence for interlaminar inhibitory circuits in the striate cortex of the cat. *Journal of Comparative Neurology, 260*, 1–23.

Koch, U., & Grothe, B. (1998). GABA-ergic and glycinergic inhibition sharpens tuning for frequency modulations in the inferior colliculus of the big brown bat. *Journal of Neurophysiology, 80*(1), 71.

Liberman, A. M., Delattre, P. C., Gerstman, L. J., & Cooper, F. S. (1956). Tempo of frequency change as a cue for distinguishing classes of speech sounds. *Journal of Experimental Psychology, 52*, 127–144.

McCasland, J. S., & Hibbard, L. S. (1997). GABAergic neurons in barrel cortex show strong, whisker-dependent metabolic activation during normal behavior. *Journal of Neuroscience 17*, 5509–5514.

McCormick, D. A. (1989). GABA as an inhibitory neurotransmitter in human cortex. *Journal of Neurophysiology, 62*(5), 1018–1028.

McCormick, D. A., Connors, B. W., Lightall, J. W., & Prince, D. A. (1985). Comparative electrophysiology of pyramidal and sparsely spiny stellate neurons of the neocortex. *Journal of Neurophysiology, 54*(4), 782.

McMollen, N. T. (1990). Preferred orientation of basket cell axonal arbors in rabbit auditory cortex: 3D reconstruction using computer microscopy. *Society of Neuroscience Abstracts, 16*, 715.

Michelson, H. B., & Wong, R. K. S. (1990). Giant IPSPs elicited by the GABAergic inhibitory circuit in hippocampus. *Society of Neuroscience Abstracts, 16*, 21.

Norris, D. (1990). A dynamic net model of human speech recognition. In G.T.E. Altman (Ed.), *Cognitive models of speech process* (pp. 87–104). MIT Press: Cambridge.

Novotny, E. J., Hyder, F., Behar, K. L., Petroff, O. A. C., & Rothman, D. (1997). Alterations in cerebral GABA and Glutamate in human epilepsy measured in vivo. *Society of Neuroscience Abstracts, 23,* 816.

Riquimareaux, H., Giaoni, S. J., & Suga, N. (1989). Functional involvement of auditory cortex in fine frequency discrimination of biosonar signals in the bat. *Journal of Acoustical Society of America, 86,* S99.

Riquimareaux, H., Giaoni, S. J., & Suga, N. (1990). Muscimol disrupts temporal discrimination by the FM- FM area of the mustached bat's auditory cortex. *Society of Neuroscience Abstracts, 16,* 795.

Riquimareaux, H., Gaioni, S. J., & Suga, N. (1992). Inactivation of the DSCF area of the auditory cortex with muscimol disrupts frequency discrimination in the mustached bat. *Journal of Neurophysiology, 68*(5), 1613–1623.

Rose, D., & Blakemore, C. (1974). Effects of bicuculline on functions of inhibition in visual cortec. *Nature, 249,* 375–379.

Rouiller, E. M., Hornung, J. P., De Ribaupierre, F. (1989). Extrathalamic ascending projections to physiologically identified fields of the cat auditory cortex. *Hearing Research, 40*(3), 233–245.

Scharff, C., & Nottebohm, F. (1991). A comparative study of the behavioral deficits following lesions of various parts of the zebra finch song system: implications for vocal learning. *Journal of Neuroscience, 11,* 2896–2899.

Schmidt, M. F., & Perkel, D. J. (1998). Slow synaptic inhibition in nucleus HVc of the adult zebra finch. *Journal of Neuroscience, 18,* 895.

Schwark, H. D., Li, J., & Fuchs, J. L. (1994). Regional distribution of $GABA_A$ receptor binding sites in cat somatosensory and motor cortex. *Journal of Comparative Neurology, 343*(3), 362–376.

Schwartzkroin, P. A., & Haglund, M. (1986). Spontaneous Rhythmic synchronous activity in epileptic human and normal monkey temporal lobe. *Epilepsia, 27*(5), 523–537.

Sillito, A. (1974). Modification of the receptive field properties of neurons in the visual cortex by bicuculline, a GABA antagonist. *Journal of Physiology (London), 239,* 36–77.

Stevens, K. N. (1972). The quantal nature of speech: evidence from articulatory-acoustic data. In E. D. David & P. Denes (Eds.), *Human Communication: a Unified View* (pp. 51–65). McGraw-Hill: San Francisco.

Stevens, K. N. (1989). On the quantal nature of speech. *Journal of Phonetics, 17,* 3.

Suga, N., Zhang, Y., & Yan, J. (1997). Sharpening of frequency tuning by inhibition in the thalamic auditory nucleus of the mustached bat. *Journal of Neurophysiology, 77*(4), 2098–2107.

Symonds, Sir C. (1962). Discussion. *Proceedings of the Royal Society Medicine, 55,* 314.

Tsumoto, T., Ecksrt, W., & Creutzfeldt, O. (1979). Modification of orientation sensitivity of cat visual cortex neurons by removal of GABA mediated inhibition. *Experimental Brain Research, 34,* 351–361.

Valley, V., & Broughton, R. (1983). The physiological (EEG) nature of drowsiness and its relation to performance defects in narcoleptics. *Electroencephalography and Clinical Neurophysiology, 55,* 243–251.

Vates, G. E., Broome, B. M., Mello, C. V., Nottebohm, F. (1996). Auditory pathways of caudal telencephalon and their relation to the song system of adult male zebra finches. *Journal of Comparative Neurology, 366,* 613.

Vates, G. E., Vicario, D. S., Nottebohm, F. (1997). Reafferent thalamo-"cortical" loops in the song system of oscine songbirds. *Comparative Neurology, 380,* 275–280.

Whaling, C. S., Solis, M. M., Doupe, A. J., Soha, J. A., Marler, P. (1997). Acoustic and neural bases for innate recognition of song. *Proceedings of the National Academy of Science USA, 94,* 12694–12698.

Winer, J. A. (1984). Anatomy of layer IV in cat primary auditory cortex (AI). *Journal of Comparative Neurology, 224,* 535–545.
Yoss, R. E., Moyer, N. J., & Hollenhorst, R. W. (1970). Pupil size and spontaneous pupillary waves associated with alertness, drowsiness, & sleep. *Neurology, 20*(6), 545–555.
Yoss, R. E., Moyer, N. J., & Ogle, K. N. (1969). The pupillogram and narcolepsy: A method to measure decreased levels of wakefulness. *Neurology, 19*(10), 921–932.

* collaborators listed alphabetically

Behavioral testing contributed by inventor who retains all proprietary rights and interests.

J. Cook, D. D. Daly, A. Hodson, J. A. Wada, & W. W. Weinberg collaborated in the work.

5

Statistical and Neural Network Models for Speech Recognition

Edmondo Trentin, Fabio Brugnara, Yoshua Bengio,[†]
Cesare Furlanello, and Renato De Mori[‡]
ITC-irst, Centro per la Ricerca Scientifica e Tecnologica - 38050 Pante' di Povo, Trento, Italy
[†]Dept. Informatique et Recherche Opérationelle, Université de Montréal, Montreal, Qc, Canada, H3C-3J7 (also, AT&T Bell Labs., Holmdel, NJ, USA)
[‡]School of Computer Science, McGill University, Montreal, Qc, Canada, H3A2A7

PROBLEM DESCRIPTION AND METHODS FOR SOLUTION

Spoken dialogue with computers is becoming a reality receiving increased attention even outside research laboratories. A collection of results obtained from research in different countries has generated valid technologies that are now used in new products. Applications in the areas of office systems (automatic call-back systems), telephone services, training, and aid to handicapped persons are now developed with more confidence than in the past.

Just in the Area of Automatic Speech Recognition (ASR), dictation systems capable of accepting continuous speech and very large vocabularies (> 10,000 words) from many speakers are now deployed in many languages (e.g., English, French, German, Italian, Spanish, Japanese, Chinese) and for a variety of application sectors in the medical, legal, political, and news fields.

In the recent years, large vocabulary word dictation systems were developed. They accepted fairly large vocabularies (a few thousand words) but were speaker-dependent (they had to be trained on each speaker who had to record a number of predetermined sentences) and required the

213

speaker to make a short pause at the end of each word. This requirement characterizes discrete word recognition systems.

Speech technologies that are acceptable today are based on a set of methods leading to technical solutions that work together in a satisfactory way in pure software systems, running on commonly available workstations and advanced personal computers (PC), with a response time close to real-time. These systems accept continuous speech, from different speakers with very large vocabularies ranging from thousands to tens of thousands of words. They use knowledge at different levels, generating and scoring hypotheses in order to recognize words and produce written texts. In addition to that, dialog systems extract conceptual representations from hypothesized words, reason about them, taking into account dialogue histories, contexts, plans and goals. Spoken messages can be produced by a dialogue unit on PCs, in real-time and in many languages with good quality.

Person–machine Communication (PMC) can be seen as an exchange of information coded in a way suitable for transmission through a physical environment. Coding is the process of producing a representation of what has to be communicated. The object of communication is structured using words represented by sequences of symbols of an alphabet and belonging to a given lexicon. Phrases are made by concatenating words according to the rules of a grammar and associated in order to be consistent with a given semantics. These various types of constraints are knowledge sources (KS) with which a symbolic version of the message to be exchanged is built. The symbolic version undergoes further transformations that make it transmittable through a physical channel.

Dictation and interpretation systems perform a decoding process using KSs to transform the message carried by a speech signal into different levels of symbolic representation. Decoding can produce word sequence or conceptual hypotheses.

Unlike person-to-person communication, PMC is expected to produce instances of computer data structures in a deterministic way. Deterministic here means that a computer system has to produce the same representation for the same signal, every time this signal is processed. So, with actual technology, speech interpretation by machine is not creative in the sense that it is performed by predesigned, predictable reactions to the data. The KSs used by machines in the decoding process are only models of the ones used by humans for producing their messages.

One of these KSs is the Language Model (LM). An LM is a collection of constraints on the sequence of words acceptable in a given language. These constraints can be represented by rules of a generative grammar G. G can be used to produce sentences of a language LG(G). G is defined as a 4-tuple: $G = (, V_T, V_N, P)$, where V_T is a set (an alphabet, in the case of Natural Language, a lexicon) of all the words of LG(G), V_N is a set of non-terminal symbols representing abstractions of language components, like, for example, syntactic categories. $\in V_N$ indicates the abstract category of all the sentences in LG(G). P is a set of rewriting generative rules of the type $\rightarrow$ where is a sequence of symbols that should contain at least one in V_N, $\in (V_T \cup V_N)$ is a string of symbols in V_T or V_N with which, starting with a rule of the type $\rightarrow$ and further rewriting the components of , it is possible to generate a sentence in LG(G). If can be only one symbol in V_N, then G and LG(G) have the property of being context-free.

An important problem in natural language (NL) analysis is that it is very difficult if not impossible to conceive a grammar G capable of generating all and only the sentences of a natural language. This is due to many factors, probably the most important one being that NL evolves in a way difficult to characterize with formal models. Nevertheless, with grammars it is possible to build very useful, but approximated LMs. Grammars with a large number of detailed rules can accurately model certain NL aspects but the same grammars can be too limited for other aspects. These grammars are said to have limited coverage. Other grammars can have a complete coverage but, being too general, they can generate sentences that do not belong to an NL. A good example of these overgenerating grammars is one that can generate every pair of words in an NL vocabulary (word pair grammar). Overgeneration can be mitigated by associating probabilities to grammar rules in such a way that undesired sentences will be generated with lower probability than legal sentences in a given NL. Some of these grammars are particularly useful for ASR because they can be represented by Stochastic Finite State Automata (SFSA) in which states correspond to symbols in V_N and arcs are labeled with words in V_T. Probabilities are associated to arcs. For example, bigram probabilities can be associated to word pairs in a stochastic word pair grammar.

Arcs in these SFSA can be replaced by other (possibly stochastic) automata, one for each word representing alternate pronunciations of each word. Arcs of these word automata are labeled with phonemes and pronunciations are obtained with a Lexical Model (LeM). In turn, each model can be replaced by a corresponding Acoustic Model (AM) relating each phoneme to distributions of acoustic parameters or features that can be observed when that phoneme is uttered.

In this way, an Integrated Network (IN) can be obtained and effectively used to generate word or interpretation hypotheses about a given speech signal.

The decoding process has to deal with ambiguity due to distortions introduced by the transmission channel, the limits of the knowledge used, and often to intrinsic imprecision of the spoken message. The imprecision is because the speaker may not intend on producing exactly an instance of the data structures belonging to the knowledge of the decoder.

To a certain extent, ambiguities can be reduced by exploiting message redundancy. In practice, knowledge is used to transform the input signal into more suitable sequences of vectors of parameters and to obtain from them various levels of symbolic representations. The first level of symbolic representation can be a word, a syllable, a phoneme, or simply an acoustic descriptor.

Interpretation is usually obtained by a search process that considers IN as the generator of an observable description $X = x_1 x_2 \ldots x_n \ldots x_N$ of the signal to be interpreted. The search process attempts to find the best sequence of IN states identifying a path through which X is generated. Competing sequence candidates are ranked based on scoring methods. Scores are used by search strategies for progressively growing partial IN paths. These candidates are often called theories. Expansion is constrained by knowledge imposing consistency among components. Redundancy can help in making coherent components more evident by boosting the score of a compound of them.

Modern systems are based on probabilistic scores for candidate hypotheses. The speech waveform is sampled and quantized (now by standard devices available in many workstations and advanced PCs). A window, displaced by fixed time steps on the time sequence of generated samples, groups them into frames. Each frame is transformed into a vector of coefficients that are more suitable than the samples for further processing. The parameter vector obtained from the n-th frame is considered as an acoustic observation x_n. A spoken sentence is thus described by a sequence X of such vectors.

A simple, popular probabilistic model for scoring hypotheses has a decoder knowledge that considers the sequence of acoustic observations $X = x_1 x_2 \ldots x_n \ldots x_N$ as the output of an information channel shown in Fig. 5.1 that receives at the input a sequence of symbols representing the intention of the speaker. If these symbols are words, then they are usually represented by the sequence $W = W_1 \ldots W_k \ldots W_K$.

X is a coded version of W. The objective of recognition is to reconstruct W based on the observation of X. This is done by using knowledge about the coding process. If the same X can be generated by different W, or knowledge is incomplete or imperfect, then reconstruction may not be successful.

In the case of dictation, ambiguity and imprecision make it necessary to consider recognition a search process that generates word hypotheses by selecting candidates for which $Pr(W \mid X)$ is maximum. If the source

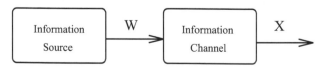

FIG. 5.1. A simple decoder model.

model provides $Pr(W)$ and the channel model provides $Pr(X \mid W)$, then the following quantity $Pr(X, W) = Pr(X \mid W)Pr(W)$ can be computed. Notice that, as $Pr(X)$ is the same for all the considered candidates W, the sequence W' for which $Pr(X, W)$ is maximum is also the sequence for which $Pr(W \mid X)$ is maximum.

$Pr(X \mid W)$ is the probability of observing X when W is pronounced. In practice, this probability cannot be computed directly from data. It has to be computed using an AM.

$Pr(W)$ is the probability of a sequence of words and is computed using a LM.

Machine dictation can be performed without understanding. The sequence of words W' that is transcribed when a sentence is uttered producing an acoustic description X is the one for which $Pr(X, W)$ is maximum with respect to all possible word sequences W.

Model parameters are estimated with imprecision from corpora of data. As imprecision is model dependent, probabilities computed with different models are weighted differently. For example, for dictation, generation of a sequence W' of word hypothesis can be based on the following score:

$$W' = \underset{W}{\operatorname{argmax}} \{\log Pr(X \mid W) + \quad \log Pr(W)\} \tag{5.1}$$

where   is a "fudge" factor that accounts for difference in model imprecision.

The (1) can also be seen as a decision criterion that combines scores for candidate hypotheses W provided by two different experts.

If the objective is understanding, then the system has to find the conceptual representation C' that maximizes $Pr(C \mid X)$ over all the possible conceptual representations C. This can be expressed as:

$$C' = \underset{C}{\operatorname{argmax}} Pr(C \mid X) \tag{5.2}$$

$$= \underset{C}{\operatorname{argmax}} \sum_{W} Pr(C, W \mid X)$$

$$= \underset{C,W}{\operatorname{argmax}} Pr(C, W \mid X)$$

$$= \underset{C,W}{\operatorname{argmax}} Pr(X \mid C, W)Pr(C, W)$$

$$= \underset{C,W}{\operatorname{argmax}} Pr(X \mid W)Pr(C, W).$$

$Pr(C, W)$ can be expressed as $Pr(C \mid W)Pr(W)$ where $Pr(W)$ is computed by the LM and $Pr(C \mid W)$ is computed by a semantic model.

The choice of KSs and the way they are used in a system determines the system architecture. System architecture design should be based on a number of performance indices; the most important of them are now briefly reviewed.

A first requirement that has already been discussed is coverage. The system has to be able to recognize virtually all the sentences that can be pronounced.

Another requirement is precision. KSs and methods for their use should produce the lowest recognition or understanding error rates.

A third requirement is acceptable computational complexity, both in terms of time and space. This has an impact on the central memory requirements for the hardware system. Having responses close to real-time is a necessary condition. This implies methods based on algorithms with linear time-complexity or with polynomial time complexity only if the input size is very small.

Knowledge can be manually compiled or obtained by automatic learning from a corpus of data. Coverage and precision of manually derived knowledge are often limited. The best results so far have been obtained using component models having a simple, manually decided structure. Statistical parameters of these models are estimated by automatic training. Complex knowledge structures are obtained by composition of basic models.

STATISTICAL ACOUSTIC MODELS

Modern ASR systems generate a sequence of word hypotheses from an acoustic signal acquired by a microphone directly connected to the Analog to Digital (A/D) converter, available in many modern workstations. The most popular algorithms implemented in these architectures are based on statistical methods (Rabiner, 1989). A general block diagram for ASR is shown in Fig. 5.2. Other approaches can be found in (Waibel & Lee, 1990) where a collection of papers describes a variety of systems with historical reviews and mathematical foundations.

A vector y_t of acoustic features is computed every 10 msec. Details of this component can be found in (Waibel & Lee, 1990). Various possible choices of vectors together with their impact on recognition performance are discussed in (Haeb-Umbach, Geller, & Ney, 1993).

Sequences of vectors of acoustic parameters are treated as observations of acoustic word models used to compute $\Pr(x_1^T|W)$,[1] the probability of observing a sequence x_1^T of vectors when a word sequence W is pronounced.

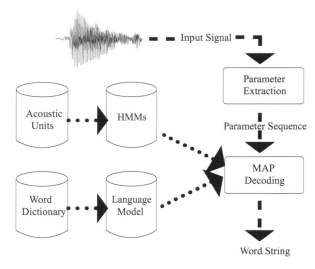

FIG. 5.2. Block diagram of a Speech Recognition System.

As outlined in the introduction, recognition is based on the search for the sequence of words having the maximum a-posteriori (MAP) probability with respect to the observations. For large vocabularies, search is performed in two steps. The first generates a word lattice or the N best word sequences with simple models to compute approximate likelihoods in real-time. In the second step more accurate likelihoods are compared with a limited number of hypotheses. Some systems generate a single word sequence hypothesis with a single step. The search produces an hypothesized word sequence if the task is dictation. If the task is understanding then a conceptual structure is obtained with a process that may involve more than two steps. Ways for automatic learning and extracting these structures are described in Kuhn and De Mori (1995).

In a statistical framework, an inventory of elementary probabilistic models of basic linguistic units (e.g., phonemes) is used to build word representations. A sequence of acoustic parameters, extracted from a spoken utterance, is seen as a realization of a concatenation of elementary processes described by Hidden Markov Models (HMMs). An HMM is a composition of two stochastic processes, a "hidden" Markov chain, which accounts for temporal variability, and an observable process, which accounts for spectral variability. This combination has proven to be powerful enough to cope with the most important sources of speech ambiguity, and flexible enough to allow the realization of recognition systems with dictionaries of tens of thousands of words.

Structure of a Hidden Markov Model

A Hidden Markov Model is defined as a pair of stochastic processes (S, X). The S process is a first-order Markov chain, and is not directly observable, while the X process is a sequence of random variables taking values in the space of acoustic parameters, or "observations."

By letting $y \in \mathcal{X}$ be a variable representing observations and $i, j \in \mathcal{S}$ be variables representing model states, assumptions for formal definition of an HMM are expressed as follows:

$$\Pr\left[S_t = i \mid S_0^{t-1} = i_0^{t-1} \right] = \Pr\left(S_t = i \mid S_{t-1} = i_{t-1} \right) \quad (5.3)$$

$$\Pr\left[X_t = y \mid S_0^{T} = i_0^{T}, X_1^{t-1} = x_1^{t-1} \right] = \Pr\left[X_t = x \mid S_{t-1}^{t} = i_t^{t} \right] \quad (5.4)$$

where the probabilities at the right-hand side of the above equations are independent of time t.

Equation 5.3, known as "first-order Markov hypothesis," states that history has no influence on the chain's future evolution if the present is specified. Equation 5.4, known as "output independence hypothesis," states that neither chain evolution nor past observations influence the present observation if the last chain transition is specified.

The model can be represented by the following parameters:

$A \qquad a_{i,j} \mid i, j \in \mathcal{S} \quad$ "transition probabilities"
$B \qquad b_{i,j} \mid i, j \in \mathcal{S} \quad$ "output distributions"
$\Pi \qquad \{ _i \mid i \in \mathcal{S} \} \quad$ "initial probabilities"

with the following definitions:

$a_{i,j} \qquad \Pr\left(S_t = j \mid S_{t-1} = i \right)$
$b_{i,j}(x) \qquad \Pr\left(X_t = x \mid S_{t-1} = i, S_t = j \right)$
$_i \qquad \Pr\left(S_0 = i \right)$

An interesting tutorial on the topic can be found in (Rabiner, 1989).

Types of Hidden Markov Models

HMMs can be classified according to the nature of the elements of the B matrix, which are distribution functions.

Distributions are defined on finite spaces in the so-called discrete HMMs. In this case, observations are vectors of symbols in a finite alphabet of N different elements. For each one of the Q vector components, a discrete

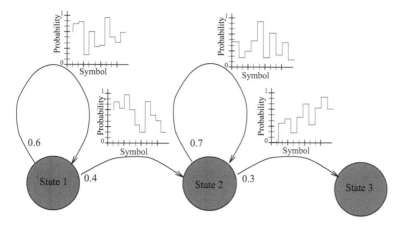

FIG. 5.3. Example of a discrete HMM. A transition probability and an output distribution on the symbol set is associated with every transition.

density $\{w(k)|k = 1\ldots N\}$ is defined, and the distribution is obtained by multiplying the probabilities of each component:

$$b_{i,j}(x) = \prod_{q=1}^{Q} w_{i,j}^{q}(x^q)$$

Noticethat this definition assumes that the different components are independent. Figure 5.3 shows an example of a discrete HMM with one-dimensional observations. Distributions are associated with model transitions.

Another possibility is to define distributions as probability densities on continuous observation spaces. In this case, strong restrictions have to be imposed on the functional form of the distributions, in order to have a manageable number of statistical parameters to estimate. The most popular approach is to characterize the model transitions with mixtures of base densities g of a family G having a simple parametric form:

$$b_{i,j}(x) = \sum_{k=1}^{N_{i,j}} w_{i,j}^{k} g_{i,j}^{k}(x)$$

Acoustic phonetic knowledge is represented by the model topology that reflects an assumption about the temporal structure of phonemes and by probability distributions of acoustic parameters. The assumption is that every value of an acoustic measure can be measured for a phoneme, but a given value has different probabilities to be associated to each phoneme.

The base densities $g \in G$ are usually gaussian or laplacian, and can be parameterized by the mean vector and the covariance matrix. HMMs with these kinds of distributions are usually referred to as continuous HMMs. In order to model complex distributions in this way a rather high number of base densities have to be used in every mixture. This may require a very large training corpus of data for the estimation of the distributions parameters. Problems arising when the available corpus is not large enough can be alleviated by sharing distributions among transitions of different models. In semicontinuous HMMs (Huang, Ariki, & Jack, 1990), for example, all mixtures are expressed in terms of a common set of base densities. Different mixtures are characterized only by different weights as shown in the following equation:

$$b_{i,j}(x) = \sum_{k=1}^{N} w_{i,j}^k g^k(x).$$

A common generalization of semicontinuous modeling consists of interpreting the input vector x as composed of several components $x[1] \ldots x[Q]$, each of which is associated with a different set of base distributions. The components are assumed to be statistically independent, hence the distributions associated with model transitions are mixtures of gaussian distributions of the form:

$$b_{i,j}(x) = \prod_{q=1}^{Q} \left(\sum_{k=1}^{N_q} w_{i,j}^{q,k} g_q^k(x[q]) \right)$$

Computation of probabilities with discrete models is faster than with continuous models; nevertheless, it is possible to speed up the mixture densities computation by applying vector quantization on the gaussians of the mixtures (Bocchieri, 1993).

Parameters of statistical models are estimated by iterative learning algorithms (Rabiner, 1989). in which the likelihood of a set of training data is guaranteed to increase at each step.

WORD AND UNIT MODELS

Words are usually represented by networks of phonemes. Each path in a word network represents a pronunciation of the word.

The same phoneme can have different acoustic distributions of observations if pronounced in different contexts. Allophone models of a phoneme are models of that phoneme in different contexts. The decision on how many allophones should be considered for a given phoneme may depend on many factors (e.g., the availability of enough training data to infer the model parameters). In practice, this number varies between a few hundreds and a few thousands.

A conceptually interesting approach is that of poliphones (Talamazzini, Niemann, Eckert, Kuhn, & Rieck, 1992). In principle, an allophone should be considered for every different word in which a phoneme appears. If the vocabulary is large, it is unlikely that there are enough data to train all these allophone models, so models for allophones of phonemes are considered at a different level of detail (word, syllable, triphone, diphone, context independent phoneme). Probability distributions for an allophone having a certain degree of generality can be obtained by mixing the distributions of more detailed allophone models. The loss in specificity is compensated by a more robust estimation of the statistical parameters due to the increase of the ratio between training data and free parameters to estimate.

Another approach consists of choosing allophones by clustering possible contexts. This choice can be made automatically with Classification and Regression Trees (CART). A CART is a binary tree having a phoneme at the root and, associated with each node n_i, a question Q_i about the context. Questions Q_i are of the type: Is the previous phoneme a nasal consonant? For each possible answer (*YES* or *NO*) there is a link to another node with which other questions are associated. There are algorithms for growing and pruning CARTs based on automatically assigning questions to a node from a manually determined pool of questions. The leaves of the tree may be simply labeled by an allophone symbol.

Papers by Bahl, de Souza, Gopalakrishnan, Nahamoo, & Picheny, 1991, and Hon and Lee, 1991 provide examples of the application of this concept and references to the description of a formalism for training and using CARTs.

Each allophone or "phone" model is an HMM made of states, transitions, and probability distributions. In order to improve the estimation of the statistical parameters of these models, some distributions can be the same or tied. For example, the distributions for the central portion of the allophones of a given phoneme can be tied reflecting the fact that they represent the stable (context-independent) physical realization of the central part of the phoneme, uttered with a stationary configuration of the vocal tract.

In general, all the models can be built by sharing distributions taken from a pool of, say, a few thousand cluster distributions called senones. Details on this approach can be found in Hwang and Huang, 1993.

Word models or allophone models can also be built by concatenation of basic structures made by states, transitions, and distributions. These units, called fenones, were introduced by Bahl, Brown, de Souza, Mercer, & Picheny, 1993b. Richer models of the same type but using more sophisticated building blocks, called *multones*, are described in (Bahl et al., 1993a).

Another approach consists of having clusters of distributions characterized by the same set of gaussian probability density functions. Allophone distributions are built by considering mixtures with the same components but with different weights (Digalakis & Murveit, 1994).

LANGUAGE MODELS

The probability $Pr(W)$ of a sequence of words $W = w_1 \ldots w_L$ is computed by an LM. In general $Pr(W)$ can be expressed as follows:

$$Pr(W) = Pr(w_1) \prod_{k=2}^{L} Pr(w_k | w_1, \ldots, w_{k-1}) = \prod_{k=1}^{L} Pr(w_k | H_k)$$

where H_k is the "history" of the words preceding w_k.

A popular approximation is used in a bigram language model, and is defined as follows:

$$Pr(w_1, \ldots, w_L) = Pr(w_1) \prod_{k=2}^{L} Pr(w_i | w_{i-1}). \tag{5.5}$$

In the fist search step, bigram probabilities are used in the LM in order to have structures on which search can be performed rapidly. More complex but more accurate LMs are used in successive search steps.

These probabilities can vary in time to take into account speaker preferences for different topics. Details on the use and the estimation of LM probabilities can be found in Ney, Essen & Kneser, 1994.

GENERATION OF WORD HYPOTHESES

Generation of word hypotheses can result in a single sequence of words, in a collection of the N best word sequences, or in a lattice of partially overlapping word hypotheses.

This generation is a search process in which a sequence of vectors of acoustic features is compared with word models. In this section, some distinctive characteristics of the computations involved in speech recognition algorithms will be described, first focusing on the case of a single-word utterance, and then considering the extension to continuous speech recognition.

In general, the speech signal and its transformations do not exhibit clear indication of word boundaries, so word boundary detection is part of the hypothesization process carried out as a search. In this process, all the word models are compared with a sequence of acoustic features. In the probabilistic framework, "comparison" between an acoustic sequence and a model involves the computation of the probability that the model assigns to the given sequence. This is the key ingredient of the recognition process. In this computation, the following quantities are used:

$_t(x_1^T, i)$: probability of having observed the partial sequence x_1^t and being in state i at time t

$$_t(x_1^T, i) \qquad \begin{array}{ll} \Pr(S_0 = i), & t = 0 \\ \Pr\ S_t = i, X_1^t = x_1^t, & t > 0 \end{array}$$

$_t(x_1^T, i)$: probability of observing the partial sequence x_{t+1}^T given that the model is in state i at time t

$$_t(x_1^T, i) \qquad \begin{array}{ll} \Pr\ X_{t+1}^T = x_{t+1}^T | S_t = i, & t < T \\ 1, & t = T \end{array}$$

$_t(x_1^T, i)$: probability of having observed the partial sequence x_1^t along the best path ending in state i at time t:

$$_t(x_1^T, i) \quad \left\{ \begin{array}{ll} \Pr(S_0 = i), & t = 0 \\ \max_{i_0^{t-1}} \Pr\ S_0^{t-1} = i_0^{t-1}, S_t = i, X_1^t = x_1^t & t > 0 \end{array} \right.$$

and   can be used to compute the total emission probability $\Pr(x_1^T | W)$ as follows:

$$\Pr(X_1^T = x_1^T) = \sum_i {}_T(x_1^T, i) \tag{5.6}$$

$$= \sum_i {}_i\ {}_0(x_1^T, i) \tag{5.7}$$

An approximation for computing this probability consists of following only the path of maximum probability. This can be done with the   quantity:

$$\Pr\ (X_1^T = x_1^T) = \max_i {}_T(x_1^T, i). \tag{5.8}$$

The computations of all the above probabilities share a common framework, employing a matrix called a *trellis*, depicted in Fig. 5.4. For the sake of simplicity, we can assume that the HMM in Fig. 5.4 represents a word and that the input signal corresponds to the pronunciation of an isolated word.

Every trellis column holds the values of one of the just introduced probabilities for a partial sequence ending at different time instants, and every

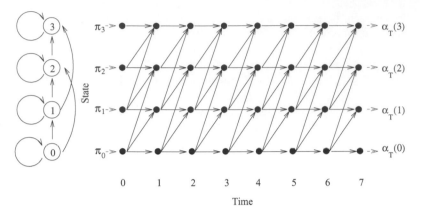

FIG. 5.4. A state-time trellis. See the text for a description.

interval between two columns corresponds to an input frame. The arrows in the trellis represent model transitions composing possible paths in the model from the initial time instant to the final one. The computation proceeds in a column-wise manner, at every time frame updating the scores of the nodes in a column by means of recursion formulas that involve the values of an adjacent column, the transition probabilities of the models, and the values of the output distributions for the corresponding frame. For and coefficients, the computation starts from the leftmost column, whose values are initialized with the values of $_i$, and ends at the opposite side, computing the final value with (6) or (8). For the coefficients, the computation goes from right to left.

The algorithm for computing coefficients is known as the Viterbi algorithm, and can be seen as an application of Dynamic Programming for finding a maximum probability path in a graph with weighted arcs. The recursion formula for its computation is the following:

$$_t(x_1^T, i) = \begin{cases} _i, & t = 0 \\ \max_j {_{t-1}}(x_1^T, j) a_{j,i} b_{j,i}(x_t), & t > 0 \end{cases}$$

By keeping track of the state j giving the maximum value in the previous recursion formula, it is possible, at the end of the input sequence, to retrieve the states visited by the best path, thus performing a sort of time-alignment of input frames with models states.

All these algorithms have a time complexity $O(MT)$, where M is the number of transitions with non-zero probability and T is the length of the input sequence. M can be at most equal to $\mid S \mid^2$, where $\mid S \mid$ is the number of states in the model, but is usually much lower, since the transition probability matrix is generally sparse. In fact, a common choice in speech recognition is to impose severe constraints on the allowed state sequences, for example $a_{i,j} = 0$ for $j < i, j > i + 2$, as is the case of the model in Fig. 5.4.

In general, recognition is based on a search process, which takes into account all the possible segmentations of the input sequence into words, and the a-priori probabilities that the LM assigns to sequences of words.

Good results can be obtained with simple LMs based on bigram or trigram probabilities. As an example, let us consider a bigram language model. This model can be conveniently incorporated into a finite state automaton as shown in Fig. 5.5, where dashed arcs correspond to transitions between words with probabilities of the LM.

After substitution of the word-labeled arcs with the corresponding HMMs, the resulting automaton becomes a big HMM itself, on which a Viterbi search for the most probable path, given an observation sequence, can be carried out. The dashed arcs are to be treated as "empty transitions" (i.e., transitions without an associated output distribution). This requires some generalization of the Viterbi algorithm. During the execution of the Viterbi algorithm, a minimum of backtracking information is kept to allow the reconstruction of the best path in terms of word labels. Note that the solution provided by this search is "suboptimal," in the sense that it gives

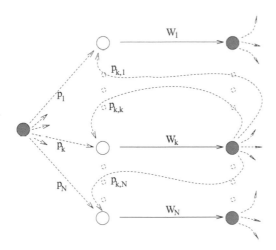

FIG. 5.5. Bigram LM represented as a weighted word graph. $p_{h,k}$ stands for $\Pr(W_k|W_h)$, p_h stands for $\Pr(W_h)$. The leftmost node is the starting node, rightmost ones are finals.

the probability of a single state sequence of the composite model, and not the total emission probability of the best word model sequence. In practice, however, it has been observed that the path probabilities computed with the previously mentioned algorithms exhibit a dominance property, consisting of a single state sequence accounting for most of the total probability (Merhav & Ephraim, 1991).

The composite model grows with the vocabulary and can lead to large search spaces. Nevertheless the uneven distribution of probabilities among different paths can help. It turns out that, when the number of states is large, at every time instant, a large portion of states have an accumulated likelihood that is much less than the highest one, so that it is very unlikely that a path passing through one of these states would become the best path at the end of the utterance. This consideration leads to a complexity reduction technique called beam search (Ney, Mergel, Nell, & Paesler, 1992), consisting of neglecting states whose accumulated score is lower than the best one minus a given threshold. In this way, a lot of computation needed to expand "bad" nodes is avoided. It is clear from the naivety of the pruning criterion that this reduction technique has the undesirable property of being not admissible, possibly causing the loss of the best path. In practice, good tuning of the beam threshold results in a gain in speed by an order of magnitude, while introducing a negligible amount of search errors.

When the dictionary is of the order of tens of thousands of words, the network becomes too big, and others methods have to be considered.

At present, different techniques exist for dealing with very large vocabularies. Most of them use multipass algorithms. Each pass prepares information for the next one, reducing the size of the search space. Details of these methods can be found in Alleva, Huang, & Hwang, 1993; Aubert, Dugast, Ney, & Steinbiss, 1994; Kubala et al., 1994; Murveit, Butzberger, Digilakis, & Weintraub, 1993.

In a first phase a set of candidate interpretations is represented in an object called word lattice, whose structure varies in different systems: It may contain only hypotheses on the location of words, or it may carry a record of acoustic scores as well. The construction of the word lattice may involve only the execution of a Viterbi beam- search with memorization of word scoring and localization, as in Aubert et al., 1994, or may itself require multiple steps, as in Alleva et al., 1993; Kubala et al., 1994; or Murveit et al., 1993. Since the word lattice is only an intermediate result, to be inspected by other detailed methods, its generation is performed with a bigram language model, and often with simplified acoustic models.

The word hypotheses in the lattice are scored with a more accurate language model, and sometimes with more detailed acoustic models. Lattice rescoring may require new calculations of HMM probabilities (Murveit et al., 1993), may proceed on the basis of precomputed probabilities only (Alleva et al., 1993; Aubert et al., 1994), or may even exploit acoustic models that are not HMMs (Kubala et al., 1994). In Alleva et al., 1993, the last step is based on an A search (Nilsson, 1971) on the word lattice, allowing the application of a "long distance language model" (i.e., a model where the probability of a word may not only depend on its immediate predecessor). In Aubert et al., 1994, a Dynamic Programming algorithm, using trigram probabilities, is performed.

A method that does not make use of the word lattice is presented in Paul, 1994. Inspired by one of the first methods proposed for continuous speech recognition (Jelinek, 1969), it combines both powerful language modeling and detailed acoustic modeling in a single step, performing an A-based search.

COMMENTS ON STATISTICAL MODELS

Interesting software architectures for ASR have been recently developed. They provide acceptable recognition performance, almost in real-time, for dictation of large vocabularies (more than 10,000 words). They are speaker-dependent or speaker-independent and accept continuous speech. Pure software solutions require, at the moment, a considerable amount of central memory. Special boards make it possible to run interesting applications on PCs.

Different groups performed experiments in 1994 on a corpus known as North American Business (NAB) that contains 248 million words.

The corpus contained a large test set of sentences read from many male and female speakers with almost no background noise and no hesitation.

Some important problems emerging from these experiments are discussed in the following.

1. **Vocabulary size and proportion of Out of Vocabulary (OOV) words** By building IN and using in successive search steps a basic dictionary of 20,000 words, 2.4% of OOV where observed (IBM). This fact contributed to the overall Word Error Rate (WER) measured as the percentage of Word Insertions (I), Deletions (D), and Substitutions (S) over all the words in the test set.

2. **Language models** With a multiple step search, it was possible to use LMs with increasing complexity in successive search steps.
The overall WER varied between 9% and 22% considering all sites involved in the experiments.

3. **Acoustic models** Almost all sites used semicontinuous or continuous context-dependent HMMs with very simple (3 or 4 states) models.

Context dependency was extended up to 5 phonemes at Cambridge University (CU).

Various types of sharing were used from sets of gaussians to complete distributions.

Usually gender-dependent thousands of models were used.

A number of up to 100,000 different gaussian distributions in a system was used, with four to a few tenths gaussians per mixture.

Cross word phoneme models were separately trained in some systems.

There are aspects of the best current systems that still need improvement. The best systems do not perform equally well with different speakers and different speaking environments. They have difficulty in handling out of vocabulary words, hesitations, false starts, and other phenomena typical of spontaneous speech. Rudimentary understanding capabilities are available for speech understanding in limited domains (Kuhn & De Mori, 1995). Key research challenges for the future are acoustic robustness, use of better acoustic features and models, use of multiple word pronunciations and efficient constraints for the access of a very large lexicon, sophisticated and multiple language models capable of representing various types of contexts, rich methods for extracting conceptual representations from word hypotheses, and automatic learning methods for extracting various types of knowledge from corpora.

NEURAL NETWORK MODELS

Artificial Neural Networks (ANNs) are learning machines trainable from examples, loosely inspired from principles of data processing in the brain. Machine learning algorithms are not limited to ANNs training but are also used in statistics and probabilistic modeling (HMMs, linear regression, time-series auto-regressive and moving average models, non-parametric statistical models, and many others), and in Artificial Intelligence (decision trees, rule induction, etc.). They have been applied in various aspects of ASR, with results comparable to those obtained with HMMs in large vocabulary dictation systems. Interesting results were obtained in some speech processing specific phoneme and feature recognition tasks.

SIMPLE LINEAR PERCEPTRONS AND
THE WIDROW-HOFF ALGORITHM

For the sake of simplicity, let us introduce a feed-forward connectionist model trainable with supervision by providing for each training input sample, the corresponding desired output. This means that input vectors are presented at the input of the network one at a time. Based on the input, the network computes an output vector. An application of this device could be feature extraction. The input vector could have as components the spectral energies obtained with a filter bank, and the outputs could be places of articulation. An effective connectionist feature extractor is discussed in Bengio et al., 1992.

Let us consider the training set $T = \{(x_k, y_k) \mid k = 1, \ldots, N\}$, where N input samples (e.g., vectors of energies) $x_1, \ldots, x_N$ have been previously labeled with their corresponding desired (target) outputs $y_1, \ldots, y_N$ (e.g., feature values; close to 1 if the feature is present in the speech segment represented by the input, close to zero otherwise). The aim is to build a model able to compute for each input of the training data an output close to the desired one, according to some optimality evaluation criterion. A particular family of such models is represented by Simple Linear Perceptrons (see Fig. 5.6).

A simple Linear Perceptron has a set of input units S_I acting as placeholders for the components of the current input vector. Each input unit is fully connected with all the neurons of the output units set S_O, via direct links or connections (synapses) characterized by a specific connection weight (synaptic strength), denoted with $w_{i,j}$ in the figure (in the following figures, connection weights are not explicitly shown). The inputs are propagated forward along the connections and multiplied by the corresponding connection weight. All the incoming weighted signals to a given output unit are summed together to form the input to the unit itself. The unit reacts by producing an activation response which is equal to its input. This model is usually referred to as a layered network, with the obvious meaning that units are arranged into subsequent layers: The computation proceeds from one layer to the one that immediately follows in the bottom-up order, but

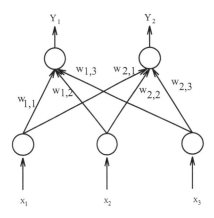

FIG. 5.6. Simple Linear Perceptron.

never in a lateral or backward manner. For this reason the network is called "feed forward."

The family of models considered in this section fits the training data as summarized by the following equation (written for the generic i-th output component):

$$f_i(\mathbf{x}) = \sum_{j \in S_I} w_{ij} x_j. \tag{5.9}$$

The Equation (5.9) is a homogeneous linear transformation (an additive bias can be easily added to the model). Simple Linear Perceptrons can thus be seen as linear regression models or linear discriminators for classification. Nevertheless, the way these networks learn from the training set is quite general, and can be extended to the study of other, more complex, ANN architectures. If it is used for detecting acoustic features, we can assume that the speech knowledge used for extracting these features has been acquired automatically by the training algorithm and is stored into the connection weights.

Once a training set T and a Simple Linear Perceptron are given, with the obvious assumption that the number of input and output units matches the dimensionality of the input and target vectors, respectively, the learning problem can be stated as the search for the network weights $\mathbf{w}$ that allow to optimally fit the data, according to a certain criterion. The latter is usually expressed as a functional of the training data (and of the model) that represents a gain to be maximized or a loss (or risk) to be minimized. A sound and common choice for the criterion function is the sum of squared differences between target outputs and actual outputs:

$$C = \frac{1}{2} \sum_{n=1}^{N} \sum_{k \in S_O} (y_{kn} \quad \hat{y}_{kn})^2 \tag{5.10}$$

where y_{kn} is k-th component of n-th target, $\hat{y}_{kn}$ is output of k-th output unit when the network is presented with the n-th input vector, and the multiplicative factor $1/2$ is introduced for computational convenience, as we shall see below. The minimization of (5.10) is known as least square criterion. A general and broadly used optimization technique for the minimization of expression (5.10) is the gradient descent method. Most network training algorithms are based on it. Although it is not guaranteed that the approach will eventually reach the absolute minimum of the criterion function, these techniques often produce practically useful behavior. It is worth noting that the estimation of the coefficients of a linear transformation that will minimize a least squares criterion on a training set using gradient descent is an instance of the well-known *Widrow-Hoff algorithm*, used to perform discriminant linear analysis for classification. We will see that gradient descent iterative algorithms are used also for training more complicated ANN architectures.

The iterative approach can be developed in the following way. Given the vector **w** of the connection weights at a certain iterative step of the algorithm, with an arbitrary choice at the initial step, a new weight vector **w'** is computed according to the expression:

$$\mathbf{w'} = \mathbf{w} + \Delta\mathbf{w} \tag{5.11}$$

where $\Delta\mathbf{w}$ denotes the weight-change vector, that in turn satisfies the following relation:

$$\Delta\mathbf{w} \propto \nabla_{\mathbf{w}}C. \tag{5.12}$$

In expression (5.12) the symbol $\nabla_{\mathbf{w}}C$ represents the gradient vector of the error functional computed with respect to the weights **w**. The algorithm takes a move away from the current weights along the direction opposite to the gradient, by prescribing:

$$\Delta\mathbf{w} = \quad \nabla_{\mathbf{w}}C \tag{5.13}$$

or, equivalently, if individual variations of weights are expressed in terms of the corresponding partial derivatives:

$$\Delta w_{ij} = \quad \frac{\partial C}{\partial w_{ij}} \tag{5.14}$$

where   is the so-called learning rate, a small constant that controls the rate of convergence of the algorithm (i.e. the length of the step away from the current point in weight space). Larger values of   allow for faster convergence, however, if the value is too large, the algorithm can diverge (C increases). The optimal value of   depends on the largest eigenvalue of the Hessian matrix of second-order derivatives of the cost function with respect to the weights (see the next section). In any case, the above iterative step is repeated, starting from the initial weights and evolving along an ideal trajectory into the weight space, until convergence to a minimum of the criterion function is reached, or when a stopping criterion is met. The latter can be related to the availability of computational resources, or can be expressed in terms of an estimation of generalization performance at each iteration (early stopping). From a theoretical point of view, the gradient descent technique can always reach a minimum of the criterion function (if the learning rate is reduced during training, that is if $\sum_{t=1}^{\infty}{}_t = \infty$ and

$\sum_{t=1}^{\infty} \frac{2}{t} < \infty$), but it can get stuck in local minima without reaching the global minimum. Starting the algorithm from different initial weights for a few times is a common practice.

In practical cases, instead of computing the gradient of function (5.10), with a summation over all the training samples (batch mode), an on-line variant of the algorithm is used, by taking the partial derivatives of the following error functional:

$$C = \frac{1}{2} \sum_{k \in S_O} (y_k \quad \hat{y}_k)^2 \tag{5.15}$$

which is locally computed over each training pair $(\mathbf{x}, \mathbf{y})$, and the weight changes are still determined using Equation (5.14) every time the network is presented with a new input vector. This approach, also known as stochastic gradient descent, proves to be quite effective when the number of training patterns is large (> hundreds). The whole training set is repeatedly fed through the net for a certain number of *epochs*. An important consequence of stochastic gradient is the ability of incremental training, since the network can potentially learn more from new examples without requiring a complete, batch retraining. This is an historical reason why the terms learning or adaptation, other than optimization, are often used to describe this process. Stochastic gradient descent has also proven to be more effective than standard gradient in many cases, particularly for its generalization ability.

In order to obtain an explicit form for Equation (5.14) suitable for an efficient implementation, the partial derivatives of Equation (5.15) with respect to a generic weight w_{ij} have to be computed. We can write:

$$\frac{\partial C}{\partial w_{ij}} = \frac{1}{2} \sum_{k \in S_O} \frac{\partial (y_k \quad \hat{y}_k)^2}{\partial w_{ij}} \tag{5.16}$$

$$= \frac{1}{2} \frac{\partial (y_i \quad \hat{y}_i)^2}{\partial w_{ij}}$$

$$= (y_i \quad \hat{y}_i) \frac{\partial \hat{y}_i}{\partial w_{ij}}.$$

Recalling Equation (5.9) we can now write the partial derivative of the output $\hat{y}_i$ from the i-th output unit with respect to the weight w_{ij} as:

$$\frac{\partial \hat{y}_i}{\partial w_{ij}} = \frac{\partial f_i(x_i)}{\partial w_{ij}} \tag{5.17}$$

$$= \frac{\partial \sum_{l \in S_I} w_{il} x_l}{\partial w_{ij}}$$

$$= x_j$$

where x_i denotes the input to output unit i. Substituting Equations (5.16) and (5.17) into Equation (5.14) we obtain:

$$\Delta w_{ij} = (y_i - \hat{y}_i)x_j \qquad (5.18)$$

that gives the weight changes for each connection weight of the network in terms of the product of the component of the current input vector to the connection, by the difference between the desired and the actual output from the corresponding neuron. If the difference is small (i.e. the network response strictly resembles the target value), only a small adjustment of the weight is performed. Larger differences imply heavier modifications of the synaptic strengths.

If we define the quantity δ_i as:

$$\delta_i = y_i - \hat{y}_i \qquad (5.19)$$

we can rewrite Equation (5.18) in the form:

$$\Delta w_{ij} = \delta_i x_j \qquad (5.20)$$

which is known as the delta rule and provides a more compact representation of the learning rule (5.18).

Equation (5.20) can be written as the difference of two terms as follows:

$$\Delta w_{ij} = y_i x_j - \hat{y}_i x_j \qquad (5.21)$$

where the first term is a typical example of Hebbian learning, which expresses the tendency to strengthen the synaptic weight whenever the input and the desired output of a neuron (pre- and post synaptic activations) are high together. The second term, on the contrary, is referred to as anti-Hebbian learning, with the intuitive opposite meaning.

A direct and important extension to the Simple Linear Perceptron model uses a more general activation functions $f_i()$ of the output units. The only constraint that must be imposed, if the gradient descent technique is still used, is that the activation functions must be continuous and differentiable functions. In this general case Equation (5.17) must be rewritten in the following form:

$$\frac{\partial \hat{y}_i}{\partial w_{ij}} = \frac{\partial f_i(x_i)}{\partial w_{ij}} \qquad (5.22)$$

$$= \frac{\partial f_i(x_i)}{\partial x_i} \frac{\partial x_i}{\partial w_{ij}}$$

$$= f_i'(x_i)\frac{\partial \sum_{l \in S_I} w_{il} x_l}{\partial w_{ij}}$$

$$= f_i'(x_i)x_j$$

where $f_i'(x_i)$ is the derivative of the activation function computed over the current input x_i to i-th unit, and Equation (5.14) now becomes:

$$\Delta w_{ij} = (y_i \quad \hat{y}_i) f_i'(x_i) x_j \qquad (5.23)$$

that easily reduces to Equation (5.18) in the linear case. It is still possible to define the quantity $_i$ to be:

$$_i = (y_i \quad \hat{y}_i) f_i'(x_i) \qquad (5.24)$$

that, in turn, is a straight generalization of Equation (5.19) and includes the latter as a special case, leading to:

$$\Delta w_{ij} = _i x_j \qquad (5.25)$$

that is identical to Equation (5.20). In the next section the above concepts are further developed in the context of multilayered networks and, surprisingly enough, the computation of the learning algorithm for these models will lead to expressions substantially identical to the delta rule.

MULTILAYER PERCEPTRONS AND
THE BACK-PROPAGATION ALGORITHM

The most popular neural network architecture is the Multilayer Perceptron (MLP), also known as feed-forward neural network. This is an extension of the Simple Linear Perceptron with additional layers of units, called hidden layers. In the hidden layers an internal, intermediate representation of data is formed and temporally stored. The motivation for introducing this model is that Simple Linear Perceptrons cannot perform many useful classification functions. An MLP is fed by an input vector and subsequent computations are passed from layer to layer in the usual feed-forward manner. This produces an output vector of values of the units of the last (output) layer of the network. Activation functions associated to hidden and output units can be linear or nonlinear, and can be different for different units. Input units still act as placeholders for the components of the current input vector. A training algorithm estimates a set of weights to be assigned to the connections between each pair of units belonging to adjacent layers, in order to optimize a training criterion.

Training is supervised. Let us consider a labeled training set $T = \{(\mathbf{x}_k, \mathbf{y}_k) \mid k = 1, \dots, N\}$. The learning problem for MLPs is to find the

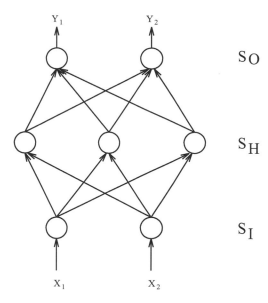

FIG. 5.7. Multilayer Perceptron.

weights that result in a (generally nonlinear) model that best fits the training data, given a certain criterion function. The most common choice for the criterion is the sum of squared differences between target and actual outputs, just as in the case of Simple Linear Perceptrons. We illustrate an on-line gradient descent technique (Le Cun, 1986; Rumelhart, Hinton, & Williams, 1986; Werbos, 1974) to minimize the cost function:

$$C = \frac{1}{2} \sum_{n \in S_O} (y_n - \hat{y}_n)^2 \tag{5.26}$$

computed as a consequence of the presentation of a certain input pattern $\mathbf{x}$ associated with a desired output vector $\mathbf{y}$ of a layered network with a set of input units S_I, hidden units S_H, and output units S_O. An example of such a network is shown in Fig. 5.7. Extension to more hidden layers is straightforward.

The learning algorithm is similar to the one for Simple Linear Perceptrons. The weight change Δw_{ij} of the connection strength between the j-th hidden unit and the i-th *output* unit is computed as follows:

$$\Delta w_{ij} = -\frac{\partial C}{\partial w_{ij}}. \tag{5.27}$$

The calculation begins as in Equation (5.16), by writing:

$$\frac{\partial C}{\partial w_{ij}} = \frac{1}{2} \sum_{n \in S_O} \frac{\partial (y_n - \hat{y}_n)^2}{\partial w_{ij}} \tag{5.28}$$

$$= \frac{1}{2} \frac{\partial (y_i - \hat{y}_i)^2}{\partial w_{ij}}$$

$$= (y_i - \hat{y}_i) \frac{\partial \hat{y}_i}{\partial w_{ij}}$$

where the term $\frac{\partial \hat{y}_i}{\partial w_{ij}}$ can be calculated as:

$$\frac{\partial \hat{y}_i}{\partial w_{ij}} = \frac{\partial f_i(a_i)}{\partial w_{ij}} \tag{5.29}$$

$$= \frac{\partial f_i(a_i)}{\partial a_i} \frac{\partial a_i}{\partial w_{ij}}$$

$$= f_i'(a_i) \frac{\partial \sum_{l \in S_H} w_{il} \hat{y}_l}{\partial w_{ij}}$$

$$= f_i'(a_i) \hat{y}_j$$

where $f_i'(a_i)$ still denotes derivative of the activation function computed over the current input a_i to the i-th unit. We define

$$\partial_i = (y_i - \hat{y}_i) f_i'(a_i) \tag{5.30}$$

and we write:

$$\Delta w_{ij} = \partial_i \hat{y}_j \tag{5.31}$$

as in the delta rule for Simple Perceptrons. Let us now consider a unit of the hidden layer, say j. The variation of a weight w_{jk} associated to a connection between the k-th input unit and the j-th hidden unit

$$\Delta w_{jk} = -\frac{\partial C}{\partial w_{jk}} \tag{5.32}$$

can be computed considering that:

$$\frac{\partial C}{\partial w_{jk}} = \frac{1}{2} \sum_{n \in S_O} \frac{\partial (y_n - \hat{y}_n)^2}{\partial w_{jk}} \tag{5.33}$$

$$= -\sum_{n \in S_O} (y_n - \hat{y}_n) \frac{\partial \hat{y}_n}{\partial w_{jk}}.$$

(5.33) resembles (5.28), but exploits the consequences that changes in weight w_{jk} have on the whole set of output units (i.e. each hidden unit affects all of the outputs in some way). Now we can write:

$$\frac{\partial \hat{y}_n}{\partial w_{jk}} = \frac{\partial f_n(a_n)}{\partial w_{jk}} \qquad (5.34)$$

$$= \frac{\partial f_n(a_n)}{\partial a_n} \frac{\partial a_n}{\partial w_{jk}}$$

$$= f_n'(a_n) \frac{\partial a_n}{\partial w_{jk}}$$

where a further development of term $\frac{\partial a_n}{\partial w_{jk}}$ leads to:

$$\frac{\partial a_n}{\partial w_{jk}} = \frac{\partial \sum_{l \in S_H} w_{nl} \hat{y}_l}{\partial w_{jk}} \qquad (5.35)$$

$$= \sum_{l \in S_H} w_{nl} \frac{\partial \hat{y}_l}{\partial w_{jk}}$$

$$= w_{nj} \frac{\partial \hat{y}_j}{\partial w_{jk}}$$

and, in turn,

$$\frac{\partial \hat{y}_j}{\partial w_{jk}} = \frac{\partial f_j(a_j)}{\partial w_{jk}} \qquad (5.36)$$

$$= \frac{\partial f_j(u_j)}{\partial a_j} \frac{\partial a_j}{\partial w_{jk}}$$

$$= f_j'(a_j) \frac{\partial \sum_{m \in S_I} w_{jm} x_m}{\partial w_{jk}}$$

$$= f_j'(a_j) x_k.$$

Substituting Equations (5.33), (5.34), (5.35), and (5.36) into Equation (5.32) we finally obtain:

$$\Delta w_{jk} = \sum_{n \in S_O} (y_n - \hat{y}_n) f_n'(a_n) w_{nj} \; f_j'(a_j) x_k \qquad (5.37)$$

$$= \left\{ \sum_{n \in S_O} w_{nj} (y_n - \hat{y}_n) f_n'(a_n) \right\} f_j'(a_j) x_k$$

$$= \left(\sum_{n \in S_O} w_{nj} \, _n \right) f_j'(a_j) x_k$$

where $_n$ is defined as in Equation (5.24), for each output unit. For a generic unit j in the hidden layer we can similarly define:

$$_j = \left(\sum_{n \in S_O} w_{nj} \;_n \right) f'_j(a_j) \qquad (5.38)$$

that brings to evidence the fact that the deltas for hidden units can no longer be computed as a direct function of the difference between the desired target output and the actual network output, because the units themselves have an indirect influence on it. The deltas can rather be expressed as a weighted sum of the deltas already computed at the upper layer, thus back-propagating deltas from one layer to the next (lower) one. In summary, the current input vector is propagated forward through the network, obtaining an output. The error, that is a squared difference between the obtained and the target output, is computed and used to determine deltas at the output layer. Weight changes for the weights of the output layer are immediately computable, according to the delta rule. These deltas are then propagated backward to the hidden layer, allowing for the computation of weight changes by application of Equation (5.37). This is usually referred to as error backpropagation, and the resulting algorithm is known as the Back-Propagation (BP) algorithm (Rumelhart et al., 1986). The compact formulation of the latter can be written as:

$$\Delta w_{jk} = \;_j x_k \qquad (5.39)$$

that, when used together with Equation (5.31) , is called the Generalized Delta Rule. If more than one hidden layer is present, the calculation proceeds exactly in the same way, back-propagating the deltas down to the next (lower) hidden layer and yielding a rule identical to Equation (5.39). The BP algorithm is the most popular training technique for neural networks, and it has been successfully used in a wide range of applications. The ability of MLPs to model a linear or nonlinear discriminant function for classification tasks, or a regressor in multivariate spaces, makes the feedforward connectionist approach a suitable method for many applications in speech processing. In Elman and Zipser, 1988b, an MLP was used as a static classifier of consonant-vowel syllables, yielding a 5% error rate for the consonants and a 0.5% error rate for the vowels on a single speaker dataset. MLPs were also used in Lippmann and Gold, 1987, to perform classification of 7 digits collected among 16 different speakers, providing a 7.6% error rate, that compared well with the results obtained with other statistical classification techniques. MLPs were used by Bengio and De Mori, 1988; and Bengio, Cosi, Cardin, & De Mori, 1989, in conjunction with local feedbacks in one of the hidden layers, for detecting various acoustic features starting from spectrograms obtained with an auditory model. The inputs were selected time/frequency regions of a spectrogram. One major limitation of MLPs for speech processing is that their architecture is not intrinsically suitable to the processing of sequential data. To overcome this problem, ANNs capable to deal with time sequences, such as Recurrent Neural Networks, have been successfully introduced and applied (see Gori et al., 1989). More recently, MLPs have been integrated with conventional speech processing algorithms (e.g., dynamic programming and hidden Markov models) (Bengio, 1996; Bourlard & Morgan, 1994), often resulting in improved recognition performance. More about hybrid systems will be described in the section on page 000.

UNSUPERVISED LEARNING

Let us now consider the *training set* $T = \{x_k \mid k = 1, \ldots, N\}$, where N input samples $x_1, \ldots, x_N$ have been collected, but no labeling is supposed to be available. Here, the learning task is aimed at discovering, in an unsupervised manner, inherent properties of the data and the way they are distributed in the feature space. Although the problem of learning anything from an unlabeled training set is very difficult, statistical pattern recognition techniques for unsupervised parametric mixture estimation and data clustering have been successfully proposed and applied in the last decades. Recently, different connectionist approaches to the problem have been introduced, often strictly related to the statistical ones, but sometimes indeed novel. They usually rely on statistical and geometrical properties of the given data.

Some of the most popular unsupervised networks, namely self-supervised (auto-associative) nets and competitive networks will be introduced in the following sections. Other unsupervised approaches to connectionist models are represented by ART and ART2 (Carpenter and Grossberg, 1987, 1988), Kohonen's Self-Organizing Map (SOM) (Kohonen, 1989, 1990), and Oja's and Sanger's networks (Oja, 1982, 1989; Oja and Karhunen, 1985; Sanger, 1989), which are capable of performing on-line projection of the input data along their Principal Components.

Unsupervised networks can be applied in a variety of speech processing tasks, for instance to perform feature extraction (Bourlard and Morgan, 1994), or vector quantization (Kohonen, 1986; Nasrabadi and Feng, 1988; Nasrabadi and King, 1988). For example, the latter can be used to adaptively quantize the parametric representation of signals to be used in discrete-density hidden Markov models (Rabiner, 1989). Unsupervised nets are also an adaptive alternative to clustering (Duda & Hart, 1973), for instance, in speaker identification based on the k-nearest neighbors algorithm (Duda and Hart, 1973), or in the initialization of statistical models based on mixtures of Gaussian components (e.g., Radial Basis Functions [Poggio and Girosi, 1990]).

Self-Supervised Networks

Self-supervised networks (Cottrell, Munro, & Zipser, 1987) are standard feed-forward networks, such as MLPs, trained in a supervised way (for instance using the BP algorithm discussed in an earlier section) on the training set $T' = \{(\mathbf{x}_k, \mathbf{x}_k) \mid k = 1, \ldots, N\}$ obtained from the original training set T by pairing each pattern with itself. The major constraint on the topology of the network is that one of the hidden layers is built up of a number of hidden units that must be significantly lower than the dimensionality of the input space. An illustrative example is given in Fig. 5.8.

Roughly speaking, the network is trained to reconstruct on its output units each input pattern that is fed into the input units by forcing the signal to be compressed through the low-dimensional hidden layer. This forces a low-dimensional representation of the information contained in the input data that is sufficient to reconstruct the original patterns. During the training step, the network learns low dimensional representations of the input vectors, preserving as much relevant information as possible. Once training is accomplished, the hidden layer can be used as an output

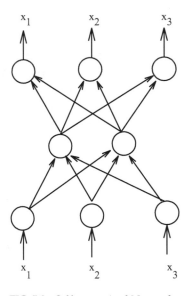

FIG. 5.8. Self-supervised Network.

layer to produce compressed patterns. This technique is an effective way to perform feature extraction (Elman and Zipser, 1988b) and, more generally, dimensionality reduction (Bourlard & Morgan, 1994; Cottrell et al., 1987) of a given signal representation. In fact, by applying the same pattern (e.g., a vector of acoustic features) at the input and at the output and using a small number of hidden units, it is possible to obtain at the output of the hidden layer a coded, compressed representation of the input. When there is only one hidden layer, this technique has been shown to be equivalent to the popular Principal Component Analysis (Baldi & Hornik, 1989; Bourlard and Kamp, 1988), that is the projection of the data along the space spanned by the principal eigenvectors (with the largest eigenvalues) of the data covariance matrix.

Competitive Neural Networks

Competitive Neural Networks (Hertz, Krogh, & Palmer, 1991) are one-layer feed-forward models similar to connectionist architectures such as ART, ART2, and SOM (Grossberg, 1976; Lippmann, 1987; Winters and Rose, 1989). These models are called competitive because each unit competes with all the others for the classification of each input pattern: The latter is indeed assigned to the winner unit, which is the closest (according to a given distance measure) to the input itself (i.e. the most representative within a certain set of prototypes). This is strictly related to the concept of clustering (Duda and Hart, 1973), where each unit represents the centroid (or mean, or codeword) of one of the clusters. The propagation of the input vector through the network consists in a projection of the pattern onto the weights of the connections entering each output unit. Connection weights are assumed to represent the components of the corresponding centroid. The aim of this forward propagation is to establish the closest centroid to the input vector (i.e. the winner unit). During training, a simple weight update rule is used to move the winner centroid toward the novel pattern, so that the components of the centroid represent a sort of moving average of the input patterns belonging to the corresponding cluster. This is basically an on-line version of several partitioning clustering algorithms (Duda and Hart, 1973). The learning rule can be derived as a consequence of maximum-likelihood estimation of the parameters of a mixture of Gaussians, under certain assumptions, and can be stated in the form:

$$\Delta w_{ij} = (x_j \quad w_{ij}) \tag{5.40}$$

where w_{ij} is the weight of the connection between input unit j and output unit i (the winner unit),   is the learning rate, and x_j is the j-th component of the pattern, of class i, presented to the network. When a new pattern is fed into the network, its distance is computed with respect to all the output units—using the connection weights as components of the corresponding mean vectors—and the pattern is assigned to the nearest unit (mixture component). The latter is referred to as the winner unit. Weight update, or learning, is then accomplished by modifying the connection weights of the winner unit by a direct application of Equation (5.40). The weights of the other units are left unchanged. This is a typical winner-take-all approach, where the units are in competition for novel input patterns. This is the rationale for using the name competitive neural networks. A detailed description of competitive learning and its relationships with statistical mixtures can be found in Nowlan, 1991. The way used here to derive the learning rule makes it clear that competitive neural networks can be seen as an on-line version of the popular *k-means* clustering algorithm (Duda and Hart, 1973). The simple, basic model can then be easily extended by introducing dynamic allocation of units or combining it with various supervised techniques. A parallel implementation is also straightforward.

ANNs FOR TIME SEQUENCES

There are problems, especially in speech processing, in which samples are temporal sequences of patterns, instead of individual independent samples. Two major classes of neural networks will be introduced, namely Time-Delay Neural Networks, and Recurrent Neural Networks. The latter generalizes the basic feed-forward architecture of MLPs by allowing arbitrary connections between units (e.g. loops and backward connections).

Time-Delay Neural Networks

Time-Delay Neural Networks (TDNN), also known as tapped delay lines, represent an effective attempt to train a static MLP for time-sequence processing by converting the temporal sequence into a spatial sequence over corresponding units. The idea is very simple, but useful in a variety of speech processing applications (Bourlard and Morgan, 1994; Waibel, 1989; Waibel, Hanazawa, Hinton, Shikano, & Lang, 1989). An example of a TDNN is shown in Fig. 5.9. The input layer has been enlarged to accept as many input patterns as the (fixed) sequence length to be processed at each time step. Input vectors enter the network from the leftmost set of input units. At each time step, inputs are shifted to the right through the unit delay line that links each set of input units to the right-adjacent one, and the next input pattern is fed into the leftmost position.

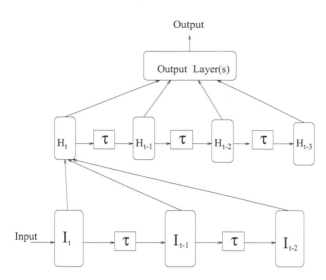

FIG. 5.9. Time-Delay Neural Network. Input is fed into the leftmost set of input units (I_t) at time t. Previous inputs (I_{t-1}, I_{t-2}) are shifted to the right, with unit delays represented by boxes labeled with τ. A similar mechanism holds in the hidden layer ($H_t, \ldots$). An integration over time of the input sequence is carried on by the leftmost set of hidden units, while the output layer of the net integrates over time the activations of the hidden units.

The same extension can also be applied to subsequent layers, introducing a tapped-delay mechanism between hidden units (e.g., only the first block of units in the tapped line actually receives input from the previous layer), introducing the ability to deal with more complicated time dependencies.

The BP algorithm can be used to train such a network. If the number of units used in subsequent layers to represent each time slot is reduced, relevant features are extracted from the original input, not based on a priori knowledge, but on a selection during the global network learning. The connections holding between adjacent layers can also be arranged in order to provide hidden units with selective inputs from groups of units in the previous layer (receptive fields). The resulting dynamics can be interpreted as a sub-sampling from the original temporal representation of the input data, with the effect of averaging over a specific time slice. In this way, different layers of the network provide the overall processing with representations of different temporal scales.

It should be noted that the TDNN can be seen as a particular case of the Convolutional Neural Network (Le Cun and Bengio, 1995) when used on "unidimensional" input (this is the case with sequences of acoustic vectors).

TDNNs have been successfully applied in speech processing. Lang and Hinton (1988) obtained a 7.8% error rate in multitalker classification of the isolated letters "B, D, E, V," using spectra collected among 100 male speakers. Waibel, Sawai, & Shikano, (1989) were able to recognize isolated consonants uttered by a Japanese speaker with a low error rate (4.1%), using a combination of specialized TDNNs. A significant 1.4% error rate in vowel recognition was obtained in the same experiments.

Recurrent Neural Networks

Recurrent Neural Networks (RNN) provide a powerful extension of feed-forward connectionist models by introducing connections bet-ween arbitrary pairs of units, independently from their position within the topology of the network. Self-recurrent loops of a unit onto itself, as well as backward connections to previous layers or lateral links between units belonging to the same layer are all allowed. An example is given in Fig. 5.10.

RNNs behave like dynamical systems. Once fed with an input, the re-current connections are responsible for an evolution in time of the internal state of the network. RNNs are particularly suited for sequence processing, due to their ability to keep an internal trace, or memory, of the past. This

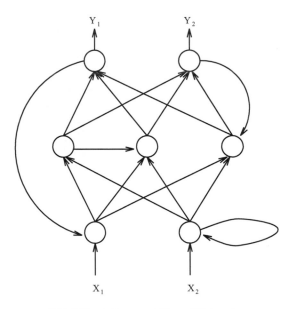

FIG. 5.10. A Recurrent Neural Network.

memory is combined with the current input to provide different output sequences when faced with different input sequences.

A first type of RNNs is applied to static patterns (i.e., the input is fixed) and its dynamic converges to specific attractors. For instance, in Boltzmann Machines (Hinton, Sejnowski, & Ackley, 1984) the recurrent connections are symmetric (bidirectional propagation of signal is allowed along the connection, i.e., pairs of adjacent units have an influence on each other). An interpretation of Boltzmann Machines in terms of statistical mechanics has been proposed, along with a learning algorithm based on simulated annealing (Kirkpatric, Gelatt, & Vecchi, 1983). An important instance of Boltzmann Machines is the Hopfield Net (Hopfield, 1982; Hopfield & Tank, 1986), basically constituted of a single layer of fully and symmetrically connected linear units, able to act as an auto-associative memory. Limitations of Boltzmann Machines reside in the requirement of symmetric (nondirectional) recurrent connections, and in the considerable computation time required to perform the simulated annealing.

Another family of RNNs is sometimes referred to as partially recurrent nets. In this case the basic architecture is that of a standard MLP, with the addition of a set of recurrent connections from the units in a given layer to the corresponding units of a previous layer (or in the same layer). Recurrent connections propagate the signal back to the units of one of the layers of the MLP, or to an additional context or state layer. An example is shown in Fig. 5.11. The units that receive signal from the recurrent connections act either as preprocessors, filtering the current (forward propagated) input with the previous signal, or as a register that keeps memory of previous history. The weights of the recurrent connections are fixed and set equal to a constant, chosen in order to calibrate the amount of previous information to be taken into account. The standard BP algorithm is used to train the underlying MLP architecture, but without the computation of the full gradient on the parameters, since the effect of the past activities through recurrent connections is not taken into account. Partially recurrent nets were introduced in Elman and Zipser, 1988a; Jordan, 1989; and Mozer, 1993 and resulted in a wide range of applications in sequence processing (both in recognition and in generation).

More generally, a recurrent neural network can have arbitrary directed connections, and all weights can be learned during the training. Different approaches to the problem of training recurrent connections have been proposed in the literature in the last years, mostly based on gradient-descent techniques. Particularly remarkable are Recurrent Back Propagation (Pineda, 1989), Back-Propagation for Sequences (BPS) (Gori, Bengio, & De Mori, 1989), Real Time Recurrent Learning (Williams and Zipser, 1989a, 1989b), and Time-dependent Recurrent Back-Propagation (Pearlmutter, 1989; Sato, 1990; Werbos, 1988).

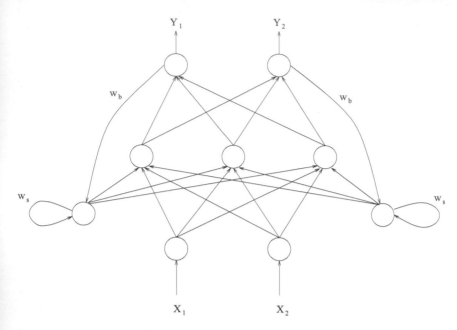

FIG. 5.11. An example of a partially recurrent neural network, with two context units with backward connections from the output layer and self-connections. The weights w_s and w_b are constant.

A training method for general recurrent architectures can be easily derived from the standard BP algorithm for feed-forward networks. In spite of its apparent simplicity, this technique is quite effective whenever the length of the sequences to be learned is not too large and is known at the beginning of the sequence itself. This is always the case when a whole training set is available (i.e., when no on-line learning is required). The algorithm is called Back-Propagation Through Time (BPTT) or unfolding in time (Minsky and Papert, 1969; Rumelhart et al., 1986).

The general idea is the following. A discrete time sequence processing task is assumed. Suppose that the activity (state) of a given unit j at time t is given by:

$$\hat{y}_j(t) = f_j \left(\sum_{l \in L_j} w_{jl} \hat{y}_{s_l}(t - d_l) + x_j(t - 1) \right) \qquad (5.41)$$

where we denoted with w_{jl} the weight of the connection between s_l-th and j-th units, with d_l the delay (number of time steps) that affects the propagation of signal between these units, and with $x_j(t - 1)$ the external input to unit j at time $t - 1$ (it is assumed to be zero if no input is applied to unit j at that time). The sum over l is extended to all the links in L_j (whose destination unit is the j-th unit). Indeed, each unit can receive external input or produce output (or neither) at certain time steps during the processing. The network is then unfolded by turning it into a feed-forward network, by introducing one copy of the original units for each time step. All forward connections present in the original net are replicated in the unfolded net. All recurrent connections are substituted by forward connections between the source unit and the copy of the destination unit in the next unfolded layer.

The unfolded net can now be trained using the BP algorithm, with the relevant constraint that all copies of a given connection w_{jk} are required to share the same weight value. This is accomplished by computing all the weight changes produced by BP at different layers, and then training using a common, unique weight change equal to the sum of the individual changes. It should be noticed that the above algorithm can deal with sequences of different lengths in the training set, by unfolding into a different number of layers for each case.

Recurrent nets have been applied in a variety of speech processing tasks. In a nasal consonant recognition experiment (Bengio, Cardin, & De Mori, 1990), a more than five-fold improvement in generalization was observed by improving the architecture of the ANN. The experiment was performed on the discrimination of nasals /m/ and /n/ in a fixed context, that of letters "m" and "n." The speech material consisted of 294 speech segments from 70 training speakers (male and female with various accents) and 38 speech segments from 10 test speakers. The speech signal was preprocessed with the auditory model and general synchrony detector, yielding 40 input features every 10 ms. Poor results were obtained with early experiments, with a simple output coding with three nodes {vowel, m, n}. A two-layer fully connected feed-forward ANN with a window of two consecutive frames at the input and 10 hidden units yielded 15% classification error on the test set.

Better results were obtained by considering observations on speech analysis showing that the most important discriminatory information for the nasal sounds is available during the transition between the vowel and the nasal. This suggested using the following output coding, with four nodes: {vowel, transition to m, transition to n, nasal}.

Since the transition was more important than the steady-state, a window of 4 frames was chosen (instead of 2 frames) at (t, t − 10 ms, t − 30 ms, t − 70 ms) at the input. To reduce the connectivity in the network, the architecture was modified to include a constrained first hidden layer with 40 units, where each unit was meant to correspond to one of the 40 spectral frequencies of the preprocessing stage. Each such hidden unit, associated to the Fth output coefficient of the auditory model synchrony detector, was connected (when possible) to input units corresponding to

auditory model coefficients $(F − 2, F − 1, F, F + 1, F + 2)$

and frames $(t, t − 10\ ms, t − 30\ ms, t − 70\ ms)$.

Experiments with the feed-forward network (40 inputs – 40 hidden – 10 hidden – 4 outputs) (network 1 in Fig. 5.12) showed that, as expected, the strongest clues about the identity of the nasal sound are those associated with the transition from vowel to nasal. Furthermore, this information is available for only a very short segment of time, just before the start of the steady part of the nasal. To extract this critical information, a second network was trained on the outputs of the first one to provide a clear discrimination during the whole duration of the nasal. This higher level network is a recurrent one with local feedback, in order to learn about the temporal structure of the task and keep the detected critical information during the length of the nasal. With the 2-network architecture as shown in Fig. 5.12, classification performance reached a plateau

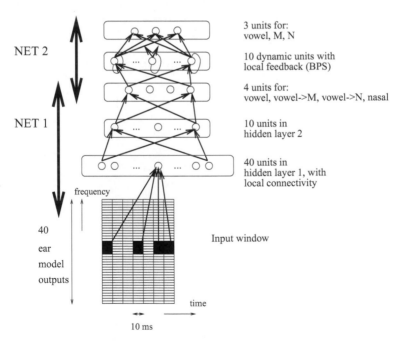

FIG. 5.12. Best architecture obtained for the recognition of nasal sounds in a fixed context. The first network is initially trained to recognize transitions from vowel to nasal. The second one models the temporal structure of the output of the first one.

of 1.1% classification errors on the training set. Generalization was very good for this task, with only a 2.6% error rate on the test set. The dramatic improvement due to the change in architecture may be enhanced by the small size of the training set. In such cases, the structural bias imposed on the network has much more effect than when the training set is very large.

Experiments on plosive recognition on a continuous speech database (TIMIT [Zue, Sereff, & Glass, 1990]) were also performed (Bengio, De Mori, Flammia, & Kompe, 1991). The task was the speaker-independent recognition of the following 7 plosive sounds in continuous speech:

$$\{/p/,/t/,/k/,/b/,/d/,/g/,/dx/\}$$

The best results for this task were obtained with a network with three layers of weights in which the first hidden layer was constrained with a local connectivity both in time and frequency, as shown in Fig. 5.13. A recurrent network performed better than a static one (Flammia, 1991). The recurrent network yielded a decrease of generalization error from 35% to 30.7% on a plosive and nasal recognition task with the TIMIT database

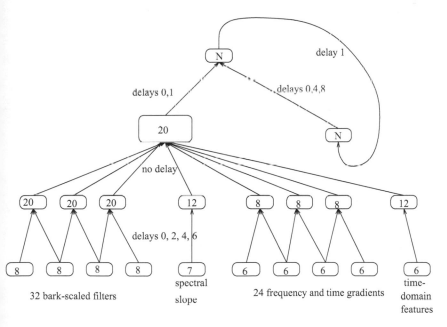

FIG. 5.13. Architecture used for the recognition of plosives, nasals, and fricatives on the TIMIT database. The first layer has a local connectivity in time and frequency. N is the number of outputs.

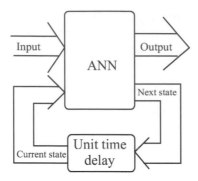

FIG. 5.14.   Scheme of Robinson's dynamic net.

and its outputs were much less noisy.[2] The output coding was based on articulatory features and representation of context.

Particularly remarkable are the results obtained by Robinson et al. (Robinson, 1994; Robinson and Fallside, 1988, 1991), where RNNs are used as state-space machines, capable of computing an output and the next state given the input and the current state. This results in a nonlinear extension of linear control theory. A schematic representation of this RNN model is shown in Fig. 5.14. The approach was successfully applied to phoneme recognition and to phone probability estimation. With such a scheme, using spectral acoustic parameters at the input, more than 70% phoneme accuracy (taking into account errors due to phoneme Substitutions, Deletions and Insertions) was obtained on the test set of the TIMIT corpus (Robinson & Fallside, 1990). Recently, Robinson et al., (1993) have integrated RNNs into a hybrid HMM/ANN speech recognizer, where the networks are used to compute posterior state probabilities (see the section on page 000). Close to 14% word error rate was achieved on a 20,000-word vocabulary, speaker-independent continuous speech task.

ANN/HMM HYBRID SYSTEMS

In order to combine the advantages of ANNs with those of HMMs, hybrids of ANNs and HMMs have been introduced. These structures may have the advantage of adding discriminative power from ANNs to HMM models or to train ANNs to perform observation transformations suitable for a given HMM type.

The majority of the proposed ANN/HMM hybrids are constructed by considering the output of an ANN as the observation of an HMM (Bengio, De Mori, Flammia, & Kompe, 1992; Franzini, Lee, & Waibel, 1990;

Haffner, Franzini, & Waibel, 1991; Levin, 1990; Tebelskis, Waibel, Petek, & Schmidbauer, 1991). ANN architectures that emulate an HMM have also been proposed (Birdle, 1990; Niles and Silverman, 1990) (see also the following sections on pages 000–000). In some of them the dynamic programming algorithm is embedded in the ANN itself (Haffner et al., 1991; Levin, Pieraccini, & Bocchieri, 1992). Alternatively, the ANN can be used to rescore the N-best hypotheses (phoneme by phoneme) produced with an HMM (Zavaliagkos, Austin, Makhoul, & Schwartz, 1993). In some cases (Bengio, 1996; Haffner et al., 1991; Tebelskis et al., 1991), the ANN outputs are not interpreted as probabilities, but are rather used as scores and generally combined with a dynamic programming algorithm akin to the Viterbi algorithm to perform the alignment and segmentation. In particular, in Bengio, 1996; and Bengio et al., 1992, the ANN is used to transform the acoustic vector in a form that is easier to model for an HMM.

The basic concept is shown in Fig. 5.15. Speech spectra or a transformation of them is the input of an ANN that performs a nonlinear transformation of the input and produces new observations for the HMM network.

The weights of the ANN specify the transformation it performs and are estimated by a joint optimization procedure with the HMM parameters in such a way that the recognition error is minimum. Thus the transformation is tailored in the specific time alignment and recognition method.

In practice the ANN is a combination of specialized ANNs, as shown in Fig. 5.16., initialized to optimize recognition on a specific class of sounds (e.g., plosives) with a class-dependent set of acoustic features. A network that combines the outputs of specialized ANNs is initialized to perform

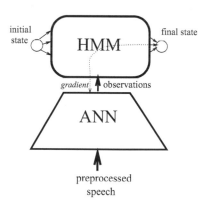

FIG. 5.15. Global optimization of a hybrid system where the ANN performs feature extraction for the HMM.

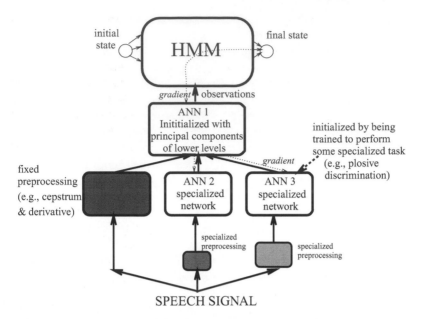

FIG. 5.16. Feature extraction by combining specialized neural models into a hybrid ANN/HMM system with global optimization.

principal component analysis. With this approach, more than 80% plosive phoneme recognition was obtained on the test set of the TIMIT corpus.

The models proposed by Bourlard et al. rely on a probabilistic interpretation of the ANN outputs (Bourlard and Morgan, 1994; Morgan, Konig, Wu, & Bourlard, 1995) (see also the section on page 000). Although the ANN and the HMM are sometimes trained separately, most researchers have proposed schemes in which both are trained together, or at least the ANN is trained in a way that depends on the HMM. There may be specialized ANNs for each phoneme class (e.g., vowels) fed by acoustic features that are effective for discrimination of phonemes within the class. Specialized ANNs can be trained separately before having their weights refined by a global optimization.

The Viterbi Net

Lippmann and Gold (1987) proposed a recurrent neural network architecture, implemented in VLSI, able to mimic the decoding behavior of the continuous-density Viterbi algorithm (Rabiner, 1989) for speech recognition of isolated words. It was called the Viterbi net. Although the recognition performance did not represent any improvement with respect to the standard HMM approach, this connectionist architecture is remarkable for historical reasons.

The Viterbi net has as many input units as the dimensionality of the acoustic vectors. Acoustic observations are fed into the network in sequence, one at a time. Inputs are propagated forward through a single, fully connected layer, and summed up before being passed to each one of a set of state-units representing the states of a corresponding left-to-right HMM. A Viterbi network is built for each word model present in the HMM. The state-units have a threshold-logic activation and a fixed delay on the output, and are laterally connected (each of them to the following one) in a way that resembles the topology of the left-to-right HMM. In addition to the summed inputs, each state-unit also receives a feedback input from an associated subnetwork, able to select the maximum between the output from the state-unit itself and the output from the adjacent state-unit on the left.

There is no actual training procedure for the Viterbi net, and this is one of its major limitations. It is initialized using the parameters of the corresponding HMM, obtained using the Baum-Welch algorithm (Rabiner, 1989). After initialization, the recurrent dynamics of the net when fed with a sequence of input vectors result in a parallel version of Viterbi decoding, producing the logarithm of the likelihood of the input sequence given the model as the final output (output from the rightmost state-unit after presentation of the last vector in the input sequence).

Experimental results on isolated word recognition tasks, performed using 12 mel cepstral coefficients and 13 differential mel cepstra as features, were satisfactory and comparable with those obtained with state-of-the-art HMMs of the time.

The Alpha Net

John S. Bridle (1990) proposed a connectionist architecture able to behave like an HMM for speech recognition. The idea underlying his approach was to look at the forward and backward phases of HMM computation, and to give them an interpretation in terms of a neural network. In fact, the model was called Alpha Net because its architecture and its dynamics were calibrated to resemble the forward computation of the alphas in the Baum-Welch algorithm.

The Alpha net is a recurrent neural network. As for the Viterbi net, its parameters are the same as those of the corresponding HMM, but in the present case a complete forward estimation of the likelihood of the observations given the models is accomplished, instead of a single best-path search as occurs with the Viterbi algorithm. Furthermore, a learning procedure, derived from the backward step of the Baum-Welch algorithm, is available. It is expressed as the backpropagation of the partial derivatives of a discriminant cost function (maximum mutual information). A recurrent architecture of the following kind is built for each unit (word) to be included in the model (and for which a corresponding HMM exists). Neurons are organized in order to represent states of the HMM. For instance, in the most common case of left-to-right HMM, each unit (neuron) is connected with a recurrent connection to itself, and with a forward connection to the unit representing the following adjacent state in the HMM. The weights of these connections are equal to the state transition probabilities between the corresponding pairs of states. The likelihoods of the emission probabilities are fed into the recurrent loops from another, a distinct part of the network, and multiplied instead of summed. The units are linear, with a unit delay, thus resulting in the computation of the product of the joint probability of transition and emission for that state at each time step. In this way, the overall behavior is consistent with the probabilistic framework of the HMM. The separate network that is responsible for computation of these likelihoods is supposed to rely, for example, on multipliers and exponentials in order to approximate as closely as possible the likelihoods generated by the Gaussian or mixture of Gaussians associated to the states of the corresponding HMM. The final output of such an architecture is the actual likelihood of the input acoustic sequence given the model, summed over all possible paths within the network.

ANNs to Compute State Posteriors

Bourlard and Morgan (1994) have proposed other HMM/ANN hybrids for continuous speech recognition. An MLP is trained to estimate posterior probabilities of HMM states, maximizing the posterior probability of a given (left-to-right) Markov model M_i given an acoustic observation sequence X. Posterior probabilities can be written as:

$$Pr(M_i \mid X) = \sum_{q_1^L} Pr(q_1^L, M_i \mid X) \tag{5.42}$$

$$= \sum_{q_1^L} Pr(q_1^L \mid X) Pr(M_i \mid q_1^L, X)$$

$$= \sum_{q_1^L} Pr(q_1^L \mid X) Pr(M_i \mid q_1^L)$$

where the model M_i is supposed to have Q states $q_1, \ldots, q_Q$, and the acoustic observation sequence $X = (x_1, \ldots, x_L)$ is assumed to be of length L. In

Equation (5.42) the sums are extended over all possible sequences q_1^L of states.

The quantity $Pr(M_i \mid q_1^L)$ does not depend on the acoustics (observation sequence X), but only on higher-level choices made in the definition of the models and can thus be computed separately.

Repeatedly applying the properties of joint probabilities, Equation (5.42) can be rewritten as:

$$Pr(M_i \mid X) = \sum_{q_1^L} Pr(q_1 \mid X)Pr(q_2 \mid X, q_1) \ldots \quad (5.43)$$

$$\ldots Pr(q_L \mid X, q_1, \ldots, q_{L-1})Pr(M_i \mid q_1^L)$$

$$= \sum_{q_1^L} \left\{ \prod_{\ell=1}^{L} Pr(q_\ell \mid X, q_1^{\ell-1}) \right\} Pr(M_i \mid q_1^L).$$

Attempts to determine analytical developments for the present formulation, similar to those adopted in the maximization of the likelihood of the observations given the model (Rabiner, 1989) and that lead us to the *Forward-Backward* and to the Viterbi algorithms, are not practicable. Bourlard's idea is then to use feed-forward neural networks as estimators of the posterior probabilities of states given the observations and the previous state sequence. Actually, an approximate version of Equation (5.43) is used, by taking:

$$Pr(M_i \mid X) = P'(M_i \mid X) \quad (5.44)$$

$$\sum_{q_1^L} \left\{ \prod_{\ell=1}^{L} Pr(q_\ell \mid \mathbf{x}_{\ell-k}, \ldots, \mathbf{x}_{\ell+k}, q_{\ell-1}) \right\} Pr(M_i \mid q_1^L)$$

that is to say, the network is trained to estimate the state posterior $Pr(q_\ell \mid \mathbf{x}_{\ell-k}, \ldots, \mathbf{x}_{\ell+k}, q_{\ell-1})$ given a fixed number $2k+1$ of acoustic vectors $\mathbf{x}_{\ell-k}, \ldots, \mathbf{x}_{\ell+k}$ (a *window* or *context* of size k centered in the current acoustic observation $\mathbf{x}_\ell$) and the previous state. This is accomplished using the BP algorithm on an MLP, which has an output unit for each state (that represents the estimate of the state posterior probability). This is a particular case of what we called Time-Delay Neural Networks (see the section on page 000). Other attempts were made to use the MLP to estimate the posteriors in different ways, for example as a function of the current observation and of the previous state only, or as a function also of previous MLP's outputs (previous states). In any case, the speech recognition performance of the resulting overall system was surprisingly poor in many experiments (Bourlard and Morgan, 1994). This was attributed to the fact that common

HMMs (with all the practical tricks required to make them effective on real-world tasks) work well within the framework of likelihoods, but not with posterior probabilities, in spite of the theory sketched above. A step backward was then made by moving the system back to likelihoods. This issue was pursued by using a somewhat standard version of the HMM, in conjunction with neural networks. The latter were trained to perform exactly the same probability estimation as in Equation (5.45), but with their outputs divided by the *a priori* probabilities of the corresponding states, in order to reduce probabilities to likelihoods normalized by the unconditional likelihood of each observation (using Bayes' theorem). Priors can be computed apart from the training data or from statistical considerations on the constraints given by the specific task. This solution was effective and allowed the system to reach the recognition performance of state-of-the-art HMM recognizers on large vocabulary continuous speech tasks, but at the expense of a loss of a theoretical framework.

One central point (and problem) with this approach concerns the training procedure. Indeed, networks are trained with BP, which would require knowledge of target values for the outputs in order to compute the gradient of the cost functional. With the exception of toy tasks, no supervised labeling of acoustic frames is actually available (labeling by hand in real-sized databases is not feasible). Bourlard et al. suggested an iterative training procedure that starts up with a linear segmentation of the acoustic observations, performs training of the networks according to the initial segmentation, then uses the Viterbi algorithm (in conjunction with the newly trained networks as estimators of the state-emission probabilities) in order to produce a new (more reliable) segmentation of the data, that in turn is used to train again the networks, and so on in an iterative fashion. Bourlard et al. argue that this is a particular instance of the Expectation-Maximization (EM) algorithm. This technique is interestingly effective, but it represents a divergence with respect to the theoretical developments that motivated the overall architecture of the system, as far as the networks are optimized over a cost function (squared differences between target and actual outputs) that is not the same one used to perform the segmentation (and the evaluation of the system performance), that is the word recognition error after Viterbi.

CONCLUSIONS

Statistical models have been found very useful for speech recognition. They are motivated by the idea that there are many realizations of features in various contexts and that it is impossible to characterize all of them by analytical rules. Instead, it is preferable and feasible to assume that, for each feature, all parameter values are possible but with different probabilities in different features. Probabilities are obtained by assuming probability distributions can be characterized by a few specification parameters that are estimated by experiments.

Models can be obtained by combining statistical elements taken from a collection of basic building blocks and allowing these blocks to be shared among different models. The number of basic blocks increases with the size and characteristics of the training data. The higher is the number of blocks, the more accurate are the models that can be built with them. Modern systems use as many as 90,000 Gaussian distributions for building models of as many as thousands of models of phonemes in various contexts. With these models, speaker-independent dictation of continuously spoken messages can be performed with vocabularies of tens of thousands of words and an error rate of about 10%. The error reduces to 2–3% for vocabularies of 1,000 words and to less than .3% for the digits. Even for large vocabularies, syntactic and semantic models are simply represented by bigram or trigram probabilities (i.e., probabilities that each word may follow any word or pair of words).

Artificial Neural Networks are other types of trainable models. In principle they are more powerful in extracting properties from raw data and in modeling time histories. It is possible to show that HMMs can be modeled with ANNs.

A detailed discussion of modeling problems at all levels of a spoken dialogue system can be found in De Mori (1998).

NOTES

1. Here and in the following, the notation x_h^k stands for the sequence $[x_h, x_{h+1}, \ldots, x_k]$.
2. Information is based on visual inspection of the network outputs.

REFERENCES

Alleva, F., Huang, X., & Hwang, M. Y. (1993). An improved search algorithm using incremental knowledge for continuous speech recognition. *Proc. ICASSP 93*, volume I, 307–310.

Aubert, X., Dugast, C., Ney, H., & Steinbiss, V. (1994). Large vocabulary continuous speech recognition of Wall Street Journal data. *Proc. ICASSP 94*, volume II, 129–132.

Bahl, L., Bellegarda, J. R., de Souza, P. V. Gopalakrishnan, P. S., Nahamoo, D., & Picheny, M. A. (1993). Multonic markov word models for large vocabulary continuous speech recognition. *IEEE Transactions on Speech and Audio Processing*, 1(3), 334–344.

Bahl, L. Brown, P. F., de Souza, P. V., Mercer, R. L., and Picheny, M. A. (1993). A method for the construction of acoustic markov models for words. *IEEE Transaction on Speech and Audio Processing*, 1(4), 443–452.

Bahl, L., de Souza, P. V., Gopalakrishnan, P. S., Nahamoo, D., & Picheny, M. A. (1991). Decision trees for phonological rules in continuous speech. *Proc. ICASSP 91*, volume S1, 185–188.

Baldi, P., & Hornik, K. (1989). Neural networks and principal component analysis: Learning from examples without local minima. *Neural Networks*, 2, 53–58.

Bengio, Y. (1996). *Neural networks for speech and sequence recognition*. London, UK: International Thomson Computer Press.

Bengio, Y., Cardin, R., & De Mori, R. (1990). Speaker independent speech recognition with neural networks and speech knowledge. In D. Touretzky, (Ed.), *Advances in neural information processing systems 2* (pp. 218–225). Denver, CO: Morgan Kaufmann.

Bengio, Y., Cosi, P., Cardin, R., & De Mori, R. (1989). Use of multi-layered networks for coding speech with phonetic features. In D. Touretzky, (Ed.), *Advances in neural information processing systems 1* (pp. 224–231). Denver, CO: Morgan Kaufmann, San Mateo.

Bengio, Y., & De Mori, R. (1988). Use of neural networks for the recognition of place of articulation. In *Proc. of ICASSP 88 (IEEE)* (pp. 103–106). New York, NY.

Bengio, Y., De Mori, R., Flammia, G., & Kompe, R. (1991). Phonetically motivated acoustic parameters for continuous speech recognition using artificial neural networks. In *Proceedings of EuroSpeech'91*, Genova, Italy.

Bengio, Y., De Mori, R., Flammia, G., & Kompe, R. (1992). Global optimization of a neural network-hidden Markov model hybrid. *IEEE Transactions on Neural Networks*, 3(2), 252–259.

Bocchieri, E. L. (1993). Vector Quantization for the efficient computation of continuous density likelihoods. *Proc. ICASSP 93*, volume II, 692–694.

Bourlard, H., & Kamp, Y. (1988). Auto-association by multilayer perceptrons and singular value decomposition. *Biological Cybernetics*, 59, 291–294.

Bourlard, H., & Morgan, N. (1994). Connectionist speech recognition. A hybrid approach. In *The Kluwer international series in engineering and computer science*, vol. 247. Boston: Kluwer Academic Publishers.

Bridle, J. (1990). Alphanets: a recurrent "neural" network architecture with a hidden Markov model interpretation. *Speech Communication*, 9(1), 83–92.

Carpenter, G., & Grossberg, S. (1987). ART2: Self-organization of stable category recognition codes for analog input patterns. *Applied Optics*, 26, 4919–4930.

Carpenter, G., & Grossberg, S. (1988). The ART of adaptive pattern recognition by a self-organizing neural network. *Computer*, IEEE-CS Computer, 21(3), March 1988, 77–88.

Cottrell, G., Munro, P., & Zipser, D. (1987). Learning internal representations from gray-scale images: An example of extensional programming. In *Ninth annual conference of the cognitive science society* (pp. 462–473). Seattle 1987. Hillsdale, NJ: Lawrence Erlbaum.

De Mori, R. (1998). *Spoken dialogues with computers*. London, UK: Academic Press.

Digalakis, V., & Murveit, H. (1994). Genones: Optimizing the degree of mixture tying in a large vocabulary hidden markov model based speech recognizer. *Proc. ICASSP 94*, volume I, 537–540.

Duda, R. O., & Hart, P. (1973). *Pattern classification and scene analysis*. New York: Wiley.

Elman, J., & Zipser, D. (1988a). Learning the hidden structure of speech. *Journal of the Acoustical Society of America*, 83, 1615–1626.

Flammia, G. (1991). Speaker independent consonant recognition in continuous speech with distinctive phonetic features. Master's thesis, McGill University, School of Computer Science.

Franzini, M., Lee, K., & Waibel, A. (1990). Connectionist Viterbi training: A new hybrid method for continuous speech recognition. *International conference on acoustics, speech and signal processing* (pp. 425–428). Proc of ICASSP 90, Albuquerque, NM.

Gori, M., Bengio, Y., & De Mori, R. (1989). BPS: A learning algorithm for capturing the dynamical nature of speech. *Proceedings of the international joint conference on neural networks* (pp. 643–644). Washington D.C. New York: IEEE.

Grossberg, S. (1976). Adaptive pattern classification and universal recoding: I. Parallel development and coding of neural feature detectors. *Biological Cybernetics*, 23, 121–134, 1998.

Haeb-Umbach, R., Geller, D., & Ney, H. (1993). Improvements in connected digit recognition using linear discriminant analysis and mixture densities. *Proc. ICASSP 93*, volume II, 239–242.

Haffner, P., Franzini, M., & Waibel, A. (1991). Integrating time alignment and neural networks for high performance continuous speech recognition. *International conference on acoustics, speech and signal processing* (pp. 105–108). Toronto.

Hertz, J., Krogh, A., & Palmer, R. G. (1991). *Introduction to the theory of neural computation.* Redwood City, CA: Addison Wesley.

Hinton, G. E., Sejnowski, T. J., & Ackley, D. H. (1984). Boltzmann machines: Constraint satisfaction networks that learn. Technical Report TR-CMU-CS-84-119. Carnegie-Mellon University, Dept. of Computer Science.

Hon, H. W., & Lee, K. F. (1991). Cmu robust vocabulary-independent speech recognition system. *Proc. ICASSP 91*, volume S2, 889–892.

Hopfield, J. (1982). Neural networks and physical systems with emergent collective computational abilities. *Proceedings of the National Academy of Sciences, USA*, 79.

Hopfield, J., & Tank, D. (1986). Computing with neural circuits: A model. *Science*, 233, 625–633.

Huang, X. D., Ariki, Y., & Jack, M. (1990). *Hidden Markov models for speech recognition.* Edinburgh: Edinburgh University Press.

Hwang, M. Y., & Huang, X. (1993). Shared-distribution hidden Markov models for speech recognition. *IEEE Transactions on Speech and Audio Processing*, 1(4), 414 420.

Jelinek, F. (1969). A fast sequential decoding algorithm using a stack. *IBM J. Res. Develop.*, 13.

Jordan, M. (1989). Serial order: A parallel, distributed processing approach. In J Elman & D. Rumelhart (Eds.), *Advances in connectionist theory: speech.* Hillsdale, NJ: Lawrence Erlbaum.

Kirkpatrick, S., Gelatt Jr., C., & Vecchi, M. (1983). Optimization by simulated annealing. *Science*, 220, 661–680.

Kohonen, T. (1986). Learning vector quantization for pattern recognition. Report TKK-F-A601. Espoo, Finland: Helsinki University of Technology.

Kohonen, T. (1989). *Self-organization and associative memory* (3rd edition). Berlin: Springer-Verlag.

Kohonen, T. (1990). The self-organizing map. *Proceedings of the IEEE*, 78(9), 1464–1480.

Kubala, F., Anastasakos, A., Makhoul, J., Nguyen, L., Schwartz, R., & Zavaliagkos, G. (1994). Comparative experiments on large vocabulary speech recognition. *Proc. ICASSP 94*, volume I, 561–564.

Kuhn, R. & De Mori, R. (1995). The application of semantic classification trees to natural language understanding. *IEEE Transactions on Pattern Analysis and Machine Intelligence*, 17(5), 449–460.

Lang, K. J., & Hinton, G. E. (1988). The development of the time-delay neural network architecture for speech recognition. Technical Report CMU-CS-88-152. Carnegie-Mellon University.

Le Cun, Y. (1986). Learning processes in an asymmetric threshold network. In F. F. Soulie, E. Bienenstock & G. Weisbuch (Eds.), *Disordered systems and biological organization* (pp. 233–240). Les Houches, France: Springer-Verlag.

Le Cun, Y., & Bengio, Y. (1995). Convolutional networks for images, speech, and time-series. In M. A. Arbib (Ed.), *The handbook of brain theory and neural networks* (pp. 255–257). MIT Press, Boston.

Levin, E. (1990). Word recognition using hidden control neural architecture. *International Conference on Acoustics, Speech and Signal Processing* (pp. 433–436). Albuquerque, NM.

Levin, E., Pieraccini, R., & Bocchieri, E. (1992). Time-warping network: a hybrid framework for speech recognition. In J. Moody, S. Hanson, & R. Lipmann (Eds.), *Advances in neural information processing systems 4* (pp. 151–158). Denver, CO: Morgan Kaufman Publishers.

Lippmann, R. (1987). An introduction to computing with neural nets. *IEEE ASSP Magazine*, 4–22.

Lippmann, R. P., & Gold, B. (1987). Neural classifiers useful for speech recognition. *IEEE Proc. first intl. conf. on neural networks*, volume IV, 417–422. San Diego, CA: IEEE.

Merhav, N., & Ephraim, Y. (1991). Maximum likelihood hidden markov modeling using a dominant state sequence of states. *IEEE Transactions on Signal Processing*, 39(9), 2111–2114.

Minsky, M., & Papert, S. (1969). *Perceptrons*. Cambridge: MIT Press.

Morgan, N., Konig, Y., Wu, S., & Bourlard, H. (1995). Transition-based statistical training for ASR. *Proceedings of IEEE automatic speech recognition workshop (snowbird)*, 133–134.

Mozer, M. C. (1993). Neural net architectures for temporal sequence processing. In A. Weigend & N. Gershenfeld (Eds.), *Predicting the future and understanding the past* (pp. 243–264). Redwood City, CA: Addison-Wesley.

Murveit, H., Butzberger, J., Digilakis, V., & Weintraub, M. (1993). Large-vocabulary dictation using sri's decipher speech recognition system: Progressive search techniques. *Proc. ICASSP 93*, volume II, 319–322.

Nasrabadi, N., & Feng, Y. (1988). Vector quantization of images based upon the kohonen self-organizing feature maps. *IEEE international conference on neural networks*, San Diego, 1988, volume 1, 101–108. New York: IEEE.

Nasrabadi, N., & King, R. (1988). Image coding using vector quantization: A review. *IEEE Transactions on Communications*, 36, 957–971.

Ney, H., Mergel, D., Noll, A., & Paesler, A. (1992). Data driven search organization for continuous speech recognition. *IEEE Transactions on Signal Processing*, 40(2), 272–281.

Ney, H., Essen, U., & Kneser, R. (1994). On structuring probabilistic dependences in stochastic language modeling. *Computer Speech and Language*, 8, 1–38.

Niles, L., & Silverman, H. (1990). Combining hidden Markov models and neural network classifiers. *International conference on acoustics, speech and signal processing*, 417–420. Albuquerque, NM.

Nilsson, N. J. (1971). *Problem-Solving Methods in Artificial Intelligence*. New York: McGraw-Hill.

Nowlan, S. J. (1991). *Soft Competitive Adaptation: Neural Network Learning Algorithms based on Fitting Statistical Mixtures*. Technical Report TR-CMU-CS-91-126. School of Computer Science, Carnegie Mellon University, Pittsburgh, PA.

Oja, E., (1982). A simplified neuron model as a principal component analyzer. *Journal of Mathematical Biology*, 15, 267–273.

Oja, E. (1989). Neural networks, principal components, and subspaces. *International Journal of Neural Systems*, 1, 61–68.

Oja, E., & Karhunen, J. (1985). On stochastic approximation of the eigenvectors and eigenvalues of the expectation of a random matrix. *Journal of Mathematical Analysis and Applications*, 106, 69–84.

Paul, D. B. (1994). The Lincoln large-vocabulary stack-decoder based HMM CSR. *Proc. ARPA workshop on human language technology*, 374–379.

Pearlmutter, B. (1989). Learning state space trajectories in recurrent neural networks. *Neural Computation*, 1, 263–269.

Pineda, F. (1989). Recurrent back-propagation and the dynamical approach to adaptive neural computation. *Neural Computation*, 1, 161–172.

Poggio, T., & Girosi, F. (1990). Networks for approximation and learning. *Proceedings of the IEEE*, 78(9), 1481–1497.

Rabiner, L. R. (1989). A tutorial on hidden Markov models and selected applications in speech recognition. *Proceedings of the IEEE*, 77(2), 257–286.

Robinson, A., & Fallside, F. (1988). Static and dynamic error propagation networks with application to speech coding. In D. Anderson (Ed.), *Neural information processing systems* (pp. 632–641). Denver, CO. American Institute of Physics, New York.

Robinson, A. J., & Fallside, F. (1990). Phoneme recognition from the TIMIT database using recurrent error propagation networks. Technical Report CUED/F-INFENG/TR.42, Cambridge University Engineering Department.

Robinson, T. (1994). The application of recurrent nets to phone probability estimation. *IEEE Transactions on Neural Networks*, 5(2), pp. 298–305.

Robinson, T., Almeida, L., Boite, J. M., Bourlard, H., Fallside, F., Hochberg, M., Kershaw, D., Kohn, P., Konig, Y., Morgan, N., Neto, J. P., Renals, S., Saerens, M., & Wooters, C. (1993). A neural network based, speaker independent, large vocabulary, continuous speech recognition system: The wernicke project. *Proc. of Eurospeech93*, Berlin, Germany.

Robinson, T., & Fallside, F. (1991). A recurrent error propagation network speech recognition system. *Computer Speech and Language*, 5(3), 259–274.

Rumelhart, D., Hinton, G., & Williams, R. (1986). Learning internal representations by error propagation. In D. Rumelhart & J. McClelland (Eds.), *Parallel distributed processing*, volume 1, chapter 8 (pp. 318–362). Cambridge: MIT Press.

Sanger, T. (1989). An optimality principle for unsupervised learning. In D. Touretzky (Ed.), *Advances in neural information processing systems 1* (pp. 11–19). Denver, CO: Morgan Kaufmann, San Mateo.

Sato, M. (1990). A real time learning algorithm for recurrent analog neural networks. *Biological Cybernetics*, 62, 237–241.

Talamazzini, E. G. S., Niemann, H., Eckert, W., Kuhn, T., & Rieck, S. (1992). Acoustic modeling of sub-word units in the isadora speech recognizer. *Proc. ICASSP 92*, volume II, 577–580.

Tebelskis, J., Waibel, A., Petek, B., & Schmidbauer, O. (1991). Continuous speech recognition using linked predictive networks. In R. P. Lippman, R. Moody, & D. S. Touretzky (Eds.), *Advances in neural information processing systems 3* (pp. 199–205). Denver, CO: Morgan Kaufmann, San Mateo.

Waibel, A. (1989). Modular construction of time-delay neural networks for speech recognition. *Neural Computation*, 1, 39–46.

Waibel, A., Hanazawa, T., Hinton, G., Shikano, K., & Lang, K. (1989). Phoneme recognition using time-delay neural networks. *IEEE Transactions on Acoustics, Speech, and Signal Processing*, 37, 328–339.

Waibel, A., & Lee, K. F. (1990). *Readings in speech recognition*. San Mateo, CA: Morgan Kaufmann.

Waibel, A., Sawai, H., and Shikano, K. (1989). Modularity and scaling in large phonemic neural networks. *IEEE Transactions on Acoustics, Speech, and Signal Processing*, 37, 1888–1898.

Werbos, P. (1974). *Beyond regression: New tools for prediction and analysis in the behavioral sciences*. PhD thesis, Harvard University.

Werbos, P. (1988). Generalization of backpropagation with application to a recurrent gas market model. *Neural Networks*, 1, 339–356.

Williams, R., & Zipser, D. (1989a). Experimental analysis of the real-time recurrent learning algorithm. *Connection Science*, 1, 87–111.

Williams, R., & Zipser, D. (1989b). A learning algorithm for continually running fully recurrent neural networks. *Neural Computation*, 1, 270–280.

Winters, J., & Rose, C. (1989). Minimum distance automata in parallel networks for optimum classification. *Neural Networks*, 2, 127–132.

Zavaliagkos, G., Austin, S., Makhoul, J., & Schwartz, R. (1993). A hybrid continuous speech recognition system using segmental neural nets with hidden Markov models. *Int. Journal of Pattern Recognition and Artificial Intelligence* (pp. 305–319). Special Issue on Applications of Neural Networks to Pattern Recognition (I. Guyon Ed.).

Zue, V., Seneff, S., & Glass, J. (1990). Speech database development: Timit and beyond. *Speech Communication*, 9(4), 351–356.

6

The Roots and Amalgams of Connectionism

Hugh W. Buckingham
Louisiana State University

The primary purpose of this chapter is to present a historical sketch of the continuity and change in associative reasoning from Aristotle to the modern day connectionist paradigm in cognitive psychology. There are numerous investigations that demonstrate the links between association-ism and behaviorism, and as I tried to demonstrate over a decade ago, there are links as well between associationism and the cerebral connectionism of the diagram makers from Charles Bastian and Karl Wernicke to Norman Geschwind (Buckingham, 1984).

I believe it can be shown similarly that many of the basic tenets of as-sociationism are submerged in the working hypotheses and epistemology of modern network connectionism, both functional and computational. Along this line I disentangle the so-called "good old fashion artificial intelligence" (Boden, 1991, p. 3) of symbol manipulation from non-symbol manipulating networks that are involved in the connectionist paradigm.

THE FORERUNNERS OF ARISTOTLE

As with everything in history, there are "forerunners"; Aristotle had his. Aside from the basic notions of similarity, contiguity, cause/effect, con-trast, and a few others that are woven into the fabric of associationism, the constructs of force, energy, power, and strength are ubiquitous. The forces, so to speak, brought about change and movement, not only in the outside world, but also in the inside world of the animal.

It has been pointed out (Clagett, 1955, p. 52) that the concept of "force" was appreciated as early as the fifth century BC with Empedocles's (490–435 BC) postulation of two opposing forces: love and strife. In the same time period, Anaxagoras thought of "nous," or mind, as an external force causing motion. An important Hippocratic principle was that to find the fundamental nature (physis) of a thing, we must examine its "power" or "dynamis." The capacity of acting or of being acted on became a pivotal issue for the Hippocratic writers. Quite obviously, the early speculations on mechanics dealt with systems of power and movement. The Aeonian, Thales of Miletus (624–536/652–548), was quoted by Aristotle as having, "conceived soul as a cause of motion," because Thales had evidently claimed that lodestone must have possessed a soul since it was capable of moving iron. Thales considered (Hunt, 1993, p. 15) that the soul (or mind) was the source of human behavior and its mode of action was a kind of physical force inherent in it. Similarly, Plato, Aristotle's teacher, claimed that motion is the essential quality of the soul and that psychological activities were related to its inner motions.

It did not take long for the dynamism of forces and motion to transfer from outside the organism to inside the organism. Robinson (1995, p. 19–20) writes that "Socrates ... directed philosophical inquiry away from the heavens and toward human concerns: that he shifted attention from cosmos to anthropos." Democritus of Abdera (460–370 BC), from his theory of atoms, claimed that objects gave off or imprinted on the atoms of the air images of themselves, which traveled through the air, reaching the eyes of the beholder, and there interacting with its atoms. The product of that interaction in turn passed to the mind and there interacted with its atoms. The ancient Greeks ultimately came to appreciate inner soul movements and forces as something close to what in modern terminology would be "mental processes," the word process carrying with it motion.

In addition to energy, strength, and force, associationist thinking co-opted the notions of similarity and contiguity. Before Aristotle, Plato had "almost casually" (Warren, 1921, p. 23) suggested in the Phaedo that the act of recollecting some past event or object involved the appreciation of similarity or contiguity. Furthermore, one of the major metaphors for memory had been appreciated long before Aristotle. In De Anima, Aristotle invoked the metaphor of the wax tablet to discuss memory and recollection; Finger (1994, p. 332) has traced that metaphor back to Homer, Plato, Socrates, Zeno, and Cicero—among others. Suffice it say, therefore, that several pieces of the associationist puzzle antedate Aristotle.

ARISTOTLE

Most of what can be found by Aristotle (384–322 BC) on associationism comes from his work entitled, *De Memoria et Reminiscentia*. Little if any comes from his rather large work *De Anima*. In varying degrees, thinkers before Aristotle believed that knowledge came from without. Idealists such as Plato allowed that much of knowledge nevertheless came from nonexternal knowledge that the organism brought to the learning situation. Not so believed the realists, such as Aristotle. Says Aristotle (p. 608), "Without a presentation, intellectual activity is impossible." So, first, there must be perception. The perception is laid down, so to speak, and conditioned by a lapse of time, becoming a memory, trace. Objects and events, and their traces in memory, may by their very nature be of like quality (i.e., be similar). They will associate accordingly. Objects and events may occur together in time or space by custom or habit being presented in some fixed sequential order frequently enough such that they will become tightly fastened as memory traces. In this way, Aristotle could say (p. 613), "as a rule, it is when antecedent movements [understood as "mental processes"—HWB] of the classes here described have first been excited, that the particular movement implied in recollection follows." Recollection, for Aristotle, involved the attempt "to obtain a beginning of movement whose sequel shall be the movement which he desires to reawaken." Only Man can recollect, according to Aristotle; all animals can recognize, which is simply a product of the perceptual abilities. Presumably, no animal other than Man could run through a recollection activity such as the "Tip-of-the-tongue" phenomenon. It is extremely important to see the two-part process in Aristotle's scheme. First, the recollector must "endeavor to get some initial experience" (Warren, 1921, p. 26) or "must try to obtain a beginning of movement" (Aristotle, p. 613). If this first operation is successful, then the associative reawakening will take place and the succeeding event, object, or whatever will be forthcoming. Often, if one can retrieve the first element (letter or phoneme) of the word that's on the tip of the tongue, that word will spring forth. The more frequently the two have been presented and used in sequence, the quicker and more successful will be the reawakening: the cornerstone of behavioral theories of learning and memory. This has been referred to as the law of use in modern terminology (Boden, 1991, p. 7). As we will see, this notion from Ancient Greece became a common tennet of the British empiricists, of the nineteenth century diagram makers, in the psychology of William James, and in practically all twentieth century behavioral learning theories. It is now a cornerstone in modern connectionist model learning.

Aristotle's work *De Memoria et Reminiscentia* (Chapter II, p. 451b) is most often quoted by scholars investigating his theories of associative memory. Some historians, such as Howard C. Warren (1921, pp. 25–26), provide a long and all-inclusive quotation from section 10 to section 35; others provide various parts of that long quotation. Warren's is most instructive, since he has gone to the trouble of providing the most inclusive quotation with a footnote containing the complete ancient Greek version and commentary on several English translation issues.

Aristotle often used physical terminology when discussing mentality. For example, although the ancient Greek verb "kine?ou"literally meant "to move, to set in motion, to urge on" (mostly used intransitively by Aristotle), Aristotle used its noun form "kinesis" in the sense of "movement" or "energy." Warren and his translator suggest that psychologists will find "experience" or "mental process" closer to what Aristotle was getting at. Finger's (1994, p. 333) quote concentrates on Aristotle's framing of the Law of Contiguity, while Hunt's (1993, p. 32) quote highlights contiguity, but also includes the Aristotelian principles of similarity and opposition. Finger's (1994, p. 333) quote is the following:

> Acts of recollection, as they occur in experience, are due to the fact that one movement has by nature another that succeeds it in regular order. If this order be necessary, whenever a subject experiences the former of two movements thus connected, it will (invariably) experience the latter [i.e., associative learning].

Hunt quotes (p. 32) from a bit later in the long section cited by Warren. There, Aristotle writes:

> Whenever we try to recollect something, we experience certain of the antecedent movements [i.e., memories—added by Hunt] until finally we come to the one after which customarily comes the one we seek. This is why we hunt up the series, having started in thought either from a present intuition or some other [how one starts in thought from some intuition appears to be unexplored by Aristotle—HWB], and from something either similar or contrary to what we seek or else from that which is contiguous to it.

These two quotations cover the major aspects of Aristotle's theories on associationism: contiguity, similarity, and opposition. In addition to these notions, Aristotle writes that the process of knowledge acquisition and memory begins with the perception of impressions from the outside world and that traces and their associates are etched on the waxy mind in varying degrees of fixedness depending on frequency of successive pairings in the case of contiguous elements or on the very nature of the similarity or opposition between two associates. Aristotle, therefore, merits recognition for this very early contribution to the history of association psychology.

It should be pointed out at this juncture that these basic Aristotelian tenets—contiguity, similarity, contrast—relate to a whole host of phenomena in the language sciences. Contiguity relates to what occurs together and is at the heart of issues treating syllable structure phonotactics, cloze procedures, and lexical relations such as syntagmatic collocation. Syllable structure conditions are made of restrictions of which kinds of segments can occur next to each other or in close approximation. Similarity is the quality involved in semantic relatedness, co- hyponymic groupings, and phonological feature sharing among phonemic segments. Hardly a study of language production errors (in normals or in aphasics) goes by without the observation that most kinds of error/target pairs bear some type of similarity. Lexical errors are often close semantic associates, and phonemic errors most often differ from the specified target by only one (or very few) feature. That is, error interactions are quite often among similarity pairs. Contrast relates to modern linguistic notions of sonority, modulation, antonymic relations, and dissimilation. There is a preferred maximum contrast between contiguous items, which enhances perceptibility. In addition, a strong semantic relation holds between two contrasting antonymic forms. When modern connectionist studies model many of the above linguistic relations and processes, the Aristotelian associative roots become quite evident.

BETWEEN ARISTOTLE AND HOBBES

Warren (1921) lists several writers between Aristotle and Hobbes who, albeit minimally, wrote about or otherwise commented on associative memory. Both Epicurus (342–270 BC) and Carneades (ca. 215–129 BC) spoke of "successive association" and the chaining of thoughts as laid down in memory through habit and custom. St. Augustine (354–430 AD) placed primary emphasis on association by contiguity. In addition, he was well aware of the difference between loss of memory and access to memory. In his *Confessions, Book X,* he argued that "recognition" of some previously unretrievable item "comes not as something new, but as something familiar." (Warren, 1921, p. 30). He reasons that were the memory trace "utterly blocked out of the mind, we should not remember it, even when reminded." (Warren, 1921, p. 30).

From the death of St. Augustine, through the Dark Ages and up to the end of the thirteenth century, little if any is reported on association theory. Luis Vives (1492–1540), a Spanish Aristotelian apologist, commented at large on the above cited passages from *De Memoria et Reminiscentia.*

According to Warren (1921, pp. 31–32), Vives outlined a broad spectrum of trains of thought among various sorts of logical and associated relationships stored in memory: cause to effect to instrument; part to whole; situation to participants (and vice versa); from something to its opposition; and from something to something else of shared likeness. However, Vives did not analyze any of these in psychological terms. Finally, even Rene Descartes (1596–1650), the Rationalist, makes an occasional statement to the effect that "things experienced together tend to be recalled together," (Warren, 1921, p. 33) which is contiguity, or, "an experience will recall an earlier experience which partly resembles it," which is similarity. Descartes even felt that the evocation of an associate "is made easier through habit, and is accomplished through the 'vestiges' of the former experience in the brain" (Warren, 1921, p. 33). This brings us to Thomas Hobbes.

THOMAS HOBBES

Hobbes, with his two major works *Human Nature* (1650) and *Leviathan* (1651), is considered "the first" British empiricist. He echoed Aristotle's views that the cognitive powers of the mind dealt only with material given by the senses. The epistemological commitment here is obvious. Like Aristotle, Hobbes placed primary emphasis on custom and habit, whereby strong memory traces resulted from frequent presentation to the senses. Of the three Aristotelian associative principles, Hobbes highlights but one, contiguity, which he refers to as "coherence." In *Human Nature*, Chapt. 5, Hobbes writes that "custom hath so great a power that the mind suggesteth only the first word, the rest follow habitually and are not followed by the mind" (Warren, 1921, p. 36). For Hobbes, "contiguous" elements in memory cohere in varying degrees of "strength" depending on the frequency with which the associates have been presented to the senses in successive order. Associative processes spread reflexively ("not followed by the mind") for Hobbes.

JOHN LOCKE

In his *Essay on Human Understanding*, Book II, Chapter 33 (1690), Locke (1632–1704) presents his contribution to the continuing saga of associationism, his being the principal statement of the British empiricists. Assuming the Aristotelian/Hobbesian tradition, Locke writes that "knowledge arises from experience alone."(Warren, 1921, p. 36). Departing somewhat, however, from the Aristotelian tradition, Locke admits of deriving certain forms of knowledge from the powers of "reflection," and thus, as Warren (1921, p. 40) puts it, "abandons the pure sensationalism of Hobbes." Reflective powers were a major innovation of Locke, and they significantly advanced the cognitive power of human mentality. There was now a level of processing that lay between input stimuli from the outside world and output behavioral manifestation, whereby the human could reflect on certain stimuli, vary attentional focus, reason about and make judgments on stimuli, and internally form distinct associations from those strictly bonded to inputs and outputs. Connectionist "hidden" units bear some conceptual resemblance to Locke's internal reflective powers (see Bechtel & Abrahamsen, 1991, pp. 102-3 for additional comments to this effect).

For Locke, associative connections are of two kinds: (1) natural correspondences and (2) chance or custom correspondences. The Aristotelian principles of "similarity" or "likeness" and "contrast" are, in a sense, built in naturally, associative bonding thereby forged. Under "natural correspondences," Locke includes "cause and effect" as well, and consequently, for Locke, "cause and effect" is in a "natural" bonding category, where associative strength is not formed by habit but rather by degree of likeness, opposition, or causality. For Locke, the pair of "cause/effect" events occur in space at once and fuse naturally into one.

In contradistinction, "chance" correspondences are formed through the "law of contiguity," the bonds accruing "strength," "power," or "energy" through frequent presentation and use. Habit, custom, and frequency are the sine qua non of contiguous association. Locke drew some further important distinctions in his discussion of "contiguity." He distinguished "successive" contiguous chains (the so-called Lockean trains) from "simultaneous" association. In a temporal sense, two items may be uniquely simultaneous, but there is always an aspect of contiguity with spatial simultaneity, since two objects or events considered simultaneously in space will, of necessity, be next to each other. Time obviously does not admit this; only space does. Space naturally goes with the sense of vision and touch, whereas time aligns more reasonably with the sense of hearing. Although we can hear two sounds simultaneously, we do not consider that they are "next to each other." When we see two objects simultaneously (in space) they must of necessity be "next to each other." Associations can go both ways, and in modern structuralist terminology we talk of "paradigmatic" and "syntagmatic" bondings, paradigmatic being closer to time and syntagmatic being closer to space. The notion of "simultaneity" of course was important for Locke, since he was developing the concept of the "complex" idea—structured as it was out of a simultaneous combination of associatively bonded interconnections of simple ideas. The modern concept of the network has its seeds, therefore, in the work of Locke. In addition, Locke proposed that the power of "abstraction" involved the paring down of the complexity to the "general idea," separated accordingly from all other ideas that accompany the general idea in its real existence, the general idea becoming the abstract category.

John Locke, in sum, rightly deserves the designation of major contributor to British empiricism.

GEORGE BERKELEY

Bishop George Berkeley (1685–1745) claimed that associative processes suggest things. In his *New Theory of Vision* (1709, p. 25) Berkeley wrote that, "Without any demonstration of the necessity of their co-existence, one idea may suggest another to the mind . . . (if the two) . . . have been observed to go together." (Warren, 1921, p. 40). For Berkeley, it was obvious that similar items or items related by "cause/effect" could "suggest" one another, but "suggestion" implied that first there was one, then there was the other. Hence, for Berkeley, causality and likeness were modes of association of successive ideas, and therefore "contiguity" was involved with naturally bonded elements as well as with fortuitously bonded elements. Recall that Locke divided natural from chance, relegating chance associations alone to the law of contiguity.

On the other hand, like Locke, Berkeley outlined a theory of complex ideas that depended on the notion of "simultaneous association." But, again, for Berkeley, simultaneity with association of ideas involved the contiguity of sensations. Accordingly, Berkeley was making the further distinction between sensation and ideation, or between senses and ideas. In so doing, Berkeley became much more of an "idealist" than Locke, although Berkeley's idealism was rooted in the senses, and therefore he was considered an empiricist as well. Even more important, Berkeley's ideas were of two sorts: those of sense and those of "imagination." Berkeley writes (in *Principles of Human Knowledge*, 1710, p. 30) that, "The ideas of sense are more strong, lively, and distinct than those of the imagination; they have likewise a steadiness, order and coherence, and are not excited at random . . . but in a regular train or series." (Warren, 1921, p. 40). Ideas of imagination, on the other hand, according to Berkeley, "are more properly termed ideas or images **of things** [bold print added], which they copy and **represent** [bold print added]." (Warren, 1921, p. 40–41). The ideas of imagination are excited in the mind "at pleasure" and are "creatures of the fancy" according to Berkeley. Nevertheless, Berkeley claims that "We perceive a continual succession of ideas [both of sense and of imagination]." (Warren, 1921, p. 41). In the end, Berkeley is credited for directing metaphysical questions into a more distinctly psychological realm, but according to Warren (1921, p. 42), Berkeley's idealist metaphysics affected the trend of British thought much less than did his rooting of this idealism in the empirical domains of the senses, and it is that which keeps Berkeley in the camp of the British empiricists—not his idealism.

DAVID HUME

The majority of Hume's work on associationism is found in his *Treatise on Human Nature* (1739) and in his *An Enquiry Concerning Human Understanding* (1748). [I will be citing Anthony Flew's (1988) edited volume of that 1748 book.] As for the origin of ideas, Hume's basic position was that most everything comes from outside stimulation. But, he does take care to point to "one contradictory phenomenon, which may prove that it is not absolutely impossible for ideas to arise, independent of their correspondent impressions" (p. 66). The "idea" of the color category "red," for example, may be formed from presentations of different shades of that color from the "imagination" (p. 66). Hume was one of the earliest empiricists to claim that ideas were the "faint images" of the more forceful and lively sensory impressions. The recollections by memory of a sensation or the "imagined" (p. 64) anticipation of the sensation, "never entirely reach the force and vivacity of the original sentiment" (p. 64).

Hume had the gnawing habit of giving little or no prior credit for the theories he was developing. He writes (p. 69), "I do not find that any philosopher has attempted to enumerate or class all the principles of association. . . . To me, there appear to be only three principles of connexion [bold print added] among ideas, namely Resemblance, Contiguity (in time or place), and cause and effect." He further suggests that "contrast" may be considered some sort of coalescence of causation and resemblance. On the relationship of "contrast" with "cause and effect," Hume reasons that where two objects are contrary, the one destroys the other, or "is the cause of its annihilation." (p. 70).

Hume rightly deserves credit for casting doubt on whether or not one can ever truly show "cause and effect." He attempts to reduce the associative principle of causality to but a mere instance of the Law of Contiguity. Hume writes in his *Treatise* (1739, Book I, Part III, p. 6. [cited in Warren, 1921, p. 45]) that "reason can never show us the connection [the causal connection] of one object with another, though aided by experience and the observation of their constant conjunction in all past instances." Accordingly, Hume's principles of association reduce to two: similarity and contiguity.

Before leaving Hume, it should be pointed out that he included in this stock of memorial ideas (traces) that of movement and the association of voluntary actions. In his *Enquiry* (p. 64), he writes that, "By the term 'impression,' I mean all our more lively perceptions, when we hear, or see, or feel, or love, or hate, or desire, or will" [bold print added]. Therefore, according to Flew (1988, p. 64, ftn 13) Hume does not confine all impressions to sensory activity; he includes emotions and "acts of will." Nevertheless, in the end, the principles of similarity and contiguity were not developed by Hume in any penetrating fashion that would have integrated them clearly with the rest of his work. The seeds were there, but as Warren (1921, p. 46) wrote, ". . . it was reserved for Hartley to extend the principle of association systematically to all classes of mental phenomena."

DAVID HARTLEY

Most historians of neuropsychology give a major contributory role to the work of David Hartley (1705–1757), who published a short monograph (in Latin) in 1746 and three years later a large two-part work entitled *Observations on Man* (1749) in English (Allen, 1999; Buckingham and Finger, 1997). In these works, Hartley did not come up with any startling new association principles, rather his contribution was to probe the depth and roots of these principles, place them in the form of axioms and corollaries, and suggest a physiological substrate for their physical instantiation. That substrate consisted of the vibrations of Sir Isaac Newton. George Bower (1881, p. 24) writes, "The theory of Association of Ideas . . . was first formulated as a philosophical system, and made the serious study of a lifetime, by Hartley." Warren (1921, p. 160) observed that, "There seems abundant reason for according Hartley the title of founder of the association school, since he was the first to adopt the associative principle as the fundamental operation of psychology." Robert Young (1970, p. 97) writes that, "Although Hartley did not experiment on the brain, his principles constituted the first physiological psychology of the associationist school." Barbara Oberg (1976, p. 443) notes, "Hartley alternated between the detailed inquiry of the neurologist puzzling out the working of the brain and the nervous system, and the task of a more traditional British empiricist philosopher tracing the progress from sensation to idea. Vibrations, the physical movement, and association, the mental phenomenon, were both important to him."

Without a doubt, Hartley can be credited as being among the first to craft, in great detail, a psychophysical account of the workings of human cognition. His system was developed through a series of tightly stated propositions. I briefly outline the propositions that reflect the continuity of associative principles, which, as we have observed, began with Aristotle.

In his introduction of the reprint of Hartley's 1746 monograph entitled *Various Conjectures on the Perception, Motion, and Generation of Ideas*, Martin Kallich (1959, p. i) writes that, "Before publishing the *Observations*, Hartley sent aloft a trial balloon in the form of [a] . . . Latin [treatise]." I draw from that treatise as well as from Hartley's longer work of 1749. Hartley's anatomy was that of the mid-eighteenth century, heavily influenced by Thomas Willis (Finger, 1994). By this time, the ventricles had given way to the solid parts of the brain as the substance for cognition, but no more than the so-called medullary mass, which for most was comprised of the medulla, the pons, the basal ganglia, and the thalamus. At this point in time, the cerebral cortex was virtually terra incognito as far as sensory/motor mental function was concerned.

Propositions 1 through 7 covered the incoming sensations, their essential vibratory nature, and their individual traces in the medullary mass. In Proposition 5, Hartley presents one of the earliest formulations of the doctrine of cerebral localization on record (Aubert & Whitaker, 1996). Propositions 8 through 11 are the most crucial for Hartley's associationism.

Proposition 8 states: "Any sensations, by being often repeated, leave behind vestiges, types, or images of themselves." These vestiges in memory are referred to as "simple ideas of sensations." Proposition 9 is a virtual parallel with 8, and it represents one of the earliest clear-cut and detailed psychophysical statements in the history of psychology. It reads, "Sensory vibrations, by being often repeated, beget in the brain a disposition to diminutive vibrations corresponding to themselves respectively."

It should be pointed out that the Newtonian vibrations were not those of stretched strings (Smith, 1987). As Hartley pointed out in *Observations* (1749, pp. 11–12) in the section concerning Proposition 4 (where he specifically introduces Newton's vibrations as part of his model), these vibrations are backward and forward motions of the small medullary particles, like pendulum oscillations or, as he wrote, like "the tremblings of the particles of sounding bodies." The vibratory motions were exceedingly short and small, "so as not to have the least efficacy to disturb *or move* [Italics added] the whole bodies of the nerves or brain." Consequently, the Newtonian/Hartleyan vibrations were not whole nerve vibrations such as those of stretched strings. Hartley is clear on this, when he writes (pp. 11–12), "For that the nerves themselves should vibrate like musical strings, is highly absurd; nor was it ever asserted by Sir Isaac Newton, or any of those who have embraced his notion of the performance of sensation and motion by means of vibrations."

With Proposition 10, Hartley's associationism truly begins. Proposition 10 states that, "Any sensations A, B, C, etc., by being associated with one another a sufficient number of times get such a power over the corresponding ideas a, b, c, etc., that any one of the sensations A, when impressed alone, shall be able to excite in the mind b, c, etc., the ideas of the rest." The continuity from Aristotle to Hobbes through Locke and Hume is clear. Proposition 10 for Hartley covers the Law of Contiguity in both time and space (Bower, 1881, p. 39). Habit and custom develop the level of strength of the associative bindings, thereby linking energy and force with frequency of use of the miniature or faint traces in memory. Old notions, indeed.

Proposition 11, like 9, is the physical counterpart of the mental. It reads, "Any vibrations A, B, C, etc., by being associated together a sufficient number of times get such as power over a, b, c, etc., the corresponding miniature vibrations, that any of the vibrations A, when excited alone, shall be able to excite b, c, etc., the miniatures corresponding to the rest." Hartley labels the miniature vibrations "vibratiuncles." Propositions 12, 13, and 14 allow Hartley to develop the "complex idea," which, as seen in the work of earlier British empiricists, is a composite of simple ideas, and, as pointed out earlier, begins to approach the notion of the "network."

Propositions 15 through 22, represent for the first time the coalescence of associations and vibrations to form an account of muscular action and movement in general. It is in these propositions that we witness for the first time in the history of psychology the notions of the so-called muscle sense and the appreciation of sensory information as a guiding force for movement systems. Proposition 15 reads, "It is credible that muscular motion is performed in the same general manner as sensation and the perception of ideas." And in Proposition 16, Hartley claimed that "muscle contraction accords with the doctrine of vibrations." In his discussion of Proposition 16, Hartley (1749, p. 88) makes the interesting observation that, "the vibrations thus excited in the fibers, put into action an attractive virtue, perhaps of the electrical kind."

Proposition 20 makes the ultimate sensory-motor connection. It reads, "Whatever has been delivered above concerning the derivation of idea vibratiuncles from sensory vibrations, and concerning their association, may be fitly applied to motor vibrations and vibratiuncles." The coalescence of associative principles to garner a characterization of voluntary and involuntary movement as well as of muscle sense is a major contribution of Hartley. Bower (1881, p. 31) has schematized Hartley's major propositions as shown in Fig. 6.1.

Although we have seen most of the basic elements in Hartley's associative principles in many forerunners, he, more than anyone before him, developed a detailed mentalistic psychology out of them. And, he made

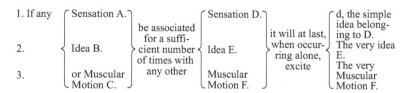

FIG. 6.1. Schematic of Hartley's muscle motion propositions.

a sincere attempt to correlate these purely functional, mental, or psychological principles with the nervous system of his milieu—the vibrations of Newton.

Hartley knew that many would balk at such psychophysical reasoning. Early on in *Observations* (p. 6), Hartley wrote, "The doctrine of vibrations may appear at first sight to have no connexion with that of association; however, if these doctrines be found in fact to contain the laws of the bodily and mental powers respectively, they must be related to each other, since the body and mind are." This belief that body and mind are related (perhaps coming from his background in medicine) guided Hartley through the relatively uncharted waters of psychophysical theory. But, he was shrewd enough to realize a certain functional autonomy to association theory. Concluding his detailed discussion of Proposition 11 in *Observations* (p. 72), he suggests that "as a vibratory motion is more suitable to the nature of sensation than any other species of motion, so does it seem also more suitable to the powers of generating ideas, and raising them by association." But, he concludes cautiously by saying, "However, these powers are evident independently, as just now observed; so that the doctrine of association may be laid down as a certain foundation, and a clue to direct our future inquiries, whatever becomes of that of vibrations" (p. 72). Similarly, at the end of Part One of *Observations* (p. 503), Hartley draws another psychophysical dissociation, arguing for functional autonomy when he writes, "And if the doctrine of vibrations be rejected, and sensation and muscular motion be supposed to be performed by some other kind of motion in the nervous parts, still it seems probable, that the same method of reasoning might be applied to this other kind of motion."

I have attempted to demonstrate that many, if not all, of the basic elements in associative reasoning were in force before David Hartley arrived on the scene: outside stimuli as the sine qua non of knowledge (the epistemological commitment of association psychology); high frequency of presentation (custom and habit) to form strong associative links; vivid sensations/faint memory traces; association by similarity, contrast, or contiguity (in time and space); and cause and effect. What Hartley did was to sharpen and to enrich these associative principles within a scientific schema of propositions and corollaries and to suggest their physiological underpinnings.

GESNER AND CRICHTON

Two very important late-eighteenth-century contributors to the history of associationism and its increased utility in describing and explaining behavioral disorders secondary to brain disease were Johann Gesner

(Benton, 1965; Benton & Joynt, 1960) and Alexander Crichton (Finger and Buckingham, 1994). Gesner, in his published major works during the period 1769–1776, described lexical and phonological paraphasias as well as neologisms in what was obviously a fluent, sensory type of aphasic, although at the time there was little if any agreed on classification of the aphasias. The speech output of Gesner's patient was so fluent and apparently so free of any arthric component that he did not think he could "better make his condition more intelligible and understandable except by saying that if a person who is not acquainted with the German language and who did not know that the patient was sick should observe him and hear him talk, he would take him for a healthy, ordinary man who is speaking an unfamiliar language" (Benton, 1965, p. 57). Gesner ruled out a general intellectual decline as well as any generalized loss of memory. Rather, Gesner felt there to be a problem with "verbal memory." By this he meant that the impairment in this specialized realm of memory consisted in the patient's inability to "associate" images or abstract ideas with their agreed on linguistic signs. Gesner's description of the jargon aphasia in this patient influenced the subsequent work of Alexander Crichton.

In 1798, Crichton (Finger and Buckingham, 1994) published a large, two-volume text describing many types of "mental derangements," by which he meant neurological disturbances of all kinds, including aphasia. He wrote specifically of what are now called sensory/fluent aphasics, who had everything from simple word-finding difficulties to a full-blown symptomatology later called Wernicke's aphasia, where patients produced lexical and segmental substitutions and jargon speech with neologisms, confabulations, and other empty forms—all fluently. As Gesner had done before him, Crichton cast his descriptions and explanations in associationistic terminology. He writes (quoted in Finger and Buckingham, 1994, p. 504), "The act of recollection is entirely dependent upon the association of ideas. In order to recollect anything, one link of the chain of ideas must be present to the mind.... The doctrine of the association of ideas is at present so generally admitted by all philosophers, that it is deemed unnecessary in this work to employ much time in illustrating the fact." Finger and Buckingham (1994) show that Crichton felt that word-finding blocks, lexical and segmental substitutions, neologisms, and others sorts of errors typical of fluent aphasic speech all involved disruptions of different sorts of associations.

NINETEENTH-CENTURY ASSOCIATIONISM

Howard Warren's (1921) detailed history of association psychology traces its extension from Hartley into the nineteenth century, especially through the continuing efforts of James Mill and J. S. Mill, whose work is linked to Alexander Bain, who in turn had a direct influence on the psychology of Herbert Spencer. Young (1970), in a major work on nineteenth-century associationism, details how the functions of associative learning and memory were harnessed to a growing understanding of physiology and brain anatomy.

Another major late-nineteenth-century psychologist whose thinking on associationism is well known is William James, who wrote "a classical chapter" on the topic in his 1890 text on psychology (Parks et al., 1991). James's wording was typically like that of the British empiricists, especially Hartley. James, for instance, writes (1890, p. 566, cited in Parks et al., 1991, p. 197) that "When two elementary brain processes have been active together or in immediate succession, one of them, on re-occurring, tends to propagate its excitement into the other." He talks of "reverberations" and "awakenings," much like the associationists before him. Parks and colleagues (1991, p. 197) point to the influence Hartley's notion (analyzed above) of "reverberations" had on James. As James put it, "nerve tracts reinforce each others' actions because they already vibrated in unison" (Parks et al., 1991, p. 197).

Tizard (1959, p. 140) cites a very interesting cautionary observation that James made concerning associations and the brain. For the purposes of this chapter I want to quote it in full, because it touches on a point that comes up repeatedly in connectionist claims, no matter what the brand of connectionism. James writes (quoted in Tizard, 1959, p. 140):

If we make a symbolic diagram on the blackboard of the laws of association between ideas, we are inevitably led to draw circles, or closed figures of some kind, and to connect them by lines. When we hear that the nerve centers contain cells which send off fibres, we say that Nature has realized our diagram for us, and that the mechanical substratum of thought is plain. In some way, it is true our diagram must be realized in the brain, but surely in no such visible and palpable way as we first suppose.

It behooves us to consider James's caveat at all times, given the ubiquitous and somewhat pernicious nature of the neural metaphor in connectionist cognitive psychology.

CLASSICAL APHASIA THEORY AND THE DOCTRINE OF LOCALIZATION

In a very real sense, the history of "classical" nineteenth-century aphasiology goes hand in hand with associative reasoning both for describing stroke patients' language and speech disruptions and for providing functional characterizations of brain physiology and anatomical localization. We have seen from the work of Locke and Berkeley that out of simple ideas, complex networks of ideas can be formed. James Mill (Bower, 1881, p. 39) was one of the first associationists to use the example of the rose to explicate the complex array of simultaneous sensations, all of which together formed the "idea" or "concept" of that flower.

In a very important paper, Theodor Meynert (1960), Karl Wernicke's mentor, reported on his work dealing with the anatomy of the white fiber system of the brain, U-shape fibers for gyral connections, as well as other fiber systems within lobes and across lobes. Wernicke received much instruction on the connective white fiber system from his collaboration with Meynert. Meynert, as Mill before him, used the example of the rose to explicate the simultaneity of multimodal sensory associations that undergirds its concept. Meynert (1960, p. 171) wrote that:

> The anatomical structure shows that as soon as the cortex functions, that is to say associates or makes conclusions, the anatomical structures of association connect all the different loci with each other, that in the memory trace of a rose, color, smell, pain of the thorns, softness of touch, and an agreeable affect are connected and that in reproducing one property of the rose we bring in other aspects, which are projected to quite different parts of the cortex, into the whole conception.

In his paper, Meynert drew heavily from the work of Charles Bell, Joannes Mueller, and Helmholtz in his characterizations of the cortex as a connectionist patchwork of white fiber systems associating the functional cortical centers in a simultaneity of mental representation. He writes (p. 160) that, "The gray and white substance of the brain can only be compared to a social grouping of living soulful beings."

As discussed in Buckingham (1984), it is not totally clear just when, how, and through whom British empiricist associationism filtered into Germany. Hughlings Jackson was well versed in associationism, which, according to Greenblatt (1970, p. 567), was "the dominant theme in the philosophical psychology of the Victorian period." Jackson's interaction with Charcot and Broca easily accounts for the entry of associationism into France; Germany was a slightly different matter. David Hume's theories could have entered Germany in the writings of Kant, who although not considered an associationist, dealt with Hume's works at length. Warren (1921), however, includes six German writers who could be called associationists, and emphasizes the contributions of Friedrich Eduard Beneke (1798–1854), who, he writes (p. 208), "stands in closest relation to associationism of all German writers." Recall, also, the contemporary work of Gesner, mentioned earlier in this chapter. Further, from studying the writing of Meynert, it is apparent that he was influenced by Mueller, who in turn used many of the notions of Sir Charles Bell and his motor/sensory connectionism.

Nineteenth-century anatomical and physiological connectionism with its functional associationism is at the heart of classical aphasia theory as developed by the "diagram makers," who at the same time were crafting their doctrine of cerebral localization. The history is well charted in Geschwind (1974) and in many other places (e.g., Eling, 1994). Nineteenth-century medical and neuroanatomical connectionism was localistic in that the associative connectivity permitted interaction between increasingly well-defined cortical "centers." Sensory/motor associative linkages took on increased importance as they were implicated in the developing models of higher cortical functions such as language production, comprehension, speech production, acoustic perception, and other systems scaffolded across language such as reading and writing. The connectionism of this nineteenth-century school of cerebral localization (Buckingham, 1984) is quite distinct from modern-day connectionism (also see Caplan, 1994, p. 1033), but the Aristotelian roots are shared as is the basic commitment of both to behaviorism and associative learning principles. One is localistic, the other not.

The Basic Tenets of Localistic Connectionism

From Charles Bastian (1869) through Wernicke (1874) to Luis Lichtheim (1885), the scientific statements of functional physiology and neuroanatomy were cast in associationist terms (Buckingham, 1982, 1984). Sensory/motor cortical association, however, flourished after the landmark paper by Fritsch and Hitzig (1960), "On the electrical excitability of the cerebrum." With the publication of this paper, the so-called Bell-Magendie principle of motor/sensory function in the nervous system was shown to reach the top of the neuraxis. Hundreds of years before, the motor/sensory dichotomy was first made at the level of the spinal cord (see Clarke & O'Malley, 1968, for an excellent historical treatment). Through years of increased experimentation in motor/sensory physiology, the dichotomous system was traced to increasingly higher structures of the nervous system (Brazier, 1957; Figlio, 1975; Walker, 1957; Young, 1970). Much before 1870, the cerebral cortex was not considered to be part of the sensory/motor system. It was considered the location of much higher level mentality, such as reason, judgment, and, most of all, memory (i.e., the intellectual faculties). Nothing so physical as raw motor or sensory phenomena was envisaged for the cerebral cortex. For this reason, in his early papers, Broca did not consider "aphemia" to be "a kind of locomotor ataxia, limited to the articulation of sounds," because, as he wrote, "Everyone knows that the cerebral convolutions are not motor organs" (Broca, 1960; reprinted in von Bonin, 1960). Rather, Broca ended up in agreement with Bouillaud, who years before had thought of "aphemia" as a disruption in the memory system for the procedures of articulation—not articulation itself. By 1870, however, the cerebral convolutions could be considered as motor organs.

Wernicke, in 1874, encouraged by Fritsch and Hitzig's (1960) paper, could therefore link up (connect) sensory and motor systems, whose centers were cortically located. This is precisely what he did in his landmark monograph "The aphasia symptom complex: A psychological study on an anatomical basis" (see translations of Wernicke's work in Eggert, 1977). Broca's area was then connected to the auditory/sensory region for speech (acoustic) perception in the temporal lobe. Classical aphasia doctrine and its localistic connectionism thus began; in one form or another it is still with us today (e.g., Caplan, 1994; Zurif & Swinney, 1994). Many of the fibrous connective tissue tracts of Wernicke's mentor, Meynert, were incorporated into the initial "diagrams," the major one being the arcuate fasciculus, that connected Broca's area with Wernicke's area. Much has been made of that tract since then. Wernicke considered it to be the sine qua non of the reverberatory linkage system that mediated sensory-motor information sharing between the two cortical centers. The procedural statements of localistic connectionism often emphasized serial operations so that for speech production, for instance, the sensory information of "heard" speech was relayed (some said it was "fed forward") to Broca's area through the arcuate fasciculus. The notion of reverberating circuitry, however, did not necessarily hold to a strict directionality, and many of the diagram makers preferred to consider the connective white fibers as simply allowing a kind of back and forth information exchange—a feedback system of sorts. White fibers don't really compute; they transmit. Although synaptic functions may certainly be considered computational, fiber tracts are considered by many to be essentially transmitters of representative information, even today (e.g., Caplan, 1994, p. 1040).

Later physiological findings revealed that the arcuate fasciculus is not only a monosynaptic and multisynaptic tract, but it is bidirectional, sending signals in both directions, running through perisylvian opercular regions of temporal, parietal, and frontal lobes. The initial reflex arc circuitry for the language system went from auditory periphery to Wernicke's area, across the arcuate fasciculus to Broca's area, and down the pyramidal system to the cranial nerves of the motor periphery for the articulators. Other posterior sensory areas and prefrontal motor regions were added to the connective system (Lichtheim, 1885), thereby incorporating semantic systems (conceptual or "Begriffe" in German), as well as the functions of reading and writing (see Fig. 6.2). The transcortical aphasias were accordingly added to the classificatory scheme (Buckingham, 1982).

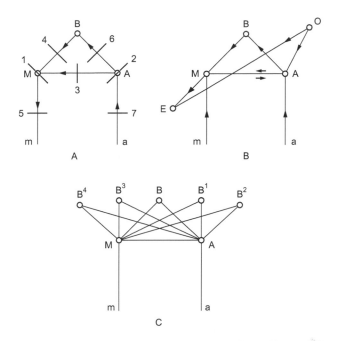

FIG. 6.2. The German word for "concepts" is "begriffe" and hence the letter "B" in the diagrams. (a) This represents Lichtheim's scheme of aphasiological categories: 1. Broca's aphasia, 2. Sensory aphasia (Wernicke's), 3. Conduction aphasia, 4. Transcortical motor aphasia, 5. Dysarthria, 6, Transcortical sensory aphasia. (b) Lechtheim's basic diagram with visual (O) and writing (E) centers added. (c) Lichtheim's diagram representing his theory that the conceptual areas were transcortical rather than simply located in one region. (From Buckingham, 1982, p. 330).

Terms from association psychology were interwoven into the functional characterizations of localistic connectionism in the work of the diagram makers. "Revival" was a crucial component of word recall, thought to involve sound "impressions" in the auditory perceptive centers of the temporal lobe. For speech production, the "will" would "call up" or otherwise "revivify" the acoustic impressions (Aristotle would have had the impressions of high-frequency words deeply chiseled into the wax of verbal memory), which would in turn be transmitted to the motor speech center at Broca's area at the foot of the third frontal convolution, and from there to the motor speech productive system for actual phonetic implementation. True to its associative roots, the learning theory embraced by the diagram makers was that of Aristotle. The "strength" of the sensory impressions (or traces, vestiges, etc.) in the cortical centers was directly correlated with the frequency with which they were introduced over time to the organism, and the motoric trace strengths were fixed to lesser or greater degrees through use. David Hartley's notion of muscle sense was put to immediate use by the diagram makers in that each time a motor gesture was produced, the feedback system involved in muscular movement recorded its action in the respective sensory region. There was little if any reference to Hartley's work by the early diagram makers, but the notion of sensory guidance and recording of movement patterns had been incorporated into association theory as a result of Hartley's contributions.

In sum, the cerebral connectionism of the nineteenth-century diagram makers was heavily localizationist, with centers in specific cortical zones connected by white matter fiber. It was not necessarily unidirectional, but the wording of its propounders often made it appear to be. The system did not necessarily have to operate in a strictly serial fashion, but, again, the paradigmatic descriptive characterizations of the diagram makers often made it seem so. Its epistomological roots were associationist and as such its learning theory was behaviorist in nature. The rather strict localization of mental functions in the cortex, looked back at phrenological theory for its justification, but was influenced as well by the positivistic trends of latter nineteenth-century science.

It should be pointed out that, although Broca was not considered to be among the diagram makers for reasons mentioned above, he nevertheless did localize verbal speech function to a specific cortical region in the frontal lobe, and, although he localized that function to the foot of the third frontal convolution and eventually to the left hemisphere only, he shared a certain affinity with Gall and Spurzheim's phrenology as did his immediate forerunners, Bouillaud and Auburtin (Buckingham, 1981).

Nonlocalization Theories

Localization theory was not without its strong opponents, however, and we must now take a look at the criticisms of the nonlocalization camp in our history of connectionism. There have been many studies on the historical development localization and nonlocalization theory (e.g., Young, 1970). For the purposes of this chapter, I concentrate on some of the basic tenets of nonlocalization thought. Karl Lashley (1950, 1951) was a major theorist in the nonlocalization camp, but his ideas were simply a modern reflection of what Pierre Flourens (1960) had outlined roughly 100 years before Lashley (Tizard, 1959). Flourens's stimulation and ablation studies of lower animals such as hens and pigeons in the early nineteenth-century had led him to believe that memory for behaviors such as moving, eating, pecking, and so forth were a product of the whole brain's action, and that when these brains were serially lesioned, the behaviors declined in a "graceful" fashion.

Flourens (1960) reported on the gradual decline of all sensory modalities in parallel subsequent to ablation of the higher nervous centers. In three pigeons with different arrays of serial extirpations he noted early on that sight and audition remained. Finally, when enough of the nervous system had been cut away, all sensory systems became extinct. Three conclusions followed (1960, p. 10):

1. One can diminish from the front or from behind or from above or from the side the cerebral lobes by a certain amount without losing their functions. Quite a small portion of these lobes suffices, therefore, for their function.

2. As this retrenchment goes on, all functions become weaker and gradually become extinct. Once certain limits are overstepped, they are completely extinct. The cerebral lobes, therefore, in their totality exercise their function.

3. Finally, when one sensation is lost they are all lost. When one faculty disappears they all disappear. There are, therefore not different seats for different faculties nor different sensations. The faculty to sense, to judge, or to want something resides in the same place as that to sense, to judge, or to want something else, and consequently, this faculty which is essentially one, resides essentially in one organ only.

The seeds of the concept of a system that is complex, holistic, and redundant, and that decays in a gradual fashion are clearly witnessed in the antilocalizationist views of Pierre Flourens. "In the last analysis," he writes (1960, p. 21):

the cerebral lobes, the cerebellum and the quadrigeminal bodies, medulla oblongata, medulla spinalis, the nerves, all these essentially different parts of the nervous system, all have specific properties, proper functions and distinct effect. And in spite of this marvelous diversity of properties, of function and of effects they constitute nonetheless a unitary system.

It was Flourens who provided the early nineteenth-century criticisms of the phrenologically driven notions of cerebral localization of function, originally developed by Franz Gall and Gaspar Spurzheim and incorporated into the localizationist theories of Bouillaud and Auburtin and ultimately to the work of Paul Broca in the 1860s (Schiller, 1979, Chapt. 10). Today's term is, of course, "graceful degradation," and it is a major tennet of modern connectionism (e.g., Bechtel & Abrahamsen, 1991, pp. 60–62;

Caplan, 1994, pp. 1031–32). The notion, however, goes back at least to the contributions of Flourens. In addition, Flourens's experiments led him to the notions, seen later in Lashley, of equipotentiality of brain power and cortical mass action (Zangwill, 1961)—all major features of connectionist thought. Parallel systems in man's brain and in the computer are in concert with these nonlocalizationist notions.

Lashley's work on cerebral mass action and graceful degradation plays a direct role in the development of modern connectionist thought. Harley (1993, p. 224) claims that this is a point of major disagreement among connectionists' conventional symbolic cognitive models, where presumably "lesioned" rules produce total disruption of processing. According to Flourens, Lashley, and modern connectionists, loss of function in man and animals is gradual because memories are at least partially distributed throughout the nervous system and that, as Lashley theorized, there is no easy one- to-one mapping between memory traces and neurons. Neuronal patterns are distributed, and therefore memory engrams are distributed. Computers can work in the same fashion. The models of the connectionist have an architecture such that the representations of words, sounds, concepts, and so on are not localized in any one unit (i.e., in any one venue) but rather are distributed as a pattern of activity among many units. When systems with this kind of structure are damaged, it is logical to expect that the functional decline will be gradual, degrading "gracefully."

EARLY MODERN CONNECTIONISM

The early modern period of connectionism began around the mid-1940s (see an excellent treatment of this history in Bechtel & Abrahamsen, 1991, Chaps. 1–3, and Boden, 1989, 1991) with Warren McCulloch and Walter Pitts's (1943) work on "a logical calculus of the ideas immanent in nervous activity" (reprinted in Boden, 1990). For the first time, the metaphors and theories of learning and memory in the Aristotelian tradition of associationism were submitted to statistical mathematical quantification, which did not take long to implement on the computer as networks of threshold logic units. And, in fact, the whole enterprise forms part of the development of computational artificial intelligence. McCulloch and Pitts set up a rather simple model of computational units (which they likened to "formal neurons") and showed how the units compute logically. The units were either "off" or "on." Units received positive or negative numerical values from other units, and these values were quickly analogized with "excitatory nerve inputs" (the positive number values) and "inhibitory nerve inputs" (the negative number values). In the words of Bechtel and Abrahamsen (1991, p. 3), "If a unit received just one inhibitory input, it was forced into the off position. If there were no inhibitory inputs, the unit would turn on if the sum of excitatory inputs exceeded its threshold." The number system could also give the appearance of what humans do when they perform the logical operations of conjunction, disjunction, and negation (AND, OR, NOT). Subsequently, researchers extended the simple pattern to a network of such units. If, in addition to the many-unit network, the system were to be supplemented with a large memory capacity, then accordingly, as McCulloch and Pitts claimed, the networks would attain equivalence to a Universal Turing machine. Margaret Boden (1989, p. 10) points out that McCulloch and Pitts's paper not only paved the way for ensuing connectionist construction of neural nets, but it also directly influenced John von Neumann's design of the digital computer.

Boden stresses the obvious fact that connectionist systems operate in ways quite different from those of von Neumann machines. But, she reasons, this does not mean necessarily that the two systems "are utterly distinct paradigms, implacable rivals in the race to understand the mind" (1991, p. 5).

A little over ten years after the McCulloch and Pitts study, von Neumann added even more complexity to networks by increasing the number of inputs any one unit could receive. Accordingly the systems would become more reliable in that the network could determine each unit's activation (or inhibition) from the statistical pattern of activations (or inhibitions) over its input units. This allowed von Neumann to follow up with what is now a major tenet of connectionist systems: "Each individual unit could be unreliable without sacrificing the reliability of the overall system" (Bechtel & Abrahamsen, 1991, p. 4).

For the first time we begin to see just how the Flourens/Lashley notions of mass action, equipotentiality, and graceful degradation could be scaffolded over connectionist networks and how the extensions to human neuropsychology followed with ease. The notions meshed with Lashley's concept of the memory system. The system was multiply distributed over an array of units, there was much redundancy in the system, a small glitch in it would not have serious consequences, and degradation in the system subsequent to lesions would be gradual (i.e., graceful).

Interestingly enough, in 1949 Donald Hebb, one of Lashley's students, used an old idea of Hartley (although this is rarely pointed out—see Parks et al. 1991) that Williams James had used to the effect that simultaneous or sequential reverberatory activity would bring about cellular rearrangements. Hartley, of course, would say that cells that vibrate together, stay together. Hebb (1949, cited in Parks et al., 1991, p. 197) wrote that:

> When an axon of Cell A is near enough to excite a Cell B and repeatedly or persistently takes part in firing it, some growth process or metabolic change takes place in one or both cells such that A's efficiency, as one of the cells firing B, is increased.

Out of this grew Hebb's contribution concerning the notion of cell "assemblies," which was an early, but rather limited, form of distributed processing. Hebb set up the cell assembly patterns as two-layer networks, with a "learning rule" (subsequently named "Hebbian learning"). That rule, again mathematical and statistical in nature, specified how much the quantity of strength ("weight") of the connection between two units should be increased or decreased in proportion to the products of their activations, and serves to extend Hartley's original notion of 200 years past that the connection between two associated items might be strengthened whenever they "fire" at the same time. According to Bechtel and Abrahamsen (1991, p. 308), Hebb's rule is an "ancestor" of the "Delta Rule," which is a learning rule that can take into consideration the "off targetness" of some actual output with some desired output, adjusting the system accordingly (i.e., changing the numerical values = "weights") to bring the output productions closer to the desired parameter. Although the Delta Rule is a form of "supervised learning," it functions between two levels of units only and can accordingly "find solutions" only if the input-output mappings are linear. An even more powerful system would admit of additional internal layers (the multilayered network), the Delta Rule generalizing to include what is called "back propagation." These units are between input and output units and are thus "hidden" in the system. As mentioned earlier in this chapter, they are not unlike what John Locke had in mind when he claimed that human mental associationist capacity included internal levels of "reflection," which added greatly to the complexity of mediating input and output parameters. In any event, with so-called back propagation, the more powerful Delta Rule can look at the error/desired target discrepancy, which is calculated at the output level, and with that knowledge can propagate back through the multilayered network of units, layer by layer, adjusting the connective numerical values (the weights) accordingly so that ultimately desired outputs will be in concert with inputs.

Obviously, the mathematics was going far beyond what was original with associationism, and with "supervised learning" the systems were going beyond simple two-layered paired associative learning. Again, though, as the systems increased in complexity in terms of numbers of inputs to units and numbers of connections across the networks, the redundancy became ubiquitous, parallel processing looked more plausible, small lesions in the system would not lead to devastating results, and breakdowns in the system would be gradual. The picture was looking more and more like the nonlocalization theories of Flourens and Lashley, who did none of the mathematics. Several recent investigations have laid out the mathematical formulae that make these systems so precise (e.g., Appendix I in Harley, 1995).

On the heels of Hebb, Frank Rosenblatt (1958) extended McCulloch and Pitts's logical calculus for pattern recognition by networks (Bechtel & Abrahamsen, 1991, p. 4). He combined McCulloch and Pitts with the added power of the generalized Delta Rule (= back propagation). In Rosenblatt's systems, which he called "perceptrons" (since he was metaphorically treating perception and constructing a model for it), one set of units gets information from the outside and either excites or inhibits (raises or lowers numerical values) another set of units, which in turn may send signals to yet a third set of units. Bechtel and Abrahamsen (1991, p. 4) write that he supplemented earlier networks by making the connective numerical values continuous rather than binary, thus increasing the range of connective weight values.

Bringing his perceptrons closer to Flourens and Lashley's notion of mass action and equipotentiality, Rosenblatt, like von Neumann, emphasized that these networks were comprised of statistical patterns over multiple units. Here is where statistical characterizations directly confronted the logic of Boole, thus carving out one of the major distinctions between connectionist theories and theories of symbolic manipulation. Accordingly, Rosenblatt argued that perceptron-like information processing systems were qualitatively different in kind from other processing automata and more in concert with a proper analogue of the biological brain. That is, it was felt that perceptron systems and those like them were closer in nature to the nonlocalizationist ideas of Flourens and Lashley: distributed over a range of units, with a good deal of redundancy, acting in parallel, and, when disrupted, breaking down with grace. Functional localization was not punctate, but rather widely distributed. These were cornerstones of a century-old theory of cortical mass action and equipotentiality, which were in direct conflict with the doctrine of cortical localization of function.

Just as Aristotle and many of the associationists after him were searching for an account of human memory, so were Lashley and Flourens, and so, indeed, were many of these early-twentieth-century connectionist theoreticians. Bechtel and Abrahamsen (1991, p. 7) note that, "Early researchers recognized that, in addition to modelling pattern recognition, networks might be useful as models of how memories were established." For instance, psychologists such as Hebb, in line with his professor, Lashley, were naturally attracted to the question of how networks might store associations between different patterns. But in the end, Hebb came up with not much more than Hartley, suggesting only that when two neurons in the brain were jointly active, the strength of the connection might be increased—a memory bond thereby being forged.

Bechtel and Abrahamsen (1991) were also correct to insist that many of these network model constructors were as much if not more interested in achieving a proper **functional** characterization of cognitive performance in general rather than directly modeling the brain. They point out that although perhaps the initial impetus for their models of cognitive performance was the growing recognition that the brain is a kind of complexly structured, interlaced network, they often settled for the modeling of cognitive phenomena in systems that exhibited some of the basic properties of neuronal structures. They were mindful of Williams James's dictate quoted above. The neural sciences were not as developed then as they are now, but it still appears that many modern connectionists are primarily interested in **functional** accounts of cognition.

SOME MODERN AMALGAMS

As with so many turf disputes and presumed paradigm disagreements in science, ultimate amalgams most often result. I believe this is the case with neural network connectionism and symbol manipulating systems. Boden (1989, 1991) finds a major amalgamating link in these two efforts by stressing the dual role of McCulloch and Pitts. It led to neural net connectionism and to symbol-manipulating von Neumann machines, for example, to PDP (and its neighbors) and to the digital computer that crunches symbols. Furthermore, both investigative efforts are major enterprises in the field of computational psychology. Neither are formal systems in the strict sense, and as Boden (1989, p. 8) points out, "Competence-analyses have no necessary connection with computational psychology, and may be produced by researchers not wedded to this approach [computational psychology]." Chomskyan generative grammar, for instance, was in no way developed by computer modeling (Chomsky, 1977, pp. 128–29). Furthermore, it goes without saying that symbol-manipulating systems can be run on analogue machines, and connectionist networks will run on digital machines. All too often, symbol-manipulating systems were cast aside because they had been initially crafted to run exclusively on the digital computer. But, this is a rather weak argument against symbol system computation. In fact, Jerry Fodor, a leading proponent of symbol manipulation, has claimed that when symbol systems can be implemented on more "neural-like" hardware with more parallel computing properties, his systems will exhibit the same virtues as connectionist systems (Bechtel & Abrahamsen, 1991, p. 215). According to Boden (1990, p. 2), however, the major amalgamating force between the two camps is their commitment to a computational psychology. That brings with it four shared philosophical assumptions: (1) Each adopts a **functional** orientation to the intelligent mind. Mental processing involves precisely specifiable procedures and mental states are defined by their **causal** relations with sensory input, movement, and other mental states. (2) All computational psychologists see psychology as the study of computational processes whereby mental representations are constructed, interpreted, and transformed. (3) All investigators view the brain as some sort of computational system. They ask what sorts of functional relations are instantiated in it rather than which cells do the actual work or how their physiological makeup allows the embodiment in the first place. (4) Although the different camps most certainly disagree about which artificial intelligence concepts and computer-modeling methodologies are likely to be the most felicitous for a proper understanding of intelligence, all share the belief that AI concepts of some kind have to play a major role in psychological theory.

Another kind of amalgamation would be to claim that strict connectionism (powerful PDP) pertains to a "subsymbolic" paradigm. For example, Paul Smolensky's (1988) connectionist machine computes units that represent nothing we would recognize but rather some very small details or "microfeatures," whose presence or absence in large numbers may correspond to something constructable as a word, a phrase, or an idea (Boden, 1991, p. 4). The symbolic computational system would account for the material that "flowed forth" from the microfeature, subsymbolic connectionist level—sort of a symbolic computational epiphenomenology as it were. Smolensky, unlike Fodor, would still claim that this subsymbolic level is a crucial component of cognition, albeit at the "micro" level.

Fodor (e.g., Fodor, 1987, 1990; Fodor & Pylyshyn, 1988; Loewer & Rey, 1991) on the other hand suggests a less kind amalgam. He is rather adamant on the issue of symbols in computational psychology. For Fodor, the issue is immutable. Without the resources of a symbolic representational system with a combinatorial syntax and a semantics, one cannot develop an adequate model of human cognition. The systems need recursive operations for the Cartesian notion of productivity. For example, human languages do not contain a finite "list" of sentences, which are selected when needed. Linguistic units are constructed de novo each time we speak, and as far as sentences go, we produce and understand many we have never encountered before. Analogies will not work because one could on analogy construct any kind of sentence, grammatical or not. Analogical reasoning and argumentation is too uncontrolled and overly powerful. It could handle all units in a language, but most certainly not only the units of a language. There also needs to be systematicity among parts of propositions, which would be quite difficult to capture in a nonsymbolic connectionist system. For example, symmetric predicates such as "similar" must in some way relate the proposition: <similar (x,y)> to <similar (y,x)>. Finally, for Fodor, nonsymbolic connectionist systems fail to account for coherent inferencing. He sees no way for them to handle the entailment from <X is a red book> to <X is a book>.

Bechtel and Abrahamsen (1991, pp. 163–74), however, make an interesting claim regarding learning (i.e., "knowing how" vs. "knowing that") how to form logical inferences, which may require Fodor to take a somewhat different approach to his argument that connectionism does not handle logic. Bechtel and Abrahamsen's point is that learning to perform logical inferences is not unlike learning to solve problems in algebra by becoming able to work out solutions to problems algorithmically without any real notion of the conceptual and theoretical undergirdings of what one is doing. The issue here of course is that models that learn to do logic may have little if anything to do with understanding the theory of logic. Everyone knows that models for how humans learn arithmetic have nothing to do with the theory of numbers. This is precisely the position that Jerrold Katz (1981) has taken regarding the generative linguist's grammar and the grammar that is acquired by humans. Katz (1981, p. 78) asks, "Why conflate the psychological study of the ideal speaker's knowledge of a language with the grammatical study of language?" Accordingly, Fodor may have to abandon arguments from the theory of logic as weapons to undermine connectionism, because why conflate the theory of logic with connectionism?

Fodor does, however, have an amalgamating compromise. It is that connectionist systems are needed, but solely at the noncognitive level of neural instantiation. Accordingly, connectionism is not pertinent for theorizing about cognition. Although Fodor and Smolensky might seem to share their relegations of connectionism to subsymbolic levels, Fodor rules out their use in the study of cognition; Smolensky does not, because for him the specification of the dynamics of the microfeatures, although not in the conscious system of awareness, is extremely important in the total layout of human cognition. Furthermore, Fodor's subsymbolic level for connectionism is all and only neural instantiation; Smolensky is not wedded to connectionism as simply the brain system over which Fodor's symbol systems are run.

Hendler (1989), through the use of microfeatures and a spreading activation process referred to as "marker-passing," has constructed a "hybrid symbolic/connectionist model." He incorporates an activation-spreading algorithm that passes symbolic information through typical connectionist systems. Here, arcs between nodes represent symbolic information rather than weight values. Hendler's model, before the amalgam, has no weighted activations between nodes, nor does it provide inhibition. As far as weight is concerned, all nodes in the purely symbolic system are equal. The amalgam essentially adds connectionist weights to the model. An account is created whereby an object's marking by the symbol system is paralleled by that same object being activated in a connectionist fashion. Accordingly, then, this activation could reverberate through the distributed memory, activating other nodes in the network. These activations must be returned to symbolic marks. According to Hendler, the coalescence is conceptually simple, but it requires a mechanism that blends two very different types of information (symbolic and mathematical). And, herein lies the amalgam: The symbolic marker-passing device manipulates discrete symbolic information, which in turn needs to propagate through the network while the distributed memory needs activation weights that propagate via threshold logic units. Hendler comes up with a mechanism to integrate the two, thereby constructing a well-motivated amalgam and demonstrating that it is possible to combine symbolic and nonsymbolic processing into a connectionist computational system.

Steven Pinker's (1991, 1994, 1995, 1999) basic amalgam of symbol computation versus connectionism has been with regard to the past tense verb system of English, a testing ground for connectionist systems launched by Rumelhart and McClelland (1986) in their "bible" (Bechtel & Abrahamsen, 1991, p. 2). The reader who is not familiar with the original Rumelhart and McClelland (1986) study should read the original book or the very detailed discussion of it in Bechtel and Abrahamsen (1991, Chapt. 6; also see Sampson, 1987). Through a two-layer pattern associator system with modifiable connections from a fixed encoding network to a decoding and binding network that outputs phonological representations of past tense forms, Rumelhart and McClelland showed that certain aspects of past tense verb morphology could be taught using the power of a Boltzmann machine with a feedforward system, Delta Rule learning for value adjustment (weight adjustment) and supervised learning, which provides output targets from the beginning that can be used as comparators during input-output matching. Root verb forms are encoded in terms of a basic set of articulatory features, scaffolded off arrays of segmental strings for each verb. For instance, the irregular verb *came* /keim/ has three segments /k/, /ei/, /m/. Each has an right/left contiguous contextual unit. /ei/, for example, is flanked by /k/ on the left and by /m/ on the right. In feature notation, for example, the /ei/ would be a series of triples: [interrupted, low, interrupted], [back, low, front], [stop, low, nasal], [unvoiced, low, voiced], and certain others. These are not "Wickelphones," but rather "Wickelfeatures," and so arguments against the incorporation of Wickelphones fail to be important ones against connectionist accounts. The features are enough to capture the notions of "classes" of contexts, however, and are built into the system with no actual rule involved. The spirit of Rumelhart and McClelland's network is that (1986, p. 217);

> Lawful behavior and judgments may be produced by a mechanism in which there is no explicit representation of the rule. Instead, we suggest that the mechanisms that process language and make judgments of grammaticality

are constructed in such a way that their performance is characterizable by rules, but that the rules themselves are not written in explicit form anywhere in the mechanism.

In a general way, the system came to simulate various aspects of past tense verb morphology learning, which had been mapped out earlier by developmental psycholinguists such as Kuczaj (1977, 1978). In Stage 1, as with children, early and high frequency verbs, which turn out to be the irregular ones, were introduced to the system and were learned as witnessed by the correct productions of these "strong" verbs from the Germanic roots of English—and some other irregular verbs of these types that came into English at later stages. The recidivism of Stage 2 was also simulated, because once regular verbs begin to be introduced to the system and the regular morphophonemics are developed, errors are now seen with past tense forms on the irregular root forms, but finally by Stage 3 most regulars and irregulars are brought under control. Within the limited goals of Rumelhart and McClelland's system, many simulations passed the Turing Test and thus comprised successful engineering feats.

Pinker, however, has pointed out some problems for the connectionist account. For the most part he is willing to allocate the rather closed system of irregular verbs to connectionist learning accounts. On the other hand (1994, p. 132), from Stage 2 on children, beginning to form the regular affixation morphophonemics of the past tense, when presented with new forms (some nonsense) such as smairf, trilb, smeej, and frilg, will produce smairf/t/, trilb/d/, smeej/d/, and frilg/d/, but the network may produce sprurice, treelilt, leefloag, and freezled for these same roots. Certainly, the Turing Test would fail here.

As we mentioned, the irregular verbs fall into several similarity classes: /ə/ - /ei/ (come/came); /ai/ - /ə/ (strike/struck); /æ/ - /ʊ/(stand/ stood); /I/ - /æ/ (sit/sat); /Iŋ/ - /əŋ/ (sting/stung); /ei/ - /oʊ/ (break/ broke); /oʊ/ - /u/ (grow/grew); /ai/ - /u/ (fly/flew); /ai/ - /oʊ/ (write/wrote); and a few others. If regulars and irregulars were truly under the control of a single system, one would expect more analogies for new coinages to follow irregular patterns, especially were those new forms to fit one of the above similarity classes for the irregulars. For example, a compound word has recently entered the English language, "to grandstand." The past tense of this form is not "grandstood." The verb "to fly out" recently coined in baseball terminology, in the past tense is as likely or even more likely to be "flied out." One would never say, "He flied an airplane for the first time." For the same reason, at a hockey game we do not claim that a player was penalized because he "high stuck" someone.

The Rumelhart/McClelland network has difficulties with homophonous forms, because their system is sound based exclusively. Lacking representations of words as lexical entries (distinct from their phonological or semantic content), their model cannot handle semantically unrelated homophones: lie/lied but lie/lay, ring/rang but wring/wrung, meet/met but mete/meted. Also, there is the interesting problem with the polysemous pair hang/hung versus hang/hanged. In general, "hanged" is preferable to "hung" as the past tense and past participle when the verb entry is that with the sense of capital punishment. In other senses of the entry of this verb, "hung" is the customary form as past tense and past participle.

Ultimately, Pinker came up with an amalgam. The past tense verb system is set up such that the irregular verb forms, catalogued as they are in their similarity classes, are acquired through something very much like paired associate learning and are thus accounted for by the architecture and dynamics of connectionist systems. Regular past tense verb morphology is best captured by a rule format, the normal allophones being conditioned by the nature of the phonological termination of the roots. This dissociation allows for the productive nature of the regular system and for the fossilized nature of the irregulars.

Pinker (1991) has also reported on some experiments that show a frequency effect for irregular verbs but not for regular verbs. In these experiments, subjects see a verb stem on a screen and are required to utter the past tense form as quickly as possible. They are significantly quicker in uttering the associated past tense form for irregular verbs with high past tense frequencies than for irregular verbs with low frequency past tense forms. This is not observed with regular verbs.

Priming experiments also reveal the qualitative differences between regular and irregular past tense systems (Pinker, 1991). A regular past tense form primes the recognition of the stem to the same degree that the stem actually primes itself. To Pinker, this suggests that people store (and therefore can only prime) the stem, thereby analyzing the regular inflected form as stem + suffix. This would then be more in line with the view that there is a rule for suffixation and not two separated lexical items. In contrast, an irregular past tense prime is not nearly as effective in priming stem recognition as is the stem itself. To Pinker, this finding suggests that stems and their irregular past tense forms are stored as separate but linked items. (See Pinker (1999) for a more recent and quite eloquent statement of his position.)

Gary Dell (1986, 1988, 1995) has constructed an amalgam as well between strict connectionist systems with and without symbols. His system is not strict parallel distributed processing, but rather operates with spreading activation. Furthermore, his system has the nodes labeled with linguistic symbols: generally limited to words and segments. Dell was a natural to adhere to connectionism, because he had spent much of his early linguistic and psychological training under Peter Reich of the University of Toronto. Peter Reich did early work under Sydney Lamb at Yale, and it was Lamb who developed a very connectionistlike model for linguistics referred to as "stratificational grammar" (see Lockwood, 1972, for a good introduction to Lamb's model). Lamb's theory consisted of a hierarchically stratified network with levels and tactics for each level. The levels were typically linguistic, and units at each level were connected with units at other levels by bidirectional links. The model was neither predicated on computer implementation nor set up to learn like Boltzman machines, for example, and the method of inquiry was not to make predictions and run programs to see if the simulations hold to the predictions. Nevertheless, if there was any linguistic model from the 1960s that would appropriately map onto modern connectionist systems, it was most certainly the Stratificational Grammar of Sydney Lamb.

Dell's early work with Reich (e.g., Dell & Reich, 1981) serves as a clear harbinger of the work Dell has produced since then. I would also note that Goldsmith's "Harmonic phonology" (Goldsmith, 1993, p. 57) has been influenced by Lamb's theories as well.

Dell's connectionist work began in the mid-1980s (1985, 1986), and later an important shorter paper was published in 1988. He has been largely interested in the analysis of slips-of-the- tongue. Space does not permit a full exposition of Dell's interactive activation work in this chapter, but see Stemberger (1985) for more detail on many of the issues involved with the simulated productions of networks that operate by spreading activation.

Briefly, though, the spreading activation model of Dell (1988, p. 129) has a lexical network (word level connected with segment level) and a word-shape network to provide syllabically structured slot-containing templates in which to order the segments. Typically there is a top-down, bottom-up connective system to allow for feedback from the segmental level back up to lexical levels. Activation in these systems starts at a word node, with an arbitrary amount of activation of numerical values (i.e., 100), while upcoming words would receive slightly less amounts. During each time step, every node sends some fraction of its activation to other directly connected nodes. Activation reaching a node increases its activation. During each time step, the activation of any node will "decay" by some factor until it reaches its so-called resting state. Dell's model assumes the resting level to be zero for phonemes but to vary according to frequency for the word nodes, phoneme frequencies being instantiated in the system of lexical nodes. Every node has the same decay rate and every connection has the same strength. Only resting levels differ with frequencies, but all nodes will obviously have higher levels immediately postactivation. In this model, the spreading process is completely linear, with only excitatory connections between the nodes. In these networks the decay rates must be somewhat faster than the spreading rates to prevent unwanted continual activation, or as Dell puts it (1988, p. 129), "to keep the network from entering a phase in which activation levels go haywire." One obviously needs to prevent rampant perseveration. Naturally, there will be some postactivation rebound, which is due to the continued activation of associated nodes, but this activation will generally diminish, and the selected node will return to this resting state.

Admittedly, connectionist models for slips-of-the-tongue have a certain preciseness about them. Simply put, in Dell's system a slip of a unit is due to the fact that that unit is more active than the target. Errors are either anticipations, perseverations, or exchanges. But, the true question then becomes: What leads the unwanted units to be more active? For instance, why would a nontargeted sound become more active? Dell reasons that spreading activation from activated word nodes creates its own interference by activating other word nodes and other segmental nodes that are not in the intended plan at all. They are often referred to as "plan external competitive errors." They compete with the target for realization. And, given the Aristotelian nature of these networks, the nonintended units, which are nevertheless activated, are unwittingly brought into the production picture to a greater or lesser extent depending on their similarity to the intended target. Thus, the very nature of the connectionist system ensures that errors will most often bear a good deal of similarity with the target.

Dell, Schwartz, Martin, Saffran, and Gagnon (1997) have extended this model to the simulation of normal and aphasic naming errors, and within aphasic errors, the authors have mathematically manipulated decay and weight values globally throughout the system as a whole to account for different types of aphasic error responses. The "Dell" model has recently been scrutinized in an in-depth study of a fluent jargonaphasic patient (Hillis, Boatman, Hart, & Gordon, 1999), and the model has undergone very extensive critical evaluation from both a mathematical and a cognitive neuropsychological perspective (Ruml & Caramazza, 2000; Caramazza, Papagno, & Ruml, 2000). The issues revolve around whether global or more focal lesioning of the model offer better accounts of the data.

The connectionist system may provide a well-motivated answer to the puzzle of the "no source" error that has been recorded by investigators (e.g., Shattuck-Hufnagel, 1979). All too often, the earlier serial models such as those of Fromkin (1971), Garrett (1975), and Shattuck-Hufnagel (1979) had only the material in the direct intended plan to draw on for error sources. It was often noted (but, in reality, not that often) that some extraneous phoneme would slip into the production that would not be in the immediate planned material. That was a puzzle. With the connectionist network, however, plan-external materials would always be in the picture, so to speak, because they are in the connective surround whether they happen to be in some intended message or not. In this realm, the connectionist account of the "no-source" error is by far the most parsimonious.

Serial models such as Garrett's can handle "plan-internal" errors a bit easier than they can handle "plan-external" errors. The clause-length material in an operating buffer for some intended sentence will contain material that may be misordered in some way, deleted, or duplicated. In terms of connectionist systems, previously spoken words or upcoming words in the intended plan are active and therefore are sources of interference, particularly, Dell (1988, p. 131) writes, if the speech rate is rapid. That is, if the decay rate does not work faster than the activation rate and resting levels are not attained in their due time, much interference will ensue and errors will crop up. Furthermore, normal synchronization of decay rates and activation rates must be achieved in order to ensure that bottom-up processing can take place, since bottom-up feedback information to lexical nodes helps filter out nonword errors in slips, serving as the "built-in" property that "edits" out errors that result in nonexisting words—at least to some extent (the so-called lexical bias).

The other source for errors would be unintended words (plan external) that might be activated by extraneous cognition or perception (e.g., Motley & Baars, 1979). Connectionist models and serial models both have to stretch their boundaries to account for these sorts of "Freudian," plan-external slips of elements that might be "on the mind" because of some extraneous "cognitive set" or because of a failure to inhibit something in the perceptual background from entering into the productive process and becoming a competitor for realization. We are in somewhat murky waters here. (See Buckingham (1999) for more discussion.)

In most of Dell's connectionist work (e.g., 1988, 1995) he draws a sharp distinction between errors that are interpreted/analyzed after the fact, and errors that one can predict deductively from the actual architecture and processing dynamics of a model. Previously observed phenomena are items such as (1) maintenance of phonotactic patterns in slips; (2) syllable position obedience; (3) only items of similar natures interact; (4) much anticipatory priming in normal slips caused by advanced planning in an activation model; (5) most sound slips involve single phonemes; (6) anticipations and perseverations of phonemes may or may not require that those phonemes exhibit their normal decay rates and quickly get back to their resting levels (if not, doublet errors will result); (7) exchanges of phonemes require that the phonemes involved return to their resting levels, otherwise the slots would not be open to receive the misplaced phoneme; (8) the built-in frequencies of words and segments will determine their vulnerability for slippage; and (9) slips are conditioned by a "lexical bias effect" and quite often by the "repeated phoneme effect."

By using his connectionist model (Dell, 1988), Dell was able to make some predictions of previously unobserved phenomena and run the program to test whether the predictions held. First, he predicted that there should be not only the typical repeated phoneme effect, where the repeated phoneme was contiguous, but there should be a nonadjacent repeated phoneme effect as well. Essentially what he found was that, induced onset consonantal exchanges in CVC words were enhanced not only if the vowel was the same in each word (deap/beem /i/), but also when the codas of the words were shared (dope/rip /p/). Obviously, the onset exchange would be enhanced were the two words to share the rime, but rime was more difficult to account for in this model because the word-shape matrices had no syllable constituent structure, but just the flat syllable structure of Onset+Vowel+Coda—a linear array with no intermediate nodes (i.e., no rime node dominating the vowel and the coda).

He also found that his model predicted speech rate interactions. When the number of time steps that pass between the encoding of each syllable (the rate) increased, there was less time to properly select phonemes, and slips occurred. Furthermore, when the rate at which the system is run sped up, there was less time for normal bidirectional reverberation between levels. Consequently, the lexical bias was not seen as frequently, and nonword slips increased. Dell found the predicted effect. Recall that only through bottom-up feedback from the phoneme level to the word level can the connectionist model account for the lexical bias effect on errors.

His model also predicted and subsequently showed that low-frequency words that are homophonic with high-frequency words inherited the heavier weights of the high-frequency counterparts. A low-frequency word like "knot" was as resistant to segmental slips as the high-frequency negative functor, "not." Subsequent corroborative simulations have shown that when decay rates are slower, perseverative errors are more likely to occur—the theory being that if resting states are not returned to with appropriate alacrity after an element is produced, that element may fire again.

Before leaving Dell, I would like to discuss one observation that has been puzzling to most investigators up to now. It has been long observed that normal slips quite often mirror fluent paraphasic errors; Freud said as much. However, there is a major imbalance in phoneme exchange errors. Many of these types of errors are observed in normal slips-of-the-tongue, but few if any are seen in paraphasias. Recall that we mentioned that for a phoneme exchange to take place, normal decay rates must be in place, a requirement that is not necessary for anticipatory and perseverative misorderings. A signpost of many aphasics is perseveration, which in connectionist terms would be a disruption in the rate at which activated elements return to their resting state (or, "checked off" in a serial model such as that of Shattuck-Hufnagel, 1979). One sees severe perseveration in many of the paraphasias of fluent aphasics (Buckingham, 1985), and one result of this is the numerous "doublet creation" errors (Buckingham,

1990), whereby right-to-left anticipatory or left-to-right carryover misorderings result in two segments, when in the target there was only one. Obviously, once the phoneme had been misactivated it did not return to its resting state (in Buckingham, 1990, the metaphor of the "checkoff monitor" of Shattuck-Hufnagel was incorporated, whereby the moved item failed to be checked off rather than failed to return to its resting level) and remained in its original slot, thereby creating the "doublet." This slowing of a return to the resting level may therefore account for why we see so few exchanges in aphasics. I know of no better explanation of this puzzle at the present than to claim that aphasics quite often have disruptions in the normal decay rates that ensure that activated elements get turned off on time.

In conclusion, one issue that has always caused Dell some concern is the difficulty in getting his connectionist network to handle word shape syllable templates that have constituent structure and to work in the associative numerical values such that, for example, the rime could take on weights that would allow it to behave as a functional unit in a way that a CV would not. Of course in an important sense, this kind of issue is tricky because, if rimes are special units in the phonological makeup of lexical items, then perhaps their structural properties would simply be built into the total vocabulary structure of the language. Connectionist simulations, therefore, may very well ultimately hold to predictions of behaviors inherent in a phonology that has an intermediate rime node. That is, simulated errors would show less mobility of codas than of onsets, because the coda is more likely to be linked to the vowel than is the onset. It is well known from several data sources that onsets are much more likely to move away from their home syllable than are codas. And, when vowels move with some consonant, that consonant is almost always the coda. VCs move together much more often than CVs. There is a much tighter licensing dynamic between codas and the syllable node than between onsets and the syllable node. Restrictions on kinds and numbers of consonants is much more apparent with codas than with onsets. In general, though, constituent structure is more difficult to handle in connectionist models. In fact, this is a general criticism that Fodor has held against connectionism for some time. For example, he writes (Loewer & Rey, 1991, p. 310), "Smolensky doesn't have what he and I agree that a connectionist explanation of systematicity would require: mental representations with constituent structure." Syllables as well as sentences must have some form of constituent structure according to Fodor. Nevertheless, Dell has come as close as anyone to constructing a connectionist system that is an amalgam of symbol systems that are connectionist, while eschewing nonsymbolic, massively parallel and distributed systems. His interactive activation models have had much success in simulating language errors in normalcy, and more recently in aphasia (e.g., Martin, Saffran, Dell, & Schwartz, 1994; Schwartz, Saffran, Bloch, & Dell, 1994). And more, he has done so without rules. Other investigators as well have developed connectionist models for aphasia (Harley, 1993, 1996; Martin & Saffran, 1992), and for related sequalae (Plaut & Shallice, 1993). But, as indicated above, the issue of globality remains unsettled.

LINGUISTIC-PHONOLOGICAL CONNECTIONISM

Rules seem to be the stuff of linguistics, but there is now a small but growing movement from within linguistics (largely from within phonology) that is attempting to move away from rules and into systems more compatible with connectionism that focus on meeting the dictates of phonotactic patterns at at least three important linguistic levels: the morphophonemic, the phonemic, and the phonetic. We may actually be witnessing "the last phonological rule" in what is now referred to as "harmonic phonology" (Goldsmith, 1993). I close my chapter with a brief discussion of this new connectionist linguistics.

During the late 1980s, Goldsmith began exploring ways to enhance the descriptive importance of the tactics of three important linguistic levels: morphophonemic, lexical, and phonemic, roughly (but, see Goldsmith's intro, 1993, p. 20). The long and complicated "derivational" mappings that linguists had set up over the decades were called into question, especially those derivations that are intermediate and that do not have any linguistic existence at a level. The major change of emphasis has been to focus exclusively on the "satisfying" of phonotactics. George Lakoff (1993), since the late 1960s, had begun to question the reality of the complex derivational machinery that seemed to be boundless in linguistic analyses. To some extent, many of these rule complexes were felt to be convenient analytical fictions by Lakoff. Goldsmith also credits Alan Sommerstein (1974) for claiming that "by and large, phonological rules can best be understood as improving the well- formedness of representations with respect to certain phonotactics." So, Goldsmith reasons, if one can construct a model to handle the phonotactics, one could go a long way in ridding the system of most of its rules, while still accounting for the most important aspects of language structure—the tactics of the principal levels. He sought for the human language faculty a "self-organizing dynamical system" (Goldsmith, 1993, p. 7).

Essentially what Goldsmith and many of his colleagues have come up with is the use of a connectionist system such as the so-called Hopfield net. These networks are (can be) feedforward, recurrent systems, and have the capacity to continue to compute subsequent to periods of activation to the point that the system has "settled into equilibrium." Settling into an equilibrium state has been referred to metaphorically as being "harmonious," and Hopfield nets have been labelled as "harmony machines." When the equilibria are the phonotactics of human languages, the process is referred to as phonotactic satisfying, or harmonic phonology. Beneath these seemingly simple metaphors is some deceptively complex mathematics, although Goldsmith (1993, pp. 11–12) says that the basic plans of the network are easy enough to grasp. He writes:

> Every unit in the network is connected to every other unit, and in the normal run of things, it is assumed that these connections are symmetrical—that is, if unit u(k) is positively connected to unit u(l) with a particular strength of connection, then unit u(l) is connected back to unit u(k) with the same strength of connection.

The very notions of "harmony" and the processes of settling into some form of equilibrium state are analogically drawn from mathematics and physics. The physical process is that of annealing, and when it takes place in computer networks, it is of course simulated annealing. Bechtel and Abrahamsen (1991, pp. 44–45) provide a good explanation of the physics. First they claim that something comparable to local minima takes place in crystal formation when incompatible sets of bonds start to form in different regions of the crystal. In turn, if these bonds are fixed, the crystal will have an imperfection. The process of annealing will avoid this situation. This procedure involves heating (thereby weakening the bonds and allowing the atoms to reorient) and then cooling very slowly, maximizing the likelihood that as the bondings are restructured the atoms will orient appropriately with each other. It's a sort of a phonotactics of crystallography—at least that is the analogy we must buy into. The idea is incorporated in connectionist networks like the Hopfield nets by treating the patterns of activation in different parts of the network as comparable to the alignment of atoms (Bechtel & Abrahamsen, 1991, p. 45). Again, the analogy is that settling into an equilibrium state where there is an optimal alignment of atoms is like settling into an equilibrium state where there is optimal phonotactics.

The reader must be aware, however, that we, as language scientists of one ilk or another, actually want to use the Hopfield net to describe or represent something **outside** of the net itself (Goldsmith, 1993, p. 12), such as conceptual connections or phonological connections with words. This is an extremely important point, and often one that is all too easily glossed over in the sometimes overzealous criticisms of connectionism. Nothing that we are interested in as language researchers is **in** the Hopfield net itself, or in any connectionist network whichever. The insides of the network are cold spaces of node interconnections of numerical values that can be fed forward, summed (averaged), activated, inhibited, brought to rest, and so forth. In humans, this is called the brain. It may or may not look much like the computer network, but neither the computer nor the brain has anything we want directly in it. According to Goldsmith (1993, p. 12), the whole "trick" is ensuring that each unit of the network corresponds to some very small aspect of the reality we want to represent. The symbols are imposed on the networks by human researchers in the social sciences; they obviously are not there otherwise.

In sum, then, the Hopfield nets are designed to do two things of interest to the linguist and to other cognitive scientists interested in language. First, they are designed to use statistical means (like other connectionist machines) to determine what the confines of well- formedness are. Here, one can easily imagine the possibility of fixing the numerical values to accord with linguistic conditions such as sonority (e.g., Larson, 1990) and other kinds of phonological and syllabic principles (e.g., Wheeler & Touretzky, 1990) that underlie phonotactic constraints. Presumably, also, one could feed enough of the lexicon of a language into a learning network in such a way that it could "discover" the patterns instantiated in the total vocabulary itself. Second, and crucial for harmonic phonology, is something more active. If we activate and hold activated only a small subset of the units of the Hopfield net (leaving others to be either on or off at the network's discretion), we will observe the network adjusting itself such that the units that we have left untouched will hold to the regularities and patterns that the network had "learned" from its training experience. In general, the connectionist focus on the universal interaction and satisfaction of structural constraints of different sorts has opened up a new research program referred to as "optimality" theory (Prince & Smolensky, 1997).

Goldsmith (1993) contains a number of stimulating and challenging chapters on connectionist phonology, much of it simply working out the logic of network characterizations in such manner that they will be plausible from connectionist points of view, the machine implementation to come later. Several chapters hold true to the spirit of generative phonology in all its complexities, though the analyses are cast in ways that "exploit a computational idiom." (Goldsmith, 1993, p. 16). Wheeler and Touretzky (1993) also have a paper in this collection, where they make maximal use of the simulated annealing with Hopfield nets. And, more recently, Wheeler and Touretzky (1997) have proposed a parallel licensing model to account for the maintenance of proper phonotactic patterns in slips- of-the-tongue and in the phonemic paraphasias and neologisms of fluent aphasic patients.

CONCLUSIONS

We must now consider our original question of whether or not connectionism and associationism are one in the same, and that, as Fodor and Pylyshyn (1988) claim, "connectionism is a return to associationism." The basic question would be then: Are connectionist systems associationist? Bechtel and Abrahamsen (1991) address precisely this issue and conclude that connectionism is not a return to, or mere, associationism, but rather that connectionism is (p. 102) "an elaboration of associationism that has benefitted from and can contribute to many of the goals of the cognitivism of the last twenty years (although) its most obvious ancestor is, indeed, associationism." Connectionism, continue Bechtel and Abrahamsen (p. 102), "can be regarded as the outcome of returning to the original vision of the associationists, adopting their powerful idea that contiguities breed connections, and applying that idea with an unprecedented degree of sophistication." They go on to say (p. 102) that:

> Among the elaborations that were not even conceived of within classical associationism are: distributed representation (particularly coarse coding), hidden units (which function to encode microfeatures and enable complex computations on inputs), mathematical models of the dynamics of associationist learning, supervised learning (in which error reduction replaces simple Hebbian learning), back propagation, and simulated annealing within a self-organizing dynamic network.

They point out that a "localist" connectionist network that incorporates Hebb's learning rule is essentially an implementation of classical associationistic learning: The system develops by either increasing or decreasing the associations between units based on their contiguity (i.e., their pairing in the same input-output case). However, the claim is that if the network is not localist but rather multilayered, then less obvious but more powerful variations on associationism can be attained. For example, hidden units can fractionate ideas into microfeatures, achieving a degree of reduction unappreciated within classical associationism. In addition, units or microfeatures can achieve contiguity [joint activation or simultaneous contiguity—HWB] by means of the propagation of activity within the network, not just by occurring together in immediate experience (e.g., within the same sensory-level input pattern). However, Bechtel and Abrahamsen (1991, p. 103) do suggest that, "This might be viewed as an implementation of the two ways that ideas can be experienced together in classical associationism (reflective thought) as well as sensation." John Locke (Warren, 1921, p. 37) had gone beyond simple sensations as the bond forgers of ideas to claim that a separate function or faculty, which he called "reflection," could transform ideas of sensations into other sorts of ideas. Moreover, the reflective faculty, according to Locke, could derive ideas alone, without outside sensation. Locke argued that one could not derive the ideas of the processes of remembrance, discerning, and reasoning from raw outside sensations. Rather, one had to reflect on it. George Berkeley had ideas of imagination as well as ideas of sensation. With reflection and imagination, of course, the boundaries of rationalism and empiricism begin to overlap somewhat, so that any machine internal process, not directly tied to input or to output, might play a role in the empiricist's depiction of the human mind as well. Reflectionism is Locke's nativism, since associations formed accordingly are exclusively internally generated. Furthermore, most empiricists felt that there had to be a priori knowledge in the human mind, since before the associationistic learning machine could initiate its operations, it had to have some idea of just what "similarity" and "contiguity" were. That is, the principles of association had to somehow be built in. In any event, Bechtel and Abrahamsen (1991, p. 103) conclude that "One is tempted to refer to connectionism as 'association with an intelligent face,'" and that, "To the extent that connectionism succeeds, the charge of mere association will lose whatever force that it currently possesses."

Finally, the whole connectionist enterprise is a relative newcomer on the cognitive horizon, and its ultimate success will depend on how often its models make and corroborate new and insightful predictions and how often its simulations pass the Turing Test, even though interpreting what the Turing Test can actually tell us is notoriously slippery business (see, Watt, 1996). In the meantime it deserves patience, respect, and serious consideration. Stuart Sutherland (1986, p. 486), in the journal *Nature*, provides some interesting commentary in his evaluation of parallel distributed processing and its affinities. He remarks that although "some members of the old guard" have been resistant to the connectionist paradigm, George Miller, "the doyen of the psychology of cognition . . . has remarked that it is the most important revolution in psychology in his day and his day includes the advent of cybernetics, information theory, generative grammar and the digital computer for simulating the mind." Miller cannot be taken lightly. Sutherland concludes by writing (1986, p. 486) that:

> As the interest and importance of these systems become more widely known we may expect the young and flexible to explore their implications in detail, using no doubt the sloppy analogies that characterize both the human mind and PDP and that are almost certainly the foundation of creative thinking.

Long live youth, flexibility, sloppy analogies, and creative thinking.

REFERENCES

Allen, R. C. (1999). *David Hartley on human nature*. Albany, NY: State University of New York Press.

Aristotle. (1931). De memoria et reminiscentia. In W. D. Ross (Ed.), *The works of Aristotle*, Book 3. Oxford, England: Clarendon Press.

Aubert, D., & Whitaker, H. A. (1996). David Hartley's model of vibratiuncles seen as a contribution to the localization theory of brain function. *History and Philosophy of Psychology Bulletin, 8*, 14–16.

Bastian, H. C. (1869). On the various forms of loss of speech in cerebral disease. *British Foreign Med. Chir. Rev. 43*, 209–236, 470–492.

Bechtel, W., & Abrahamsen, A. (1991). *Connectionism and the mind*. Oxford, England: Blackwell.

Benton, A. L. (1965). Johann A. P. Gesner on aphasia. *Medical History, 9*, 54–60.

Benton, A. L., & Joynt, R. J. (1960). Early descriptions of aphasia. *Archives of Neurology, 3*, 205–221.

Berkeley, G. (1709). *Essay towards a new theory of vision*. Dublin: A. Rhames.

Berkeley, G. (1982). *A treatise concerning the principles of human knowledge*. Indianapolis, IN: Hacket Pub. Co. (Original publication date, 1710).

Boden, M. A. (1989). *Artificial intelligence in psychology: Interdisciplinary essays*. Cambridge, MA: MIT Press.

Boden, M. A. (Ed.) (1990). *The philosophy of artificial intelligence*. New York: Oxford University Press.

Boden, M. A. (1991). Horses of a different color. In W. Ramsey, S. P. Stich, & D. E. Rumelhart (Eds.), *Philosophy and connectionist theory* (pp. 3–19). Hillsdale, NJ: Erlbaum Associates, Publishers.

Bower, G. S. (1881). *Hartley and James Mill* (reprinted 1990). Bristol, U.K.: Thoemmes Antiquarian Books Ltd.

Brazier, M. A. B. (1957). Rise of neurophysiology in the 19th century. *Journal of Neurophysiology, 20*, 212–226.

Broca, P. P. (1960). Remarks on the seat of the faculty of articulate language, followed by an observation of aphemia. In G. Von Bonin (Ed.), Remarques sur le siège de la faculté du langage articulé suivies d'une observation d'aphémie. (Trans.), *Some papers on the cerebral cortex* (pp. 49–72). Springfield, IL: Charles Thomas. (Original work published in 1861).

Buckingham, H. W. (1981). A pre-history of the problem of Broca's aphasia. In R. H. Brookshire (Ed.), *Clinical aphasiology: Proceedings of the conference* (pp. 3–16). Minneapolis, MN: BRK Publishers.

Buckingham, H. W. (1982). Neuropsychological models of language. In N. J. Lass, L. V. McReynolds, J. L. Northern, & D. E. Yoder (Eds.), *Speech, language, and hearing*: Vol 1. *Normal processes* (pp. 323–347). Philadelphia, PA: W. B. Saunders Company.

Buckingham, H. W. (1984). Early development of association theory in psychology as a forerunner to connection theory. *Brain and Cognition, 3*, 19–34.

Buckingham, H. W. (1985). Perseveration in aphasia. In S. Newman & R. Epstein (Eds.), *Current perspectives in dysphasia* (pp. 113–154). Edinburgh: Churchill Livingstone.

Buckingham, H. W. (1990). Principle of sonority, doublet creation, and the checkoff monitor. In J. L. Nespoulous & P. Villiard (Eds.), *Morphology, phonology, and aphasia* (pp. 193–205). New York: Springer-Verlag.

Buckingham, H. W. (1995). *Connectionism from Aristotle to Hartley*. Paper presented at the meeting of the History of the Neurosciences, Univ. of Quebec at Montreal, May 13.

Buckingham, H. W. (1999). Freud's continuity thesis. *Brain and Language, 69*, 76–92.

Buckingham, H. W., & Finger, S. (1997). David Hartley's psychobiological associationism and the legacy of Aristotle. *Journal of the History of the Neurosciences, 6*, 21–37.

Caplan, D. (1994). Language and the brain. In M. A. Gernsbacher (Ed.), *Handbook of psycholinguistics* (pp. 1023–1053). San Diego, CA: Academic Press.

Caramazza, A., Papagno, C., & Ruml, W. (2000). The selective impairment of phonological processing in speech production. *Brain and Language, 75*, 428–450.

Chomsky, N. (1977). *Language and responsibility.* New York: Pantheon Books.

Clagett, M. (1955). *Greek science in antiquity.* New York: Collier Books.

Clark, A. (1993). *Associative engines.* Cambridge, MA: The MIT Press.

Clarke, E., & O'Malley, C. D. (1968). *The human brain and spinal cord.* Berkeley: Univ. of California Press.

Dell, G. S. (1985). Positive feedback in hierarchical connectionist models: Application to language production. *Cognitive Science, 9*, 3–23

Dell, G. S. (1986). A spreading activation theory of retrieval in sentence production. *Psychological Review, 93*, 283–321.

Dell, G. S. (1988). The retrieval of phonological forms in production: Tests of predictions from a connectionist model. *Journal of Memory and Language, 27*, 124–142.

Dell, G. S. (1995). Speaking and misspeaking. In L. R. Gleitman & M. Liberman (Eds.), *Language: An invitation to cognitive science* (2nd ed.) Vol 1 (pp. 183–208). Cambridge, MA: MIT Press.

Dell, G. S., & Reich, P. A. (1981). Stages in sentence production: An analysis of speech error data. *Journal of Verbal Learning and Verbal Behavior, 20*, 611–629.

Dell, G. S., Schwartz, M. F., Martin, N., Saffran, E. M., & Gagnon, D. A. 1997. Lexical access in aphasic and nonaphasic speakers. *Psychological Review, 104*, 801–838.

Dictionary of National Biography. (1921–22). Vol. IX. Oxford, U.K.: Oxford University Press.

Eggert, G. H. (1977). *Wernicke's works on aphasia: A sourcebook and review.* The Hague: Mouton Publishers.

Eling, P. (ed.) (1994). *Reader in the history of aphasia: From [Franz] Gall to [Norman] Geschwind.* Amsterdam: John Benjamins Publishing Co.

Figlio, K. M. (1975). Theories of perception and the physiology of mind in the late eighteenth century. *History of Science, 13*, 177– 212.

Finger, S. (1994). *Origins of neuroscience.* New York: Oxford University Press.

Finger, S., & Buckingham, H. W. (1994). Alexander Crichton (1763–1856): Disorders of fluent speech and associationist theory. *Archives of Neurology, 51*, 498–503.

Flew, A. (ed.) (1988). *An enquiry concerning human understanding by David Hume* (with introduction, notes, and editorial arrangement). LaSalle, IL: Open Court.

Flourens, P. (1960). Investigations of the properties and the functions of the various parts which compose the cerebral mass. In G. Von Bonin (ed.) Recherches expérimentales sur les propriétés et les fonctions du système nerveux dans les animaux vertébrés. (Trans.), Some papers on the cerebral cortex (pp. 3–21). Springfield, IL: Charles Thomas. (Original work published in 1824).

Fodor, J. A. (1987). *Psychosemantics.* Cambridge, MA: MIT Press.

Fodor, J. A. (1990). *A theory of content and other essays.* Cambridge, MA: MIT Press.

Fodor, J. A. (1995). West coast fuzzy: Why we don't know how minds work. [Review of P. M. Churchland's *The engine of reason, the seat of the soul*]. *Times Literary Supplement*, Aug. 25, 5–6.

Fodor, J. A., & Pylyshyn, Z. W. (1988). Connectionism and cognitive architecture: A critical analysis. In S. Pinker & J. Mehler (Eds.), *Connections and symbols* (pp. 3–71). Cambridge, MA: MIT Press.

Fritsch, G., & Hitzig, E. (1960). On the electrical excitability of the cerebrum. In G. Von Bonin (ed.) Op. Cit., (pp. 73–96). (Original work published in 1870 trans über die elektrische Erregbarkeit des Grosshirns.)

Fromkin, V. A. (1971). The non-anomalous nature of anomalous utterances. *Language, 51,* 696–719.

Garrett, M. F. (1975). The analysis of sentence production. In G. Bower (Ed.), *The psychology of learning and motivation* (Vol. 9) (pp. 133–177). New York: Academic Press.

Geschwind, N. (1965). Disconnexion syndromes in animals and man. *Brain, 88,* 237–294, 585–644. (Reprinted in Geschwind, 1974).

Geschwind, N. (1974). Selected papers on language and the brain. In R. S. Cohen & M. W. Wartofsky, (Eds,) Vol. XVI *Boston Studies in the Philosophy of Science.* Dordrecht, Holland: D. Reidel Publishing Co.

Gleitman, L. R., & Liberman, M. (Eds.). (1995). *Language: An invitation to cognitive science.* Vol. 1. [Daniel N. Osherson, general editor]. Cambridge, MA: MIT Press.

Goldsmith, J. (Ed.). (1993). *The last phonological rule: Reflections on constraints and derivations.* Chicago: University of Chicago Press.

Greenblatt, S. H. (1970). Hughlings Jackson's first encounter with the work of Paul Broca: The physiological and philosophical background. *Bulletin of the History of Medicine, 44,* 555–570.

Hackman, W. D. (1986). *Apples to atoms: Portraits of scientists from Newton to Rutherford.* London: National Portrait Gallery.

Harley, T. A. (1993). Connectionist approaches to language disorders. *Aphasiology, 7,* 221–249.

Harley, T. A. (1995). *The psychology of language: From data to theory.* East Sussex, UK: Erlbaum (UK) Taylor & Francis.

Harley, T. A. (1996). Connectionist modelling of the recovery of language functions following brain damage. *Brain and Language, 52,* 7–24.

Hartley, D. (1746). *Various conjectures on the perception, motion, and generation of ideas.* Trans. by R. E. A. Palmer, with Introduction and notes by Martin Kallich. Reprinted by the Augustan Reprint Society, No. 77–8. William Andrews Clark Memorial Library, UCLA, 1959.

Hartley, D. (1749). *Observations on man.* London: Charles Hitch & Stephen Austen. Reprinted with introduction by Theodore L. Huguelet by Scholars' Facsimiles & Reprints, Delmar, New York, 1976.

Hebb, D. O. (1949). *The organization of behavior.* New York: Wiley.

Hendler, J. A. (1989). Marker-passing over microfeatures: Towards a hybrid symbolic/connectionist model. *Cognitive Science, 13,* 79–106.

Hillis, A. E., Boatman, D., Hart, J., & Gordon, B. (1999). Making sense out of jargon: A neurolinguistic and computational account of jargon aphasia. *Neurology, 53,* 1813–1824.

Hobbes, T. (1650). *Human nature or the fundamental elements of policy.* London: Printed by T. Newcomb, for Frai Bowman of Oxon.

Hobbes, T. (1651). *Leviathan, or the matter, form and power of a common-wealth, ecclesiasticall and civill.* London: Printed for A. Cooke at the Green Dragon in St. Paul's Churchyard.

Hume, D. (1739). *A treatise of human nature* (Reprinted 1896). Oxford: Clarendon Press.

Hume, D. (1748). *An enquiry concerning human understanding.* Introduction, notes, and editorial arrangement by Antony Flew. (Reprinted 1988). La Salle, IL: Open Court.

Hunt, M. (1993). *The story of psychology.* New York, NY: Doubleday.

Jaynes, J. (1973). The problem of animate motion in the Seventeenth Century. In M. Henley, J. Jaynes, & J. J. Sullivan (Eds.), *Historical conceptions of psychology* (pp. 166–179). New York: Springer Publishing Co.

Kallich, M. (1959). Introduction and Notes. In D. Hartley (1746/1959) *Various conjectures on the perception, motion, and generation of ideas.* The Augustan Reprint Society. Los Angeles, CA: William Andrews Clark Memorial Library of the Univ. of California at Los Angeles.

Katz, J. J. (1981). *Language and other abstract objects.* Totowa, NJ: Rowman & Littlefield.

Kuczaj, S. (1977). The acquisition of regular and irregular past tense forms. *Journal of Verbal Learning and Verbal Behavior, 16,* 589–600.

Kuczaj, S. (1978). Children's judgments of grammatical and ungrammatical past-tense forms. *Child Development, 49,* 319–326.

Lakoff, G. (1993). Cognitive phonology. In J. Goldsmith (Ed.), The last phonological rule: Reflections on constraints and derivations (pp. 117–145). Chicago: University of Chicago Press.

Larson, G. N. (1990). Local computational networks and the distribution of segments in the Spanish syllable. In M. Ziolkowski, M. Noske, & K. Deaton (Eds.), *The parasession on the syllable in phonetics and phonology* (Vol. 2) (pp. 257–272). Papers from the 26th regional meeting of the Chicago Linguistic Society. Chicago: Chicago Linguistic Society.

Lashley, K. S. (1950). In search of the engram. *Society of Experimental Biology Symposium* (No. 4): *Physiological mechanisms in animal behavior* (pp. 454–482). Cambridge, U.K.: Cambridge University Press.

Lashley, K. S. (1951). The problem of serial order in behavior. In L. A. Jeffress (Ed.), *Cerebral mechanisms in behavior: The Hixon Symposium* (pp. 112–146). New York: Wiley.

Lichtheim, L. (1885). On aphasia. *Brain, 7,* 433–484.

Loewer, B., & Rey, G. (Eds.). (1991). *Meaning and mind: Fodor and his critics.* Oxford, U.K.: Blackwell.

Locke, J. (1690). *Essay concerning human understanding.* 5th ed, London: Dent, 1961. [Cited in Warren, 1921.]

Lockwood, D. G. (1972). *Introduction to stratificational linguistics.* New York: Harcourt Brace Jovanovich, Inc.

Martin, N., & Saffran, E. M. (1992). A computational account of deep dysphasia: Evidence from a single case study. *Brain and Language, 43,* 240–274.

Martin, N., Saffran, E. M., Dell, G. S., & Schwartz, M. F. (1994). Origins of paraphasias in deep dysphasia: Testing the consequences of a decay impairment to an interactive spreading activation model of lexical retrieval. *Brain and Language, 47,* 609–660.

McClelland, J. L., & Rumelhart, D. E. (Eds.). (1986). *Parallel distributed processing.* Vols. I & II. Cambridge, MA: The MIT Press.

McCulloch, W. S., & Pitts, W. H. (1943). A logical calculus of the ideas immanent in nervous activity. *Bulletin of Mathematical Biophysics, 5,* 115–133. Reprinted in M. A. Boden (ed.) 1990. *The philosophy of artificial intelligence.* Op. Cit. (pp. 22–39).

Meynert, T. (1960). On the collaboration of parts of the brain. In G. Von Bonin (Ed.), Op. Cit. (pp. 159–180). (Original work published in 1891, Über das zusammenwirken der Gehirntheile).

Motley, M. T., & Baars, B. J. (1979). Effects of cognitive set upon laboratory induced verbal (Freudian) slips. *Journal of Speech and Hearing Research, 22,* 421–432.

Oberg, B. B. (1976). David Hartley and the association of ideas. *Journal of the History of Ideas, 37,* 441–454.

Parks, R. W., Long, D. L., Levine, D. S., Crockett, D. J., McGeer, E. G., McGeer, P. L., Dalton, I. E., Zec, R. F., Becker, R. E., Coburn, K. L., Siler, G., Nelson M. E., & Bower, J. M., (1991). Parallel distributed processing and neural networks: Origins, methodology and cognitive functions. *International Journal of Neuroscience, 60,* 195–214.

Pinker, S. (1991). Rules of language. *Science, 253* (Aug 2): 531–535.

Pinker, S. (1994). *The language instinct.* New York: William Morrow and Company, Inc.

Pinker, S. 1995. Why the child holded the baby rabbits: A case study in language acquisition. In L. R. Gleitman & M. Liberman (Eds.), *Language: An invitation to cognitive science* (Vol. 1) Op. Cit. (pp. 107–133).

Pinker, S. 1999. *Words and Rules: The Ingredients of Language.* New York: Basic Books.

Plaut, D. C., & Shallice, T. (1993). Perseverative and semantic influences on visual object naming errors in optic aphasia: A connectionist account. *Journal of Cognitive Neuroscience, 5,* 89–117.

Prince, A., & Smolensky, P. (1997). Optimality: From neural networks to universal grammar. *Science, 275,* 1604–1610.

Rand, B. (1923). The early development of Hartley's doctrine of associationism. *Psychological Review, 30,* 306–320.

Riese, W. (1959). *A history of neurology.* New York, NY: MD Publications, Inc.

Robinson, D. N. (1995). *An intellectual history of psychology* (3rd ed.). Madison: University of Wisconsin Press.

Rosenblatt, F. (1958). The perceptron: A probabilistic model for information storage and organization in the brain. *Psychological Review, 65,* 368–408.

Rumelhart, D. E., & McClelland, J. L. (Eds.). (1986). *Parallel distributed processing.* Cambridge, MA: MIT Press.

Ruml, W., & Caramazza, A. (2000). An evaluation of a computational model of lexical access: Comments on Dell, et al. (1997). *Psychological Review, 107,* 609–634.

Sampson, G. (1987). Review of *Parallel distributed processing,* Vols. 1 & 2., ed. by Rumelhart & McClelland. *Language, 63,* 871–886.

Schiller, F. (1979). *Paul Broca: Founder of French Anthropology, explorer of the brain.* Berkeley: Univ. of California Press. (2nd ed., 1992).

Schwartz, M. F., Saffran, E. M., Bloch, D. E., & Dell, G. S. (1994). Disordered speech production in aphasic and normal speakers. *Brain and Language, 47,* 52–88.

Searle, J. 1990. The battle over the university. *New York Review of Books, 37,* 34–42.

Sevald, C. A., & Dell, G. S. (1994). The sequential cuing effect in speech production. *Cognition, 53,* 91–127.

Shattuck-Hufnagel, S. (1979). Speech errors as evidence for a serial-ordering mechanism in speech production. In W. E. Cooper & E. C. T. Walker (Eds.), *Sentence processing: Psycholinguistic studies presented to Merrill Garrett* (pp. 295–342). Hillsdale, NJ: Erlbaum Associates, Publishers.

Smith, C. U. M. (1987). David Hartley's Newtonian neuropsychology. *Journal of the History of the Behavioral Sciences, 23,* 123–136.

Smolensky, P. (1988). On the proper treatment of connectionism. *Behavioral and Brain Sciences, 11,* 1–74.

Sommerstein, A. (1974). On phonotactically motivated rules. *Journal of Linguistics, 10,* 71–94.

Stemberger, J. P. (1985). An interactive activation model of language production. In A. W. Ellis (Ed.), *Progress in the psychology of language* (Vol. 1) (pp. 143–186). London: Erlbaum Associates, Publishers.

Sutherland, S. (1986). Parallel distributed processing. *Nature, 323,* (9 October): 486.

Tizard, B. (1959). Theories of brain localization from Flourens to Lashley. *Medical History, 3,* 132–145.

Von Bonin, G. (Ed.). (1960). *Some papers on the cerebral cortex.* Springfield, IL: Charles Thomas.

Walker, A. E. (1957). Stimulation and ablation: Their role in the history of cerebral physiology. *Journal of Neurophysiology, 20,* 435–449.

Walls, J. (1982). The psychology of David Hartley and the root metaphor of mechanism: A study in the history of psychology. *The Journal of Mind and Behavior, 3,* 259–274.

Warren, H. C. (1921). *A history of the association psychology.* New York, NY: Charles Scribner's Sons.

Watt, S. N. K. (1996). Naive psychology and the inverted Turing Test. *PSYCOLOQUY, 7* (14) turing-test.1.watt

Wernicke, K. (1874). The aphasia symptom complex: A psychological study on an anatomic basis. Translated in E. G. Eggert (Ed.), *Op. Cit.* (pp. 91–145).

Wheeler, D. W., & Touretzky, D. S. (1990). From syllables to stress: A cognitively plausible model. In M. Ziolkowski, M. Noske, & K. Deaton, (Eds.), *Op. Cit.* (pp. 413–427).

Wheeler, D. W., & Touretzky, D. S. (1993). A connectionist implementation of cognitive phonology. In J. Goldsmith (Ed.), Op. Cit. (pp. 146–172).

Wheeler, D. W., & Touretzky, D. S. (1997). A parallel licensing model of normal slips and phonemic paraphasias. *Brain and Language, 59*, 147–201.

Willis, T. (1681). *The anatomy of the brain.* (Reprinted by USV Pharmaceutical Corp, Tucahoe, NY, 1971.)

Young, R. M. (1970). *Mind, brain and adaptation in the nineteenth century.* Oxford, U.K.: Clarendon Press. (2nd ed., 1990).

Zangwill, O. L. (1961). Lashley's concept of cerebral mass action. In W. H. Thorpe & O. L. Zangwill (Eds.), *Current problems in animal behavior* (pp. 59–86). Cambridge, U.K.: Cambridge University Press.

Ziolkowski, M., Noske, M., & Deaton, K. (Eds.). (1990). *Papers from the 26th regional meeting of the Chicago Linguistic Society.* Vol 2: *The parasession on the syllable in phonetics and phonology.* Chicago: Chicago Linguistic Society.

Zurif, E., & Swinney, D. (1994). The neuropsychology of language. In M. A. Gernsbacher (Ed.), *Handbook of psycholinguistics* (pp. 1055–1074). San Diego, CA: Academic Press.

Subject Index

A

Accommodation, 7, 8–10, 21, 46, 64, 101
Agrammatism, 127
analogy, 291
ANN – Artificial Neural Networks, 230
annealing (simulated), 302, 304
anomia, 130, 131, 136
Anomic aphasia (Anomia)
    Acquired naming disorder, 151, 155, 158,
        159, 160, 169, 170, 171, 172, 173, 174,
        176, 178, 179
Anticontrol, 136
aphasia, 127
aphemia, 281
apraxia, 128
arcuate fasiculus, 158, 282
articulation, 126
artificial intelligence, 265, 291
assimilation, 7, 8, 9, 21, 101
association
    cause and effect, 265, 271–273
    contiguity (law of use), 265–275, 305
    force, 265, 266
    similarity, 265–274, 305
    vibrations, 274–276
    vibratiuncles, 276
attractors, 116, 118–123, 125, 129, 130, 133,
        134, 137
    strange, 120, 121, 124
auditory cortex
    columns-slabs, 198
    cortical activity, 198
    GABA, 197
    neuroanatomy, 195, 196
auditory processing
    ANN connectionist models of, 206

Three categories, 206, 207
automatic speech recognition, 213
autoorganization, 123, 130

B

back propagation, 236, 288, 289
Bbts
    echolocation, 190
    phonation, 190
BDAE (Boston Diagnostic Assessment Test),
    150
Begriffe, 282, 283
Bell-Magendie principle, 281
Bird song perception, 189
Blend, 127, 135
Boltzmann machine, 293, 296
Boolean logic, 289
Bottom-up (processing), 124
British Empiricism, 270–274, 279, 280
Broca
    aphasia, 151, 158
    aphasia (non fluent), 127, 133
    area, 114, 128, 151, 282, 283

C

canonical, 4, 48, 89–91
cascade, 171
cascade processing, 117
category periphery effects, 179
category-specific effects, 179
cholinergic systems, 135
classical aphasia doctrine, 150, 151, 158, 282,
    283
classification and regression trees, 223
cognitive, 1, 2, 7, 12–22, 27–34, 48, 51, 60, 61